Review of
Hemodialysis
for **Nurses**
and **Dialysis Personnel**

$\mathcal{H}$ Review of emodialysis
for Nurses
and Dialysis Personnel

SEVENTH EDITION

Judith Z. Kallenbach, MSN, RN, CNN
Regional Director of Education
Fresenius Medical Services North America
Akron, Ohio

C.F. Gutch, MD, FACP
Professor Emeritus, Department of Internal Medicine
University of South Dakota School of Medicine
Sioux Falls, South Dakota

Martha H. Stoner, RN, PhD
Associate Professor Emeritus
School of Nursing
University of Colorado at Denver and the Health Sciences Center
Denver, Colorado

Anna L. Corea, RN, MN, CNAA
Former Assistant Clinical Professor
School of Nursing
University of California—Los Angeles
Los Angeles, California

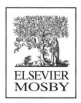

ELSEVIER
MOSBY

ELSEVIER
MOSBY

11830 Westline Industrial Drive
St. Louis, Missouri 63146

ISBN-13: 978-0-323-02871-4
ISBN-10: 0-323-02871-3

Executive Publisher: Darlene Como
Developmental Editor: Barb Watts
Publishing Services Manager: Jeffrey Patterson
Senior Project Manage: Mary G. Stueck
Designer: Teresa McBryan

Working together to grow
libraries in developing countries

www.elsevier.com | www.bookaid.org | www.sabre.org

ELSEVIER   BOOK AID
International   Sabre Foundation

Printed in the United States of America

Last digit is the print number: 9 8 7 6 5 4 3

*This book is dedicated to my family
Keith, Michael, and Maeve
With thanks and appreciation for
your never-ending support and encouragement.*

Global Review by

LYNDA K. BALL, RN, BSN, CNN
Quality Improvement Coordinator
Northwest Renal Network
Seattle, Washington

Preface

As with previous editions, the seventh edition of *Review of Hemodialysis* provides the reader with a practical approach to providing care to the chronic kidney disease patient. This edition has been updated to reflect changes in the National Kidney Foundation Kidney Disease Outcomes Quality Initiative (NKF-K/DOQI) guidelines, American Association of Medical Instrumentation (AAMI) standards, medication guidelines, and dialysis modalities. Expanded sections on the causes of chronic kidney disease, intradialytic complications, vascular access, and renal anatomy and physiology can also be found.

It is my hope that this edition will be valuable to the beginning practitioner in nephrology, and to those practitioners already dedicated to utilizing best practice standards to provide care to our renal patients.

Special thanks to Tracy Flitcraft for his profusion of ideas and expertise on dialysis delivery, principles, and quality, and to Elena Kubetin for her thoughts on peritoneal and home therapies. Thank you also to Lynda Ball for her expert review and suggestions, Martha Stoner for her guidance in directing me to this project, and to Michelle Trope and Barb Watts at Elsevier, for their help and support throughout.

Acknowledgments

The publisher and authors wish to thank the contributors of past editions: Kathy Bender, RN, BSN, CNN; Lowanna S. Binkley, RN, MA, CNN; Christopher R. Blagg, MD, FRCP; Eileen D. Brewer, MD; Linda S. Christensen, RN, CNN; Kenneth E. Cotton, MA, MBA, MPA; Helen Currier, RN, CNN; Jim Curtis, CHT, CNCT; Lesley C. Dinwiddie, RN, MSN, FNP, CNN; Ronald Emerson, AD, CHT; Nancy Gallagher, RN, BS, CNN; Peter W. Gardner; Susan K, Hansen, RN, MBA, CNN; Mara Hersh-Rifkin, MSW, LCSW; Margaret S. Holloway, RN, MN; Martin V. Hudson, CNBT; Kathy Laws, RN, BS, CNN; Mary M. Macaluso, RN, BSN, CPDN, CNN; Gwen Elise McNatt, RN, MS, CNN, CFNP; Allen R. Nissenson, MD, FACP; Patt Peterson, RN; Eileen Peacock, RN, MSN, CNN, CIC, CPHQ; Ginnette Pepper, RN, PhD; Christy A. Price, RN, MSN; Georgina Randolph, RN, MSN, MBA, CNN; Karen Robbins, RN, MS, CNN; Mark Rolston, CHT; Karen Schardin, RN, BSN, CNN; Sandra Smolka-Hill, RN, MSN, CNN; Julia Walsh Starr, RN, MSN; Beverly Wells Storck, RN, BSN; Jo Anne E. Strutz, RN; Cedric Tuck-Sherman, MBA; Philip M. Varughese, BS, CHT; Susan C. Vogel, RN, MHA, CNN; Ron Wathen, MD, PhD; Susan E. Weil, RD, CS; Mary Ann Wierszbiczki, RN, MN; and Gail S. Wick, BNS, RN, CNN. We are grateful for your commitment and desire to share your expertise with the nephrology community.

Contents

1

The Hemodialysis Team

Dialysis, the process of cleansing the blood of accumulated waste products, is a complex treatment requiring a team of highly trained individuals with a variety of skills. For this chronic treatment to be successful, the interdisciplinary team must work with the patient and family, supporting them in the areas of clinical need, psychosocial needs, and religious beliefs. Team members will include, but not be limited to, the physician, nurse, technician, dietitian, social worker, and administrator. Other team members might include a biomedical technician, psychologist, dentist, child development specialist, pharmacist, physician's assistant, and vocational rehabilitation counselor, member of the clergy, nurse practitioner, and clinical nurse specialist, or others who have special skills needed to help the patient reach maximum potential. The patient and family members are integral components of the dialysis team; without them, all the efforts of the other team members would be fruitless.

STRUCTURE OF THE DIALYSIS FACILITY

Every dialysis facility has a medical director who is ultimately responsible for medical care in the facility. Each dialysis facility has written policies and procedures that guide staff members in the clinical practice and patient care, and that monitor established standards of care, quality assurance, equipment and maintenance standards, reuse, and any pertinent medication or treatment protocols. These policies are written by the team and approved by the facility and nursing administrator, as required by the Joint Commission on Accreditation of Healthcare Organizations (JCAHO) for a special care unit. Freestanding facilities do not fall under the aegis of JCAHO. However, their policies and procedures must be approved by the facility's governing body, which includes the medical director, director of nursing, and administrator and be in accordance with the laws of that state and the Centers for Medicare and Medicaid Services (CMS) rules. Whenever a patient in acute renal failure or a severely uremic patient is dialyzed in the hospital setting, a physician should be readily available to handle crises or complications of the treatment.

ROLE OF THE PHYSICIAN

The nephrologist assesses the patient and determines when end-stage renal disease (ESRD) has been reached and requires the initiation of dialysis treatment. A nephrologist is an internist with further specialty training of 2 to 3 years in the field of nephrology. Evidence points increasingly to the importance of having patients seen and followed by a nephrologist early in the course of chronic kidney disease, and long before progression to ESRD. With early nephrologic intervention, appropriate medical therapy can be instituted, perhaps improving or at least maintaining renal function and slowing the need for dialysis.

Once the need for dialysis is determined, the nephrologist is responsible for writing the orders for the dialysis prescription—those components of the procedure that make it therapeutic. These include the specific dialyzer, blood and dialysate flow rates, the anticoagulation requirements, the duration or length of time of dialysis, the frequency, and whatever unique instructions may be required for the specific vascular access.

ROLE OF THE NURSE
What are the functions of the dialysis nurse?

Although nurses are responsible for the direct care of patients undergoing dialysis, technical staff perform much of this care under the nurse's supervision. Patient and family education, and ongoing reinforcement and support for self-care are more critical services provided by the nurse. In addition, the nurse is responsible for ongoing assessment of the patient and is generally the one who initiates multidisciplinary case conferences when the patient's physical, emotional, or social condition indicates the need.

Nursing administration or nursing service organizations may differ among dialysis units. In those facilities using a primary nursing model, each patient has a specifically designated primary nurse who is responsible for overall patient care. But case management is also appropriate for the care of dialysis patients. This model expands the nursing care/responsibility beyond the dialysis unit to the hospital, ambulatory care or outpatient facilities, and home. Case management ensures continuity of care from both a quality of care and an economic perspective. Whichever model is used, the goal of nursing is to serve as an advocate for those patients who require assistance and to empower them to become their own advocates.

With an increasing emphasis being placed on continuous quality improvement (CQI) as one means to ensure delivery of quality care to patients, nurses are taking the lead in this activity. Nurses are also seen in the roles of business manager, research coordinator, fiscal administrator, and chief technician in some settings.

What experience and background are essential for a nurse to be successful in dialysis?

Whereas some facilities may have different requirements for the nurses filling various positions within a dialysis facility, there are minimal qualifications required by all. A dialysis nurse should be a professional nurse with a minimum of 1 year of experience in medical-surgical nursing. A license to practice nursing in the state is required, and certification within a specialty, such as nephrology, critical care, and so on, is preferred. A background in critical care nursing or emergency department nursing is particularly useful, and for the nurse who functions in a managerial role, experience with personnel development, leadership roles, and other supervisory positions can be helpful in ensuring success in the position in a dialysis unit. Most facilities have a formal training program for newly hired registered nurses. Less experienced nurses who assume a role as a beginning practitioner need an environment that offers extensive orientation, education, close supervision, and support.

What other qualities should the dialysis nurse possess?

Other important qualifications include the ability to interact effectively with patients and personnel, as well as a demonstrated interest and skill both in patient teaching and in problem solving. Self-confidence and patience also are important in a dialysis nurse. Caring for dialysis patients and their families can be highly stressful because of the intensity of care required, the chronic nature of ESRD, and the patient's struggles with independence versus dependence. Dialysis nurses should be exemplars of the blend of the art and science of nursing. A significant scientific knowledge base and technical skill must be complemented by a caring, compassionate sensitivity; personal resiliency; and an ability to cope with stress. All are useful characteristics in a dialysis nurse.

Furthermore, some interest in teaching and an ability to teach are essential attributes. The dialysis nurse is frequently called upon to provide learning experiences for patients, family members, other dialysis personnel, diverse health care professionals, and the public. The dialysis nurse must have supervisory skills to make appropriate assignments to technicians and other personnel and to evaluate accurately the care provided by them.

What is the role of the advanced practice nurse in dialysis?

The use of advanced practice nurses (APN) in the acute and chronic dialysis settings has become more common as the patient population continues to increase. Nurse practitioners and clinical nurse specialists specializing in renal care now work in a diversity of healthcare settings covering all nephrology specialties. APNs can manage the care of chronic kidney disease patients at all stages. Some APNs function in the role of clinician, educator, consultant, administrator, or researcher. Current trends suggest an increase in the number of kidney disease patients and a decrease in the number of nephrologists available to provide their care. APNs can work collaboratively with the healthcare team to ensure that all kidney disease patients are receiving quality care.

Are there established standards of practice for dialysis nurses?

Regulations governing the administration of the ESRD program under CMS describe a number of standards and criteria related to qualifications of professional staff, acceptable patient care policies and procedures, and unit administration. However, CMS does not issue standards of practice for dialysis nurses.

Professional nursing organizations promote high standards of nephrology nursing practice. In 1987, the Nephrology Nursing Certification Commission (NNCC) was established to develop, implement, and coordinate all aspects of certification for nephrology nurses in the United States, and in 1988, the American Nephrology Nurses Association (ANNA) published its first Standards of Care. A nephrology nurse who meets the qualifications and passes the NNCC's written examination is entitled to use the initials CNN (certified nephrology nurse) as a professional credential.

Other certification options include the certified hemodialysis nurse (CHN) or certified peritoneal dialysis nurse (CPDN), available for both registered nurses and licensed practical nurses from the Board of Nephrology Examiners, Nursing and Technology (BONENT). The certified dialysis nurse (CDN) is a credentialing available to registered nurses without a baccalaureate degree from the ANNA. More recently, ANNA published the *Scope and Standards of Advanced Practice in Nephrology Nursing*. These standards describe competent APN care in nephrology and presents competent behaviors of the role. The Kidney Disease Outcomes Quality Initiative (K/DOQI), put forth by the National Kidney Foundation (NKF) in October 1997, offers some clinical practice guidelines in the areas of anemia management, hemodialysis adequacy, peritoneal dialysis adequacy, and vascular access. The intended goal of these outcomes is the improvement of the quality of care and outcomes for all persons with kidney disease and to help reduce the risk of developing kidney disease. These are practice guidelines only and are not intended to be requirements or to be specific to nursing practice, but rather they are guidelines for the general care of the CKD patient undergoing dialysis (see p. 338 for additional information on NKF-K/DOQI).

What education is available for nurses interested in dialysis?

Most dialysis units provide specialized learning opportunities for nurses as supervised on-the-job instruction during the period of orientation. Some units offer formal educational programs for dialysis personnel other than their own employees. These more formal programs include both theory and clinical practice. The curriculum should include instruction in the following areas: renal anatomy and physiology, including pathophysiology; fluid, electrolyte, and acid-base balance; dialysis theory; vascular access; dialysis procedures and techniques; recognition of complications and emergency conditions, and appropriate prevention and intervention; psychosocial problems; dietary regimens; medications; and interpersonal relations, including effective intervention in patients with chronic illness.

Some community colleges offer dialysis training programs that teach the theoretic basics of dialysis, with clinical practicums provided by the dialysis facility supporting the student. With the push for professional nurses to have a minimum of a baccalaureate degree in nursing at the entry level, interest is growing in formalizing a nephrology nursing curriculum at the graduate level. Vanderbilt University (Nashville) has offered a nephrology nursing specialty arm in its nurse practitioner program. Other schools of nursing are also addressing nephrology nursing as a specialty area in the graduate program.

Continuing education programs for dialysis nurses are available through a variety of educational and professional organizations. These include the Council on Nephrology Nursing and Technology of the National Kidney Foundation, ANNA, as well as local chapters of these organizations. In addition, the Association of Critical Care Nurses, Infection Control Nurses, and other such organizations offer some programs of interest to nephrology nurses.

What is the role of the dialysis nurse administrator?

The nursing leader responsible for patient care coordination may assume several titles, depending on the facility's structure. Whether as the nursing administrator, the director of nurses (DoN), charge nurse, or nursing coordinator, this nurse will have the primary responsibility for direct patient care. Supporting a professional practice model will ensure that patients receive optimal care.

Modeling knowledgeable, skillful care of patients is a vital aspect of the role of the nurse administrator, along with recruitment and retention of an adequate number of well-prepared patient caregivers—both nurses and technicians. It is also the responsibility of the nurse administrator to equip personnel with knowledge through learning opportunities and provide resources in the form of supplies and time, enabling staff to give the desired quality of patient care. The nurse administrator ensures high quality of care within a cost-effective environment while promoting patient and staff safety.

ROLE OF THE DIALYSIS UNIT ADMINISTRATOR

A dialysis unit administrator is responsible for ensuring the fiscal soundness of the dialysis facility. The administrator may make purchasing decisions, and it is desirable that these be made with an understanding of the clinical implications of such decisions. A unit administrator usually comes prepared with either a clinical or a fiscal background. Occasionally an administrator with a clinical background will also acquire an MBA or other fiscal or business educational preparation. This individual is thus prepared with both the clinical expertise to make decisions in the best interest of patients, as well as decisions based on what is best for the facility as a business.

ROLE OF THE TECHNICIAN

The role of the dialysis technician varies from state to state because of differences in practice regulations and mandates by different regulatory agencies. Technicians have been members of the dialysis team since dialysis programs began. Two major roles have existed for technicians: one is directed at assembly and maintenance of the equipment, and the other role focuses on patient care. In some settings, technicians combine patient and equipment care responsibilities. The timely and accurate assembly of dialysis equipment is vital to any dialysis program. Ongoing maintenance of costly equipment is a highly valued element of a dialysis program. Technicians work with all members of the dialysis team; in most settings they are most closely aligned with nurses. Patient care activities are delegated and supervised by professional nurses.

What abilities are required of the dialysis technicians?

Knowledge of mechanics and technological skill is essential for technicians who assume responsibility for equipment setup and maintenance. An understanding of the principles of physics and computer technology is desirable for technicians. Interpersonal skills are necessary for good relations with patients and their families. Patient care technicians must have some understanding of human anatomy and physiology and the pathophysiology of ESRD. The dialysis technician must have a full understanding of the theories and principles of dialysis, treatment complications, and care of the vascular access. For patient safety, a technician also must possess patient monitoring skills and clinical judgment.

Are there established standards of practice for technicians?

Dialysis technicians are bound by the standards of practice issued by the state in which they practice, if the state has practice guidelines. Different levels of regulation exist by state and include licensure, registration, or certification. States with existing legislation that requires technicians to pass a national certification exam include Arizona, California, Ohio, and Oregon. Kentucky, Georgia, New Mexico, and Texas have special training requirements but do not mandate national certification testing. Technicians are also bound by the K/DOQI guidelines, as well as by unit-specific policies and procedures. Currently, three organizations offer technician certification exams. Several credentialing programs are available to dialysis technicians.

What educational opportunities are available to dialysis technicians?

Dialysis programs offer on-the-job training for newly hired and inexperienced technicians. Some states with dialysis technician regulations mandate the minimum number of hours the dialysis technician must complete in both the clinic and the classroom in order to practice. Certificate programs for dialysis technicians are available through some community colleges, and continuing education programs are conducted by healthcare agencies, specialty organizations, and technical colleges.

The National Association of Nephrology Technicians/Technologists (NANT) offers many educational programs both locally and nationally. In addition, large nephrology meetings may provide advanced learning opportunities for the technician who is seeking an expansion of responsibilities or who is functioning in an expanded role. These include, but are not limited to, the Annual Dialysis Conference, National Kidney Foundation Clinical Meetings, the American Society of Nephrology meeting, the ANNA symposium, and the meetings sponsored by the Association for Advancement of Medical Instrumentation (AAMI).

ROLE OF THE RENAL DIETITIAN

A renal dietitian serves in a consultative role to patients and their families as well as to other members of the dialysis team. Dietitians provide an indispensable function in supporting the patient through all phases of chronic kidney disease. Dietary management is instrumental in delaying the need for dialysis. Furthermore, even once dialysis is initiated, ongoing assessment of the nutritional status of the patient and education of the patient and family are contributions made by the renal dietitian. See

Table 1-1	Credentialing Programs for Dialysis Technicians			
Credentialing agency	Certification	Eligibility requirements	Cognitive/Practice domains	Measures
The Nephrology Nursing Certification Commission (NNCC)	Certified clinical hemodialysis technicians (CCHT)	Minimum 6 months' experience in nephrology technology	Clinical, 50% Technical, 23% Environmental, 15% Role, 12%	Basic competency for hemodialysis patient care technicians
The Board of Nephrology Examiners Nursing and Technology (BONENT)	Certified hemodialysis technician/ technologist (CHT)	Minimum 12 months' experience in nephrology technology	Patient care, 65% Machine technology, 10% Water treatment, 5% Dialyzer reprocessing, 5% Education/personal development, 15%	Technical proficiency for all hemodialysis technicians
The National Nephrology Certification Organization (NNCO)	Certified clinical nephrology technologist (CCNT)	Minimum 12 months' experience in nephrology technology	Principles of dialysis, 25% Machine preparation and operation, 20% Patient assessment, 20% Treatment, 35%	Competence in the specialized area of practice of patient care for hemodialysis technicians
	Certified biomedical nephrology technologist (CBNT)		Principles of dialysis, 25% Scientific concepts, 15% Electronic applications, 10% Water treatment, 20% Equipment functions, 20% Environmental/regulatory issues, 10%	Competence in the specialized area of practice of biomedical hemodialysis

From National Association of Nephrology Technicians (NANT): *Position Statement on the Recognition and Support of Three Credentialing Programs for Dialysis Technicians*, Dayton, OH, April 22, 2001, NANT.

Chapter 14 for a more detailed description of the role of nutrition and the renal dietitian in the care of the person with chronic kidney disease.

ROLE OF THE SOCIAL WORKER
What are the main goals of the nephrology social worker?

Chronic kidney disease patients experience multiple losses and require significant psychosocial intervention at various stages throughout their illness trajectory. Two major activities have been described by the Council of Nephrology Social Workers:
- To develop awareness of the psychosocial aspects of chronic renal disease
- To develop and carry out methods for dealing with these problems and needs as key to the role of the renal social worker

How does the social worker achieve these two goals in a treatment center?

The social worker assists the patient and family in their adjustment to the illness. This involves a psychosocial assessment, provision of emotional support, and educational reinforcement. A thorough working knowledge of all available resources is essential. The social worker participates with other treatment team members in short- and long-term planning with the patient and his or her family. Evaluation of the patient's social background is important in successful development of the treatment plan. The social worker apprises other team members of special facets of patient or family behavior, history, and functioning that may influence the individual patient's care and course of treatment.

What are the necessary qualifications of the nephrology social worker?

A qualified social worker is defined by ESRD regulations as a person who is licensed, if applicable, by the state in which practicing and who meets at least *one* of the following conditions:
- Has completed a course of study with specialization in clinical practice and holds a master's degree from a graduate school of social work accredited by the Council on Social Work Education
- Has served for at least 2 years as social worker, 1 year of which was in a dialysis unit or transplant program before September 1, 1976, and has established a consultative relationship with a social worker who qualified under item 1.

Continuing education programs are available through the Council of Nephrology Social Workers.

Should psychiatric resources be available to the patient?

An awareness of one's own mortality and a life restricted by dependence on a machine are just two of the issues that confront the dialysis patient. The social worker assists patients and families in adapting to illness-imposed lifestyle changes, such as alterations in family and societal roles. Psychiatric consultation or team conferences with psychiatric staff are an important resource for the social worker and dialysis team for several reasons.

First, most dialysis patients are subjected to situational stress. Despite this fact, psychiatric intervention may be perceived by the patient as an unnecessary and unwelcome intrusion. The social worker assists patients in resolving problems and in dealing with crises but should have psychiatric resources available for consultation or referral when needed.

Second, some patients become increasingly dependent or noncompliant during periods of their illness. During such times, the social worker should work with the patient, family, and other team members to help understand the behavior. Ultimately, the patient is responsible for much of his or her own management, and this should be emphasized by the social worker.

Finally, because sexual dysfunction can be a problem for patients undergoing maintenance dialysis, the social worker may be the team member whom the patient and/or family approaches for counseling.

ETHICS, RIGHTS, AND RESPONSIBILITIES

For the ESRD patient and family, life with maintenance dialysis requires major changes in activity and lifestyle. These disruptions are sometimes unpleasant as well as unanticipated. Frequently the dialysis unit and involved personnel are perceived by the patient as a cause of his or her unsatisfactory situation. Frustration and conflict are prone to develop and must be resolved.

Is written consent necessary before starting dialysis?

Informed written consent for any invasive procedure, including dialysis, is always required. For emergency dialysis, if the patient is too ill, the next of kin or another person who has durable power of attorney may sign the consent for treatment.

It is important that staff members, as well as patients and families, understand the importance of informed consent, because patients and families often have misconceptions or unrealistic ideas about dialysis and what procedures may be involved. The exact format of the consent form is determined by the unit or institution's legal adviser. It should clearly document that an adequate discussion and explanation of benefits, complications, risks, and alternatives are provided and understood by the patient. Separate consent is necessary for access procedures or modification. Update of the dialysis consent form is necessary if there is a significant change in procedure that might affect the patient, such as dialyzer reuse.

What are some of the rights of the patient?

- To be fully informed about his or her illness
- To be informed as to the nature of the treatment and the usual risks

- To be fully informed about alternative methods of treatment
- To know that personal privacy will be respected and professional confidentiality maintained
- To have input into the treatment regimen

May a patient voluntarily decide to discontinue dialysis?

Many professionals, but not all, believe that a rational adult who, for reasons that are valid to him or her, elects to stop treatment with full understanding of the consequences should have that right. The ethical and legal issues are complex; not all ESRD workers agree, and in some instances courts have ordered dialysis to be continued.

What are some responsibilities of personnel to patients?

- To make the patient as fully informed as possible, as long as it is consistent with high-quality care
- To ensure that all safeguards are met fully and to provide high-quality dialysis service
- To be supportive of patient and family in their adjustment to the illness, its treatment, and the accompanying changes in their lives. This involves teaching them about the disease and its treatment so that they can make informed decisions and set realistic goals.

What are some patient responsibilities?

- To understand and to follow the instructions of the physicians, nurses, and other personnel providing care
- To strive for a high degree of independence through learning and to assume responsibility for self-care as far as possible
- To respect the rights and privacy of other patients

What are some additional personnel responsibilities?

- One person, usually a nurse, must be in charge. Problems should be taken to this individual to prevent misconceptions or ambiguity.
- All personnel must carry out assigned responsibilities to the best of individual ability, provide the best possible patient care, and contribute to the overall smooth operation of the unit.
- All personnel should strive for a pleasant environment that allows for interaction among patients, personnel, and visitors while maintaining an appropriate level of efficiency and professionalism.

2 Basic Chemistry of Body Fluids and Electrolytes

Normal kidneys maintain the balance between body water and the substances dissolved in it within the narrow limits necessary for life. Kidneys also excrete the waste products of protein metabolism. Dialysis partially substitutes for these two important functions when the normal kidneys fail. Fundamental to understanding the processes used by the kidney—natural or artificial—is a basic knowledge of the chemistry involved and the measurements used.

METRIC SYSTEM

A solid review of the basic system of measurement is necessary because the metric system is used in chemical and physical measurements that relate to body physiology. Length is expressed by the basic unit of the meter. The basic unit of mass is the gram, and the liter is the basic unit of volume. Table 2-1 lists common metric terms and their interrelationship.

The metric system is entirely decimal. Prefixes indicate smaller or larger units (Table 2-2).

To relate the metric system to more familiar uses, the following approximations may be helpful:

- A man who is 6 feet 4 inches tall is about 1.95 m in height.
- A dime is about 1 mm thick.
- A 154-pound person weighs 70 kg.

The following are commonly used conversion factors to change metric units to the English system of pounds, inches, and quarts.

- 1 meter (m) = 39.37 inches (in)
- 1 inch (in) = 2.54 centimeters (cm)
- 1 liter (L) = 1.057 quarts (U.S.) (qt)
- 1 gallon (gal) = 3.785 liters (L)
- 1 kilogram (kg) = 2.2 pounds (lb)
- 1 ounce (oz) = 28.35 grams (g)
- 1 fluid ounce (fl oz) = 29.57 milliliters (mL)

Temperature is expressed in degrees centigrade. Zero degrees centigrade is the freezing point of water and 100° C is its boiling point. The following is a comparison of some centigrade temperatures with the Fahrenheit scale:

Table 2-1	Commonly Used Metric Units		
Quantity	Unit	Symbol	Relationship of units
Length	Millimeter	mm	1 mm = 0.001 m
	Centimeter	cm	1 cm = 0.01 m
	Meter	m	1 m
	Kilometer	km	1 km = 1000 m
Area	Square centimeter	cm²	1 cm² = 0.0001 m²
	Square meter	m²	1 m²
	Square kilometer	km²	1 km² = 1,000,000 m²
Volume	Milliliter	mL	1 mL = 0.001 L
	Deciliter	dL	1 dL = 0.01 L
	Liter	L	1 L
	Cubic meter	m³	1 m³ = 1000 L
Mass	Milligram	mg	1 mg = 0.001 g
	Gram	g	1 g
	Kilogram	kg	1 kg = 1000 g

Table 2-2	Metric Decimal Prefixes	
Multiplication factors	Prefix	Symbol
1		
$= 10^{-1}$	deci	d
$= 10^{-2}$	centi	c
$0.001 = 10^{-3}$	milli	m
$0.000001 = 10^{-6}$	micro	μ
$0.000000001 = 10^{-9}$	nano	n
$0.00000000001 = 10^{-12}$	pica	p

	°F	°C
Boiling point of water	212	100
Normal body temperature	98.6	37
Freezing point of water	32	0

For conversion of Fahrenheit values to centigrade and vice versa, use the formula:

Fahrenheit temperature = 9/5 (centigrade temperature) + 32

Centigrade temperature = 5/9 (Fahrenheit temperature) − 32

CHEMISTRY

All physical things are composed of a finite number of kinds of matter. Matter is anything that possesses weight and occupies space. The basic kinds of matter are called elements. An element cannot be further divided without changing its chemical properties. There are 108 known elements. They may exist alone, in mixtures, or in chemical combinations (compounds). Some elements exist alone in their natural form as a solid, liquid, or gas. For instance, gold nuggets are pure, crystalline gold (Au). Metallic mercury (Hg) is a liquid under ordinary conditions. Helium (He) is a monatomic gas. The physical state depends upon the melting or boiling point. Many elements do not exist in an uncombined state, but only as compounds. Oxygen as it exists in air is not monatomic oxygen (O) but a compound of two oxygen atoms, O_2. Almost all hydrogen (H) exists in compounds, such as water (H_2O).

What is an atom?

An atom is the smallest particle of an element that retains the properties of that element. Atoms are composed of a central nucleus containing protons and neutrons and electrons that move in an orbital fashion around the nucleus. An atom resembles a miniature solar system. The sun represents the nucleus; the paths of the planets represent the orbiting electrons. Several electrons may occupy the same orbital path.

Protons are a part of all nuclei and have a positive charge equivalent to that of an electron. An electron is a particle of infinitesimal small mass with a negative charge. A neutron is equal to a proton in mass, but is electrically neutral.

What is a compound?

A compound is a chemical combination of elements. The proportion of elements is fixed for each compound. For example, water, H_2O, always exists in a 2:1 ratio of hydrogen and oxygen.

What is a molecule?

A molecule is the smallest unit of a substance that retains its chemical properties. A molecule of oxygen, O_2, has different chemical properties than an atom of oxygen, O.

What is atomic weight?

Atomic weights relate to one another based on an arbitrary scale that assigns a weight of 12 atomic mass units (amu) to the carbon isotope 12 (^{12}C). On this scale, protons and neutrons each weigh 1 amu; electrons have negligible mass. The hydrogen atom (^1H) is 1 amu, and the oxygen atom (^{16}O) is 16 amu. One atomic mass unit is sometimes called a dalton (Da), after John Dalton, an early developer of the atomic concept.

What does atomic number indicate?

The atomic number is the number of protons in the nucleus of an atom. This is a unique number that characterizes each element. This number of protons in a nucleus determines the chemical nature of the atom; by contrast, the number of neutrons affects only the weight of an atom. When two atoms with the same number of protons have different numbers of neutrons, and hence have different weights, they are called isotopes.

How does atomic weight relate to molecular weight?

To calculate molecular weight, add the weights of each atom that make up that molecule. For instance, water, H_2O, consists of two hydrogen atoms and one oxygen atom. From this, we can calculate that the molecular weight of water is 18 Da $(1 + 1 + 16)$. If the amu weight of an element is expressed in grams, it is called a gram atomic weight; for compounds, the term is gram molecular weight. This does not make calculating more complex, however. For instance, 16 g of oxygen contain the same number of particles as does 1 g of hydrogen because oxygen weighs 16 times as much as hydrogen.

What determines the physical state of a molecule?

Every molecule possesses kinetic energy, the energy of movement. The speed of a molecule depends on the temperature. An increase in temperature increases molecular speed; cooling reduces molecular speed. The rapid movement of each molecule acts to keep all particles separate from one another.

There are also powerful attractive forces between particles. These attractive forces tend to aggregate molecules. In a crystal of ice the attractive forces are greater than the separating forces, and the molecules remain trapped in the crystal structure. When heat is added, kinetic energy increases until the separative forces are greater than the attractive forces. This is the process of melting. Further addition of heat increases the kinetic energy until some molecules acquire sufficient energy to escape the liquid state entirely by boiling and producing steam.

Conversely, as cooling occurs, steam condenses into water, and then crystallizes into ice. These steps occur as kinetic energy and molecular speed are reduced, and the attractive forces become more important.

What is a solution?

A solution is a homogeneous mixture of dissolved particles (solute) and a liquid (solvent). In physiologic solutions, the solvent is usually water. Physiologic saline contains 0.85 g of NaCl in 100 mL of water.

How is the concentration of a solution measured?

Nonionized particles have been measured in terms of weight of solute per volume of solvent. Blood glucose and urea commonly have been measured as milligrams per 100 mL (mg/dL). For ionized particles it is important to know the relative number of particles present and the contribution of their charge. These are measured more precisely by the use of molarity and normality, and are usually expressed as mEq/L (milliequivalents per liter).

What are SI Units?

"SI Units" is the abbreviation for le Systeme Internationale d'Unites. This is an extension of the metric system that provides uniformity of units of measurement and easy conversion. Since 1987 *SI* has been used to report data by most clinical laboratories in the United States. In this system the amount of a substance is written as moles per liter rather than mass, such as g/L or mg/dL. See Appendix B for some common chemistry conversion factors.

What is an electrolyte?

An electrolyte is a substance that dissolves in water to form ionized particles.

What is an ion?

An ion is a particle that has an electric charge. It may be a charged atom, such as a sodium ion, or a charged compound, such as a lactate ion.

What is conductivity?

Conductivity is the ability of a solution to conduct an electric current. It is illustrated by an electrolytic cell. Fig. 2-1 shows such a cell—a container of solution with two electrodes. The electrodes are connected by wires through a battery and an ammeter; the ammeter measures flow of current through the circuit. If the only communication between electrodes is through very pure water, little or no current flows; there is no way for electrons to pass through the water.

If sodium chloride is added to the water, current will flow. Sodium ions are attracted to the negative electrode (cathode), where each ion accepts an electron. At the same time, chloride ions are attracted to the positive electrode (anode), where each gives up an electron.

The ease with which electrons flow in a solution depends on the kinds of electrolytes that are present and their concentration. Conductivity monitors are vital components of dialysis fluid delivery systems that must produce solutions of constant, precise solute content.

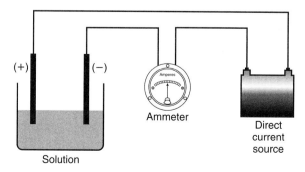

Fig. 2-1 Electrolytic cell.

Why is conductivity an important measurement in dialysis?

Dialysate is produced by mixing a concentrated solution of electrolytes with very pure water. The correct proportion of concentration of electrolytes and water is measured by the electrical conductivity of the solution. The proportion of electrolytes to water must be within certain limits to ensure patient safety. The conductivity of pure water is zero, whereas the conductivity of dialysate is dependent on the amount of sodium in the solution. A dialysate solution containing too little sodium may cause water to shift into the patient's blood cells. This may cause hypotension, cramping, and hemolysis. Too much sodium in the dialysate may cause high blood levels of sodium. When the sodium levels in the blood become too high, fluid may leave the cells, causing the blood cells to shrivel. This is known as crenation and may cause symptoms such as hypertension, profound thirst, and headache.

What is osmosis?

Osmosis is the movement of fluid from an area of low concentration of solutes to an area of high concentration of solutes (Fig. 2-2). A strong electrolyte solution has a reduced water concentration because some of the water has been replaced by solute. If two solutions of different concentrations are separated by a membrane permeable only to water, water flows from the area of greatest water concentration to the area of least water concentration. This is the same as saying that water flows from the area of least solute concentration to the area of greatest solute concentration. Only the water moves, not the solute.

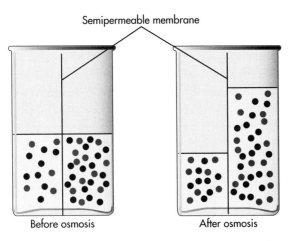

Semipermeable membrane

Before osmosis   After osmosis

Fig. 2-2 Osmosis is the process of water movement through a semipermeable membrane from an area of low solute concentration to an area of high solute concentration. *(From Lewis SM, Heitkemper MM, Dirksen SR: Medical-Surgical Nursing, ed. 6, St Louis, 2004, Mosby.)*

Membrane

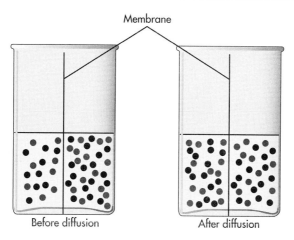

Before diffusion   After diffusion

Fig. 2-3 Diffusion is the movement of molecules from an area of high concentration to an area of low concentration. A normal pH is maintained by a ratio of 1 part carbonic acid to 20 parts bicarbonate. *(From Lewis SM, Heitkemper MM, Dirksen SR:* Medical-Surgical Nursing, *ed. 6, St Louis, 2004, Mosby.)*

What is diffusion?

Diffusion is the movement of solutes from an area of higher concentration of solutes to an area of lower concentration of solutes, so that both sides are equal (Fig. 2-3). Only the solutes move, not the water.

What is pH?

The measure either of acidity or alkalinity of a substance is expressed as pH (Fig. 2-4). The initials pH stands for "potential," or "power," of hydrogen and the value demonstrates the concentration of hydrogen ions in a solution. Normal H^+ ion concentration in human extracellular fluid is 7.35 to 7.45. If a substance has a pH value less than 7, it is an acid. A substance having a pH value greater than 7 is an alkali. If a substance has a pH value of 7, it is considered neutral. pH measures only the free H^+ in solution. If some H^+ is bound and not ionized, it does not affect the pH. The pH is maintained by the action of buffers.

What is a buffer?

Buffers are substances that, in solution, maintain a constant hydrogen ion concentration despite addition of either acid or base. Buffers minimize pH changes when acid or bases are added to a solution. Bicarbonates, phosphates, amino acids, and proteins all act as buffers. Bicarbonate is the major plasma buffer.

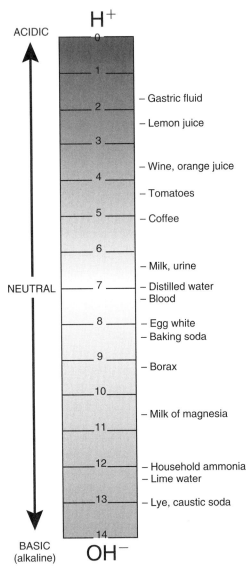

Fig. 2-4 The pH range on a logarithmic scale of 1 to 14. The actual concentration of hydrogen ions changes tenfold with each pH unit on the scale. *(From Thibodeau GA, Patton KT:* Structure and Function of the Body, *ed 12, St. Louis, 2004, Mosby.)*

Why is the hydrogen ion concentration important?

All metabolic processes of the body require this precise range of H^+ concentration. If the H^+ concentration exceeds that of pure water, the solution is acidic. If the concentration is less, it is basic, or alkaline. If the concentration becomes too great or too small, massive derangements of metabolism occur. The extremes of (H^+) compatible with life lie between 16 and 160 nmol/L (pH 7.8 to 6.8) (Fig. 2-5). Two body organs are involved in H^+ regulation: the lungs and the kidneys. The lungs eliminate carbon dioxide (the major end product of metabolism) as rapidly as it is produced, and in so doing regulate the partial pressure of carbon dioxide in blood. The kidneys regulate blood pH by reabsorbing or excreting acids or bases. Kidney failure causes retention of hydrogen ions; this is called metabolic acidosis. See Chapter 4 for further discussion.

What is an acid?

An acid is a substance that can donate a hydrogen ion, and a base is a substance that can accept a hydrogen ion. An acid may be called a proton donor, and a base a proton receptor. Remember that the hydrogen atom consists of a positively charged nucleus, or proton, and a single, negatively charged orbiting electron. The hydrogen ion (H^+) is the proton without the orbiting electron.

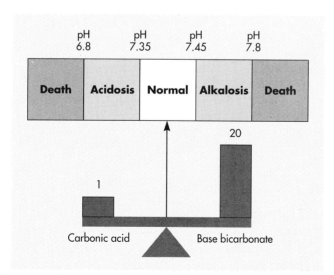

Fig. 2-5 The normal range of plasma pH is 7.35 to 7.45. A normal pH is maintained by a ratio of 1 part carbonic acid to 20 parts bicarbonate. *(From Lewis SM, Heitkemper MM, Dirksen SR: Medical-Surgical Nursing, ed. 6, St Louis, 2004, Mosby.)*

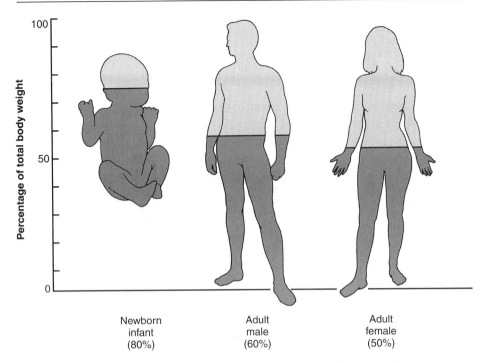

Fig. 2-6 Percentage of total body weight composed of water. *(From Thibodeau GA, Patton KT: Structure and Function of the Body, ed 12, St. Louis, 2004, Mosby [Rolin Graphics].)*

BODY WATER
How much water does the body contain?

Water is the major constituent of the body. It comprises 45% to 75% of the total body weight of an adult. The proportion varies inversely with the amount of body fat. A 70-kg man (154 lb) has about 42 L of total body water (60% of weight). Women have less. Infants and very young children have the highest proportion of body water (Fig. 2-6).

What purpose does this fluid serve?

Body tissue is made up of living cells. Complex chemical processes within these cells produce energy in the form of heat, motion, and regeneration. Oxygen and nutrients are metabolized; carbon dioxide and other wastes are produced. Water within the cell is the medium for these chemical processes.

Water also surrounds and bathes all cells, protecting them from the hazards of the external world. It is the vehicle for transportation of nutrients from—and wastes to—the outside environment.

How is water distributed in the body?

Total body water is the sum of all fluids within all compartments of the body. The total body water is distributed between two major compartments: the intracellular fluid (ICF) and the extracellular fluid (ECF). Approximately two thirds (or 40% of body weight) of the total amount of body water are contained in the intracellular fluid compartment and one third (or 20% of body weight) of the total amount of body water is contained in the extracellular compartment. The extracellular fluid can further be separated into interstitial (spaces between the cells and outside of the blood vessels), intravascular (fluid in the blood plasma), and transcellular (fluids outside of normal compartments), which includes synovial, pericardial, intraocular, peritoneal, and other body fluids that do not interchange readily (Fig. 2-7).

What are the constituents of intracellular fluid?

Intracellular fluid provides fluid to the cells to function. The composition of ICF varies with the specific tissue. Muscle values are commonly used in calculations. Potassium, the major intracellular cation, is 155 mEq/L; magnesium is 40 mEq/L, and sodium is only 10 mEq/L. Organic phosphates and protein are the important anions; chloride and bicarbonate total only 10 mEq/L.

What is the composition of extracellular fluid?

Plasma water and interstitial fluid are nearly the same. Sodium is the major cation (145 mEq/L). Chloride and bicarbonate are the major anions. About 7% of plasma volume is protein and lipid material that does not cross the capillary wall. The protein molecules are anionic; to maintain electrical neutrality, there are slightly fewer sodium and chloride ions in plasma than in interstitial fluid. Clinical calculations of electrolytes usually ignore these small differences and assume that plasma electrolytes are representative of the total ECF.

What determines the distribution of water between plasma and the interstitial compartment?

This depends on the balance among colloid (protein and lipid) osmotic pressure, intracapillary blood pressure, and tissue turgor pressure. This is known as the Starling effect.

How are the electrolyte concentrations kept different inside and outside the cell?

The cell membrane is impermeable to protein and the organic phosphate complexes, confining them inside the cell. There are metabolically active (energy-consuming) "pumps" in the cell wall that transport sodium ions from within the cell to the outside, while moving potassium ions from the exterior to the cell's interior.

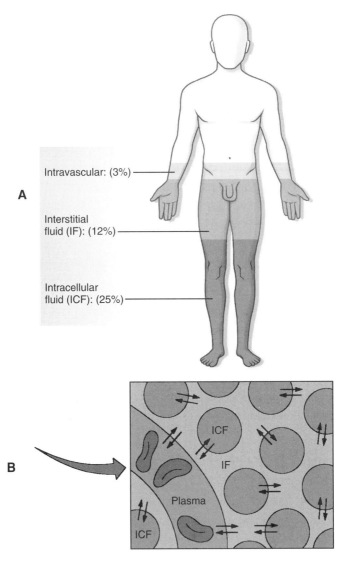

Fig. 2-7 Distribution of three types of fluid in total body water for young adult male. *(From Thibodeau GA, Patton KT:* Structure and Function of the Body, *ed 12, St. Louis, 2004, Mosby* [Rolin Graphics].)

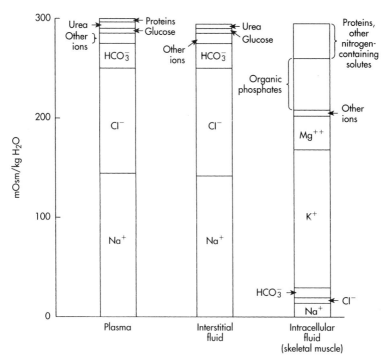

Fig. 2-8 Osmotic composition of major body fluids. *(Redrawn from Laiken ND, Fanestil DF:* Best and Taylor's Physiological Basis of Medical Practice, *ed 12, Baltimore, 1991, Williams & Wilkins.)*

Does water pass across the cell membrane?

Yes, water moves quickly in either direction to maintain total osmolar equality on both sides of the membrane (Fig. 2-8).

Are there nonelectrolytes in body fluids?

Yes. These include glucose, amino acids, and other nutrients and metabolic wastes such as urea. Their concentration is relatively low compared with the electrolytes.

Are urea and creatinine electrolytes?

No. Both urea and creatinine are soluble in water, but they do not form charged particles.

What is meant by fluid balance?

A normal diet contains 500 to 1000 mL of water in the food itself. Some 300 to 500 mL of water is produced each day by metabolism of food and from tissue breakdown. Other fluid taken in, such as coffee, tea, juice, or other beverages, obviously represents water intake and averages 1500 to 2000 mL/day.

Box 2-1		
NORMAL FLUID BALANCE IN THE ADULT		

Intake		
Fluids		1200 mL
Solid food		1000 mL
Water from oxidation		300 mL
		2500 mL
Output		
Insensible loss (skin and lungs)		900 mL
In feces		100 mL
Urine		1500 mL
		2500 mL

Between 700 and 1000 mL of water is lost each day through evaporation from the lungs and by insensible perspiration (Box 2-1). Vigorous activity or a rise in temperature causes additional loss (measurable in liters if the environmental temperature increase is severe). A minimum of 400 mL of fluid or more must be excreted as urine each day to prevent the accumulation of metabolic wastes.

The electrolyte composition, pH, osmolality, and so on are precisely maintained in the body's internal fluid environment. The kidneys keep this balance, called homeostasis. The kidney conserves fluid or excretes excess as needed. When kidney failure occurs, meticulous attention to the balance of fluid intake and losses becomes a necessity.

3 Renal Physiology and the Pathology of Renal Failure

Before any discussion of the pathology of renal failure can begin, it is important to review the following functions that normal kidneys perform (Fig. 3-1):

- Elimination of metabolic wastes and other toxic materials
- Regulation of fluid volume
- Maintenance of electrolyte balance
- Regulation of blood pH

In addition, the kidneys also have several endocrine functions, including the following:

- Production of renin, which affects sodium, fluid volume, and blood pressure
- Formation of erythropoietin, which controls red cell production in the bone marrow

A normal kidney is also a receptor site for several hormones:

- Antidiuretic hormone (ADH), produced by the pituitary, reduces the excretion of water.
- Aldosterone, produced by the adrenal cortex, promotes sodium retention and enhances secretion of potassium and hydrogen ion.
- Parathyroid hormone increases phosphorus and bicarbonate excretion and stimulates conversion of vitamin D to the active 1,25-dihydroxycholecalciferol vitamin D_3 form.

RENAL PHYSIOLOGY
Blood supply to the kidneys

The kidneys are highly vascular organs and receive 20% to 25% of the resting cardiac output, which is greater than 1000 mL/min. Cardiac output is the volume of blood pumped per minute by each ventricle of the heart. Each kidney receives blood from a renal artery that originates from the abdominal aorta, and blood leaves the kidney through the renal vein. The renal artery branches out to form the afferent arterioles, which in turn form the glomerular capillaries of individual glomeruli. The glomerular capillaries then join to form the efferent arterioles, which in turn diffuse into peritubular capillaries and the vasa recta (Fig. 3-2).

Blood flow to the kidney is dependent on hydration and cardiac output. Dehydration, blood loss, congestive heart failure, and myocardial infarction are examples of situations that would compromise blood flow to the kidney.

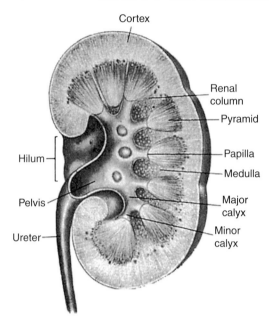

Fig. 3-1 Longitudinal section of normal kidney.

What is the difference between the peritubular capillaries and the vasa recta?

The peritubular capillaries surround the proximal and distal convoluted tubules and allow tubular secretion and reabsorption to occur. The vasa recta capillaries and branches surround the loops of Henle of the juxtamedullary nephrons and are located in the renal medulla. They play a major role in the concentration of urine as it moves through the tubules.

What is a nephron?

The nephron is the main functional unit of the kidney. There are more than a million such units in each of the two kidneys. Each nephron is a complex structure and has two main components: vascular and tubular. The vascular component consists of the afferent arteriole, glomerulus, efferent arteriole, and peritubular capillaries. The tubular portions of the nephron include Bowman's capsule, proximal tubule, loop of Henle, and the distal tubule.

The glomerulus consists of a network of thin-walled capillaries supplied by the afferent arteriole and is closely surrounded by a pear-shaped epithelial membrane called Bowman's capsule. The glomerulus and Bowman's capsule combined are called the renal corpuscle. The space between the two layers of Bowman's capsule opens into the proximal tubule, which makes a series of convolutions in the cortex of the kidney. It straightens out, and then makes a U-turn, known as the loop of Henle, in the kidney

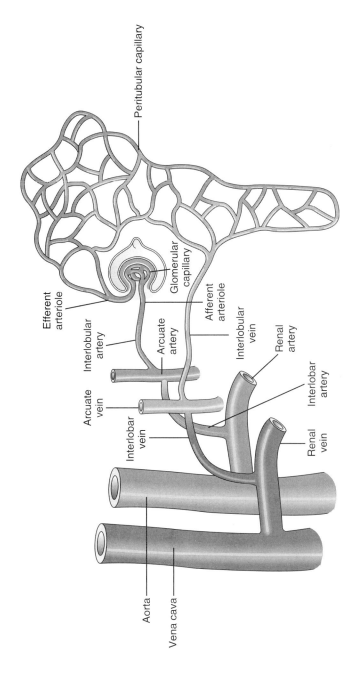

Fig. 3-2 The venous vessels of the kidney parallel the arterial vessels and are similarly named. *(From Copstead LC, Banasik JL, Pathophysiology, ed 3, St Louis, 2005, Saunders.)*

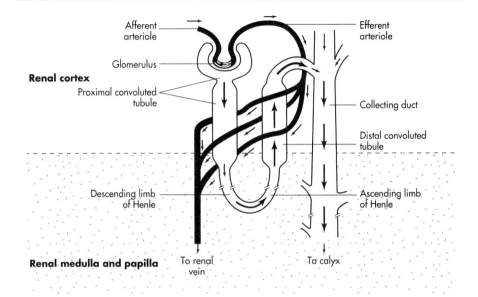

Fig. 3-3 Diagram of nephron with afferent arteriole, glomerulus, efferent arteriole, and collecting duct.

medulla. It becomes convoluted again adjacent to its own glomerulus and finally joins other distal tubules to form a collecting duct to carry the freshly formed urine to the kidney pelvis (Fig. 3-3). Each kidney pelvis funnels the urine into its ureter, which connects with the urinary bladder. The urethra conveys the urine from the bladder to the exterior.

What is the first step in urine formation?

Blood enters the glomerulus through an afferent arteriole. Because of the blood pressure in the capillaries and because of their thin walls, filtration of blood occurs. Water and dissolved solutes of molecular weight less than 68,000 Da (albumin) pass freely into Bowman's space. This essentially protein-free fluid is the glomerular filtrate, and its rate of production is the glomerular filtration rate (GFR). The GFR is the amount of filtrate the kidneys produce each minute. A man of average size has about 180 L of filtrate per day, or 125 mL/min. Ninety-nine percent of this filtrate is reabsorbed as it passes through the tubules.

Glomerular filtration is dependent on sufficient blood circulation to the glomerulus and maintenance of normal filtration pressures. The filtration of molecules depends on their shape, size, and ionic charge. As the molecular weight and size increase, the degree of filtration decreases. The glomerular basement membrane exerts a net negative charge. Substances carrying a negative charge will be repelled by the basement membrane, and its filtration will be prohibited.

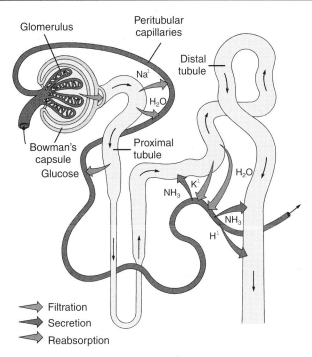

Fig. 3-4 Path of filtrate as it moves through different parts of a nephron. *(From Thibodeau GA, Patton KT:* Anatomy & physiology, *ed 5, St Louis, 2003, Mosby.)*

What happens to the filtrate as it moves through the tubules?

The main function of the tubules is reabsorption and secretion. Tubular reabsorption is the process of the filtrate moving back into the blood of the peritubular capillaries or vasa recta (Fig. 3-4). This process is very selective and depends on the body's needs at the time. Materials that are reabsorbed back into the bloodstream are ions such as sodium, potassium, chloride, bicarbonate, and calcium.

Of the 180 L of glomerular filtrate produced each day, about 2 L remain as the final urine. The rest of the water is reabsorbed along with glucose, amino acids, small proteins, and most electrolytes. The remaining filtrate becomes concentrated and begins to resemble the ultimate urine as it progresses down the tubule. Final adjustments of water-to-solute load occur in the distal tubule under the influence of ADH. The tubules conserve water and electrolytes by returning them to the blood. Hydrogen ions and metabolic wastes are excreted along with a volume of water appropriate to the total body need. The majority of reabsorption occurs in the proximal tubule; however, some reabsorption does occur in the distal tubule.

Tubular secretion adds materials to the filtrate from the blood. Tubular secretion helps to remove toxic substances from the blood and to help restore blood pH by excreting excessive hydrogen ions. Substances secreted into the tubules include potassium, hydrogen, ammonia, creatinine, and some drugs.

RENAL FAILURE
What happens in kidney failure?

Renal failure may be acute or chronic. In both there is enough loss of nephron function to upset the normal steady state of the body's internal environment. Waste products of protein metabolism accumulate.

This is termed *azotemia,* indicating retention of nitrogenous products (azote = nitrogen). Azotemia is a major component of the uremic syndrome.

What is urea?

Urea is the waste product of protein metabolism and the most abundant organic waste. Most urea is produced during the breakdown of amino acids. Its normal value in the blood is 15 to 40 mg/dL.

What is creatinine?

Creatinine is a protein produced by muscle and released into the blood. The creatinine level in the blood is determined by the rate it is being removed in the urine.

What is uremia?

Uremia, or the uremic syndrome, encompasses a complex of symptoms and findings resulting from disordered biochemical processes when kidney function fails.

Is retention of urea the cause of uremia?

Severity of the uremic symptoms roughly parallels the rise in blood urea. Urea clearly contributes to some of the symptoms—malaise, lethargy, anorexia, insomnia—but it is not the primary toxin of uremia. Numerous other substances are retained in the body when kidney function fails. More than 200 potential uremic toxins have been identified.

What is chronic kidney disease?

The National Kidney Foundation (NKF) defines chronic kidney disease (CKD) as either damage to the kidney or a GFR of less than 60 mL/min/1.73 m^2 for more than 3 months. Kidney damage is further defined as pathologic irregularities or markers of damage such as abnormalities in the blood, urine tests, or imaging studies. End-stage renal disease develops when the kidneys permanently lose most of their ability to remove waste and maintain fluid and chemical balances inside the body. This process can develop rapidly, within 2 to 3 months, or may develop slowly over 30 to 40 years.

CKD is defined according to the presence or absence of kidney damage and level of kidney function—regardless of the type of kidney disease (diagnosis). Among individuals with CKD, the stages are defined based on the level of kidney function. Identifying the presence and stage of CKD in an individual is not a substitute for accurate assessment of the cause of kidney disease, extent of kidney damage, level of kidney function, comorbid conditions, complications of decreased kidney function, or risks for loss of kidney function or cardiovascular disease in that patient. Defining stages of CKD requires "categorization" of continuous measures of kidney function, and the "cut-off levels" between stages are inherently arbitrary. Nonetheless, staging of CKD will facilitate application of clinical practice guidelines, clinical performance measures, and quality improvement.

What is the course of chronic kidney disease?

Progressive and irreversible loss of function occurs over many months or years. As the number of functioning nephrons decreases, each remaining unit must clear an increasing solute load. Eventually the limit to the amount of solute that can be cleared is reached, and the concentration in body fluids must rise. Azotemia and clinical uremia result. Fortunately the slow rate of progression allows the body to adapt somewhat. Symptoms may be relatively mild proportionate to the chemical abnormalities.

What are the stages of CKD?

CKD can be expressed in a series of stages from one to five (Table 3-1).

The stages of CKD are based on the level of the GFR, which is widely recognized and accepted as the best overall measure of kidney function.

The NKF gives the following examples of potential etiologies in the causes of chronic kidney disease: diabetes mellitus (types 1 and 2), systemic lupus erythematosus, human immunodeficiency virus (HIV), nephropathy, hepatitis B or C, hypertension, infection, stones, multiple myelomas, antibodies, and cystic diseases.

Table 3-1	Stages of Chronic Kidney Disease (CKD)	
Stage	Description	Glomerular filtration rate (GFR) (mL/min/1.73 m^2)
1	Kidney damage with normal or ↑GFR	>90
2	Kidney damage with mild ↓GFR	60-89
3	Moderate ↓GFR	30-59
4	Severe ↓GFR	15-29
5	Kidney failure	<15 or dialysis

From Sepulveda S, Davis L, Schwab S: Chronic kidney disease (CKD) practice management tool: A reference guide for best practices, *Orthobiotech Nephrology* 39(2 Suppl): 546–575, 2002; National Kidney Foundation K/DOQI, March, 2002.

The NKF recommends that all individuals be assessed to see whether they are at an increased risk for developing CKD. The evaluation should include serum creatinine levels, assessment of proteinuria, and assessment of urinary sediment or urine dipstick for white or red blood cells. The best indicators, however, of level of kidney function are the estimates of the GFR. The goal is to delay or ameliorate the progression of the disease.

The recommendations from the NKF focus on stages and not on the disease etiology or pathology. The ultimate goal is to improve outcomes by maximizing opportunities for prevention (Table 3-2).

What is end-stage renal disease (ESRD)?

In the course of chronic kidney disease the renal insufficiency often may be managed by diet, sodium restriction, phosphate control, and medication for a considerable time. As function falls to 10% to 15% of normal, the end is reached; dialysis or transplantation is necessary if the patient is to survive.

Table 3-2	Stages of Chronic Kidney Disease (CKD): Clinical Action Steps		
Stage	**Description**	**Glomerular filtration rate (GFR) (mL/min/1.73 m²)**	**Clinical action***
1	Kidney damage with normal or ↑GFR	>90	Diagnosis and treatment Treatment of comorbid conditions Slowing progression Cardiovascular (CVD) risk reduction
2	Kidney damage with mild ↓GFR	60-89	Estimating progression
3	Moderate ↓GFR	30-59	Evaluating and treating complications
4	Severe ↓GFR	15-29	Preparation for kidney replacement therapy
5	Kidney failure	<15 or dialysis	Replacement, if uremia present

*Management of CKD patients should be based on the stage of disease as defined by National Kidney Foundation. From Sepulveda S, Davis L, Schwab S: Chronic kidney disease (CKD) practice management tool: A reference guide for best practices, *Orthobiotech Nephrology* 39(2 Suppl):546-575, 2002; National Kidney Foundation K/DOQI, March, 2002.

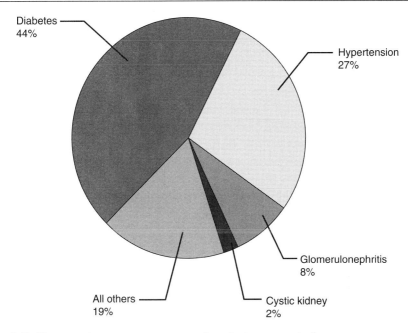

Fig. 3-5 The most common causes of end-stage renal disease.

What places a person at risk for developing CKD?

The NKF has identified older age, family history, and ethnic descent (African American, American Indian, Latino, Asian, or Pacific Islander) as factors that increase susceptibility to kidney disease. High levels of proteinuria, hypertension, poor glycemic control in diabetes, and smoking are factors that can accelerate the progression of kidney disease. The most common causes of ESRD in the United States are shown in Fig. 3-5. The number of patients diagnosed with ESRD caused by diabetes continues to climb, almost doubling from 1991 to 2001. The rates of glomerulonephritis have declined as much as 12% from 1995 to 2001. Early detection of proteinuria, a sensitive marker of kidney damage, will allow timelier introduction of therapy to slow progression of disease.

What are some glomerular causes of ESRD?

Glomerular diseases damage the glomeruli and allow proteins and red blood cells to leak into the urine. Glomerular diseases fall into two major categories: glomerulonephritis and glomerulosclerosis.

Glomerulonephritis is an inflammatory disease affecting the glomeruli of the kidney. It can be either a primary disease of the kidney or may occur as a secondary complication of another disease, such as systemic lupus erythematosus, diabetes nephritis, or Goodpasture syndrome. The glomeruli become inflamed or damaged and allow red blood cells and significant amounts of proteins to pass into the urine. Glomerulonephritis may be caused by infection involving *Streptococcus* bacteria. The glomerular damage from the strep infection is not caused by the bacteria directly affecting the kidney, but by the large production of antibodies that deposit in the glomeruli, causing the damage. As the immune system responds to infection, antigen-antibody complexes are formed. As the number of antigen-antibody complexes increase, they accumulate and block the glomeruli. The filtration capabilities of the glomerulus declines and the individuals begin to experience symptoms such as a low serum albumin, hematuria, edema, hypertension, and decreased urine output.

Glomerulosclerosis describes the scarring or hardening of the blood vessels in the kidney. Systemic diseases such as lupus and diabetes mellitus cause the glomerular cells to produce scar material. The glomerular cells may produce growth factors that stimulate this scar tissue formation, or the growth factors can be brought to the glomerulus by the circulating blood volume that enters the glomerulus.

Diabetic nephropathy can occur with both type 1 diabetes mellitus (insulin-dependent diabetes [IDDM]) and type 2 (non–insulin-dependent diabetes). The glomerular basement membrane thickens with this nephropathy. Hyperglycemia increases the speed of blood flow to the kidney, which puts a strain on the glomeruli and elevates the blood pressure. Diabetic nephropathy seldom develops before 10 years' duration of type 1 diabetes and more likely occurs in people with 10- to 20-year tenure. The treatment, complications, and specific care needs of the patient with diabetic nephropathy are examined in Chapter 18.

Are there any genetic diseases that can cause CKD?

Polycystic kidney disease (PKD) is the most common of all life-threatening genetic diseases in the United States and is the third leading cause of renal failure. The pattern of inheritance is autosomal dominant. This means that both sexes are just as likely to be affected. Because the gene is dominant, only one affected gene is needed for the disease to develop. Consequently, the likelihood of passing the affected gene to a son or daughter is one in two, or 50%. PKD is a progressive disease and causes numerous cysts to form anywhere along the nephron. These fluid-filled cysts replace normal kidney tissue and begin to enlarge and compress the surrounding nephrons and renal vessels. The compressed renal tissue eventually becomes fibrotic and causes kidney function to deteriorate. The kidneys can become quite enlarged as the cysts grow in size and number, causing the patient to experience a significant increase in abdominal girth. In some patients you will see an increased hematocrit due to increased secretion of erythropoietin. This occurs from compression of the kidneys, with increased erythropoietin being secreted from the cysts.

Symptoms vary by individual as well as the onset of ESRD in family members. Cyst development is seen in 50% of all individuals by the age of 18. Low back pain or flank pain is one of the most common symptoms of PKD. Urinary tract infections, hematuria, severe hypertension, and decreased renal function are also seen. The cysts cause the patient to be susceptible to infection as bacteria become imbedded around the cysts, making it difficult for antibiotics to penetrate to the kidneys or cysts. Nephrectomy may need to be performed when the kidneys become very painful or chronically infected. The patient with PKD may develop cysts elsewhere, such as on the ovaries, testes, pancreas, liver, or spleen.

What is amyloidosis?

Amyloidosis is a disorder that causes the body's antibody-producing cells to produce abnormal protein fibers. These antibody fibers join together and deposit in various organs. Elevated levels of these protein fibers accumulate in tissues and organs and may cause renal failure when they accumulate in the kidneys. The symptoms of amyloidosis depend on the organ or body system affected. The heart, kidneys, nervous system, and gastrointestinal tract are the most often affected. A common symptom of kidney amyloidosis is proteinuria and hypertension.

What is nephrosclerosis?

Nephrosclerosis is the term that translates as "hardening of the kidney" and describes the damage that occurs to the kidneys from prolonged, severe hypertension. Untreated hypertension leads to sclerosis of the renal arterioles, which decreases the blood supply to the nephrons. During the course of disease, some glomeruli become sclerotic, resulting in hyperfiltration to compensate for the loss of renal function. Progressive scleroses of the glomeruli occur as a result. The renal vessels thicken and hypertrophy over time and the kidneys lose their ability to produce renin, whose function is to decrease blood pressure. Because hypertension is both a cause and a symptom of chronic kidney disease, it is sometimes difficult to determine which came first. Proteinuria, hematuria, and left ventricular hypertrophy may be found in the patient with nephrosclerosis. Aggressive attempts to control the blood pressure are necessary to slow renal decline.

What are some infectious causes of renal failure?

Pyelonephritis is an infection of the kidney and renal pelvis. Bacteria spread most commonly by ascending from the lower urinary tract. Pyelonephritis usually does not progress to CKD unless there is an underlying urinary tract problem, for example, obstruction. Organisms that normally colonize the bowel such as gram-negative bacilli and enterococci are usually those involved because they prosper in the urine and then ascend to the kidneys. Kidney damage occurs by the inflammation, fibrosis, and scarring caused by the infection.

Renal tuberculosis is an infection caused by *Mycobacterium tuberculosis*. The urinary tract is the second most common site for infection after the lungs. Kidneys become damaged by lesions that cause inflammation, caseation, and eventually rupture. The infection spreads throughout the kidney and destroys the renal tissue. The kidneys become atrophied, scarred, and calcified. Tuberculosis of the kidneys usually occurs secondary to pulmonary disease. Renal tuberculosis may remain dormant for many years after pulmonary infection. Symptoms include increased urination, suprapubic pain, hematuria, and fever.

What is nephrotic syndrome?

Nephrotic syndrome is not a specific renal disease but a disorder that occurs when glomeruli are damaged and protein is permitted to leak into the urine. Glomerulonephritis, diabetes mellitus, and lupus are examples of specific diseases that cause nephrotic syndrome. Nephrotic syndrome, as it depletes the volume of protein in the blood, causes fluids to shift into the tissues, causing edema. Large volumes of protein being lost into the urine also cause the urine to become very foamy. No specific treatment exists for nephrotic syndrome other than decreasing the amount of salt in the diet to control the edema.

Can a person develop cancer of the kidney?

Renal cell carcinoma or renal cell adenocarcinoma accounts for approximately 90% of kidney cancers and 3% of all adult malignancies. Renal cell carcinoma is found more frequently in men and has a high mortality rate when detected after metastases. The disease usually affects only one kidney, although equal incidence is seen in both the right and left kidneys. The tumor may arise in any part of the kidney and compress renal tissue, which inevitably causes tissue necrosis and diminished blood flow. Metastasis often is seen in the lungs, lymph nodes, liver, and bones. The patient will exhibit hematuria, flank pain, weight loss, fever, and hypertension. A palpable mass in the flank or abdomen is sometimes seen.

What is renal artery stenosis?

Renal artery stenosis is a condition in which there is a narrowing of the lumens of the arteries that supply the kidneys. A major reduction of blood flow to the kidneys occurs, damaging the renal parenchyma. The decreased renal perfusion leads to increased rennin secretion, further damaging the kidneys.

How is acute renal failure defined?

It is any sudden, severe impairment of kidney function. Onset is rapid, over hours or a few days. Classically there is oliguria (less than 400 mL of urine per 24 hours). However, nearly half the cases are a nonoliguric variety. Nonoliguric renal failure is less fulminant and less difficult to manage than the oliguric form; dialysis is often not necessary.

What causes acute renal failure?

There are three categories of causes for kidney failure: (1) prerenal, (2) intrarenal (intrinsic), and (3) postrenal (see Box 15-1, pp. 210–211).

Prerenal causes reduced blood flow to the kidney sufficiently to impair function. The most common causes include low extracellular fluid volume (as in severe dehydration), heart failure, and blockage of the renal arteries.

Postrenal causes blocked flow of urine leaving the kidney. Obstruction may be at the ureter, bladder, or urethral level.

Identification of prerenal and postrenal causes is important because often they may be corrected quickly, without residual damage to the kidneys.

Intrinsic ARF is caused by direct damage to kidney tissue. This might occur with an acute inflammation (rapidly progressive glomerulonephritis). Much more often, it is the result of severely compromised blood flow (hemorrhagic shock) or direct toxicity to kidney parenchymal cells; this can come from some antibiotics, myoglobin, or ethylene glycol. The result is acute tubular necrosis, which causes 75% of all acute renal failure. Commonly called acute tubular necrosis (ATN), this condition is caused by injury to cells of the kidney tubules. The cell damage may be toxic (from chemicals or drugs) or ischemic (from severely reduced blood flow). Actual necrosis of cells does not always occur, but functional impairment is severe.

What brings on ATN?

The most frequent causes include surgery, trauma, sepsis, cardiovascular collapse, and nephrotoxic injury. Multisystem failure with sepsis is a frequent cause of ATN and is associated with high mortality.

Nephrotoxins include hemoglobin (from hemolysis of red cells) and myoglobin from muscle breakdown (rhabdomyolysis) as a result of crush injury, heatstroke, seizure, and so on. Many diagnostic and therapeutic agents, antibiotics (aminoglycosides especially), anesthetics, contrast media, cancer chemotherapy agents—as well as street drugs—are toxic to the kidney in varying degrees.

How is ARF recognized?

Most cases are found in hospital intensive care units. Monitoring of fluid intake/output, urine electrolytes, and serum solutes can furnish early clues. Serum creatinine may increase by 50 to 100 µmol/L, and urea may increase by 3.7 to 10.7 mmol/L each day. When tissue breakdown is extensive, serum potassium, phosphate, sulfate, and hydrogen ions rise rapidly.

What is the course of acute renal failure?

ARF from prerenal or postrenal causes reverses quickly when the precipitating factor is corrected. Most intrinsic renal failure, or ATN, is recoverable. However, other effects of the injury or the medical or surgical catastrophe that precipitated the renal failure may continue. These—with the complications of infection, sepsis, and hemorrhage—often have a very high mortality rate.

4

Clinical Manifestations of End-Stage Renal Disease (ESRD)

These are the features of a gradually developing uremic syndrome: fatigue, slowed thinking, and pruritus that occurs early. As all organ systems become involved, a wide complex of symptoms and findings evolves.

CARDIOVASCULAR SYSTEM
What cardiovascular abnormalities occur with uremia?

Patients with chronic kidney disease are the highest risk group of individuals for cardiovascular disease, and cardiovascular events are the major cause of death in dialysis patients. The cardiovascular mortality risk is increased two- to fourfold in patients with diabetes (American Diabetes Association, 2002).

Hypertension is the most common cardiovascular complication seen in patients with renal failure and affects the majority of patients (Box 4-1). Hypertension is associated with the progression of left ventricular hypertrophy (LVH), which places the patient at an increased risk for cardiovascular morbidity. Expanded extracellular fluid volume from fluid overload associated with sodium retention is the most prevalent cause. Many patients have increased plasma renin activity. Nephrectomy is an option to assist in the control of resistant hypertension, but is rarely seen today with the current pharmacologic agents available for treatment.

Fluid volume and sodium regulation by diet, antihypertensive medications, and ultrafiltration help in the management of hypertension. Patients are also encouraged to exercise with their physician's approval, and stop smoking programs or literature should be offered.

Atherosclerosis is a major factor in morbidity and mortality. A defect in liver lipoprotein lipase is a likely cause of increased serum triglycerides. Coronary artery disease, stroke, and peripheral arterial disease are increased.

Myocardial dysfunction presents as LVH resulting from hypertension, anemia, and atherosclerosis. With LVH the left ventricle grows abnormally thick, causing an interference with the normal pumping action of the heart. Signs and symptoms of LVH depend on the cause, but can include shortness of breath, chest pain, arrhythmias, dizziness, and congestive heart failure. The symptoms of LVH can be controlled or improved with the correction of hypertension and anemia. Some patients experience no symptoms at all, but progression to cardiac failure is not unusual.

Box 4-1		
CLASSIFICATION OF BLOOD PRESSURE		
Category	SBP (mm Hg)	DBP (mm Hg)
Normal	<120 and	<80
Prehypertension	120-139 or	80-89
Hypertension, stage 1	140-159 or	90-99
Hypertension, stage 2	≥160 or	≥100

DBP, Diastolic blood pressure; *SBP,* systolic blood pressure.
From Seventh Report of the Joint National Committee on Prevention, Detection, Evaluation, and Treatment of High Blood Pressure: *Classification of Blood Pressure,* Bethesda, MD, National Institutes of Health, National Heart, Lung, and Blood Institute, May, 2003.

Coronary artery calcification may occur as a result of imbalances in calcium phosphorus metabolism. Calcification of blood vessels, including the coronary arteries, which bring blood to the heart muscle, can place the patient at risk for heart attack and stroke.

Congestive heart failure (CHF) may be acute but is usually a chronic manifestation related to the retention of sodium and water. Symptoms of CHF include edema of the lower extremities, shortness of breath, and often fatigue, weakness, and the inability to perform physical activities. Weight gain from the excess fluid is another common symptom.

Pericarditis is a cardiovascular complication seen in the patient with end-stage renal disease (ESRD). Surrounding the heart is a double-membrane sac containing approximately 15 to 20 mL of fluid. This fluid provides lubrication, allowing the layers of the pericardium to glide smoothly over one another during the contraction of the heart. Uremic toxins, fluid overload, or bacterial/viral infections can all irritate the pericardial membrane, causing inflammation of the lining around the heart (the pericardium) and triggering chest pain and fluid accumulation around the heart (pericardial effusion).

Patients often present with the classic triad of symptoms: chest pain, low-grade fever, and pericardial friction rub. The chest pain is intensified by deep inspiration, swallowing, and coughing and improves when sitting and leaning forward. The pericardial friction rub is harsh and leathery and heard best at the lower left sternal border during systole as the inflamed layers of the pericardial sac rub together. Aggressive dialysis therapy (daily dialysis) with ultrafiltration to minimize uremic toxins and excess fluids is necessary. Heparin therapy during the treatment is either decreased or not given to the patient at all to minimize bleeding into the pericardial space. Antiinflammatory agents, both steroidal and nonsteroidal, may be prescribed to reduce inflammation.

Pericardial effusion can develop when increased fluid invades the pericardial space. Chest pain and elevated temperature will continue but the pericardial friction rub may be absent on auscultation. Hypotension and shortness of breath may also be seen. The fluid is usually bloody; if volume is large, tamponade may result.

Pericardial tamponade occurs when a large volume of fluid fills the pericardial space, compressing the cardiac muscle. Pericardial tamponade may have a slow or immediate onset and is associated with a high degree of mortality.

INTEGUMENTARY SYSTEM
What integumentary changes are seen in renal failure?

Patients with ESRD present with very brittle hair, nails, and skin due to a decrease in the size and activity of the sweat and sebaceous glands. Calcium may deposit in the skin, causing intractable pruritus leading to excoriations of the skin from the itching. Uremic frost is rarely seen today and only in the patient with advanced uremia left untreated. Whitish precipitates of urea crystals deposit on the skin giving it a "frosty" appearance. The skin color may appear tan-yellow from the pallor of anemia coupled with the retention of urinary pigments called *urochromes*. Ecchymosis is commonly seen due to platelet dysfunctions.

IMMUNE SYSTEM
Why are infections a problem?

Leukocyte abnormalities include reduced white blood cell (WBC) count in some patients. Granulocytes have reduced response to infection and low bactericidal activity. In fact, infection is the second most common cause of death in ESRD patients. Susceptibility is enhanced by malnutrition, immune system defects, and by the frequency of cannulation and other invasive procedures. The administration of intravenous iron has also been associated with infections in the ESRD patient. Caution must be taken when assessing body temperature because hypothermia is common and responses to infection may not be accompanied with fever. Elevated uremic levels impair phagocytosis and suppress the inflammatory response as well as hypersensitivity reactions.

Urea has an antipyretic effect and patients present with subnormal body temperatures. Poor nutrition plays a role in the diminished activity of white blood cell production. Caution must be taken to carefully assess the patient for any signs of infection or subtle changes in temperature.

GASTROINTESTINAL SYSTEM
What are some gastrointestinal manifestations of uremia?

Uremic individuals have a poor appetite and are often nauseated. Altered taste and dry mouth are common. Patients often complain of a metallic taste in their mouth, which leads to decreased appetite. The circulating uremic toxins cause nausea and vomiting which can also be aggravated by intradialytic hypotension. Gastrointestinal bleeding, often occult, is aggravated by medications (aspirin, heparin) and by the platelet defects. Uremic fetor is characteristic of the patient with kidney disease and is the smell of urine or ammonia on the breath from decomposing urea. Gastrointestinal bleeding is seen from irritation of the gastrointestinal mucosa from the uremic environment and from capillary fragility as urea in the gastrointestinal tract breaks down releasing the irritant ammonia. Diarrhea may be seen from intestinal irritation or hyperkalemia.

Functional constipation is frequent in patients on dialysis due to medications, fluid restrictions, low-potassium and low-fiber diet, and decreased activity levels. Discretion must be used in the choice of laxatives because many products used to manage constipation contain magnesium, phosphorus, or potassium.

Why is prevention of constipation important?

Because of a restricted diet, limited fluid intake, and regular ingestion of phosphate binders, ESRD patients tend to become constipated or develop fecal impactions. As older patients are taken into dialysis programs, there is more functional constipation. Such patients have a high incidence of diverticula of the colon. In addition, diverticulitis or perforation is not rare. Hematomas of the bowel and perforation caused by injudicious enemas have occurred. Cathartics and laxatives should be avoided. Stool softeners seem to work well, although they are often required in larger than usual doses. Patients should be encouraged to eat a high-fiber diet, to adhere to a program of regular exercise, and to plan a regularly scheduled time for bowel movements to reduce the problems of constipation. Severe constipation may also cause hyperkalemia because stool potassium losses account for up to 40% of total body potassium losses per day in dialysis patients (see Chapter 14).

Is peptic ulcer disease common in dialysis patients?

Some reports cite an increased incidence of peptic ulcer disease in dialysis patients, others do not. There are reports of higher than normal gastric acidity related to high blood levels of gastrin, which may relate to parathyroid overactivity. Other studies indicate low gastric acidity related to increased urea and ammonia content of gastric juice. Our own experience suggests that the incidence of ulcer disease is about the same as for the nonuremic general population.

Does ascites occur in ESRD patients?

Ascites (a massive fluid collection in the peritoneal cavity) is an infrequent problem that is very troublesome. Most cases are related to repeated fluid overload, poor nutrition, and cardiomyopathy. Although some patients overcome ascites, deterioration and death are frequent outcomes.

HEMATOLOGIC SYSTEM
What are the hematologic abnormalities?

Bleeding tendencies are seen as a result of a decrease in the quality and quantity of platelet production.

Anemia is the most common and severe hematologic defect. The hematocrit for normal men is 46% to 52%; for women it is 40% to 45%. People with uremia or on maintenance dialysis are anemic and have considerably lower hematocrit values. Anemia from diminished erythropoietin secretion occurs and results in fatigue, pallor, shortness of breath, and chest pain. The hostile uremic environment decreases the survival of red blood cells from 120 to 70 days.

What causes anemia?

Causes include (1) failure of production, or inhibition of action, of erythropoietin, a hormone produced by the kidney that stimulates the bone marrow to produce red blood cells; (2) a shortened life span of the red blood cells; (3) impaired intake of iron; (4) blood loss, including a tendency to bleed from the nose, gums, gastrointestinal tract, uterus, or skin, caused by platelet abnormalities; (5) blood loss related to the dialysis procedure itself; (6) elevated levels of parathyroid hormone (PTH), which has a suppressive effect on erythropoiesis in the bone marrow; and (7) poor nutrition and diet.

How does dialysis influence anemia?

Incomplete blood recovery after dialysis, dialyzer leaks, and frequent blood sampling contribute to anemia. The patient who is receiving adequate dialysis, is in a good nutritional state, and has adequate iron stores and intake will usually stabilize with a hematocrit between 20% and 30%. It is unusual for the hematocrit to go much higher except in people with polycystic kidney disease, in whom there may be greater than normal production of erythropoietin.

To minimize blood loss related to dialysis, particular care must be taken to (1) pretest dialyzers to prevent leaks, (2) monitor heparinization to prevent clotting, (3) return blood as completely as possible, (4) prevent damage to blood cells from incorrect pump occlusion or equipment malfunction, and (5) minimize the volume and number of blood samples drawn.

What symptoms does anemia produce in ESRD patients?

In chronic renal failure the anemia has usually been present for many weeks or months, and patients become adjusted to it. As the hematocrit improves on dialysis, they begin to feel better. These people still have considerably fewer red blood cells than normal and become dyspneic and tire easily. Other symptoms attributable to anemia include poor exercise tolerance, weakness, sexual dysfunction, anorexia, and inability to think clearly.

MUSCULOSKELETAL SYSTEM
How do the kidneys keep the bones healthy?

The kidneys keep the bones healthy by balancing the amount of calcium and phosphorus in the blood. Healthy kidneys produce a hormone called calcitriol, which enables the body to absorb calcium from the diet into the bloodstream.

During the progression of renal failure there is loss of ability to excrete phosphate. Phosphate ions accumulate in the body fluids and lead to a reciprocal decrease of serum calcium. The parathyroid glands seek to maintain a normal concentration of calcium in body fluid and respond by increasing production of PTH. This causes calcium to be

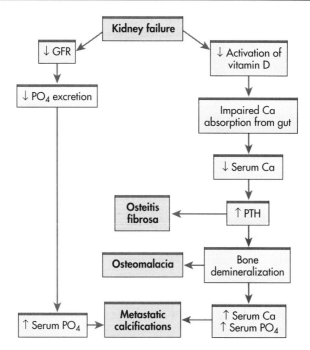

Fig. 4-1 Pathogenesis of renal osteodystrophy. *(From Lewis SM, Heitkemper MM, Dirksen SR:* Medical-Surgical Nursing, ed 6, St Louis, 2004, Mosby.)

resorbed from the bones, resulting in loss of bone density and strength. In addition, the active form of vitamin D, needed for normal bone metabolism, is manufactured in the kidney and is deficient in ESRD patients. Dialysis does not fully correct the disordered calcium-phosphorus metabolism, and progressive renal osteodystrophy (the term for several bony manifestations) is a serious problem for many ESRD patients (Fig. 4-1).

What other factors are involved in the bone disorder?

The absorption of dietary calcium from the intestinal tract is decreased in end-stage renal failure. There is resistance to the action of PTH, which normally enhances the resorption of calcium from bone. Chronic acidosis enhances calcium reabsorption from bone, further contributing to loss of bone density. In addition, the aluminum-containing phosphate-binding gels cause a form of renal bone disease. The aluminum in these gels is absorbed and deposited in bone, leading to a form of osteomalacia.

What are the bony changes seen in osteodystrophy?

These include adynamic bone, osteomalacia, osteitis fibrosa, osteoporosis, osteosclerosis, and growth retardation (in children); in addition, metastatic calcification also occurs. Adynamic bone is bone with little or no metabolic activity; osteomalacia is deficient calcification of bone; osteitis fibrosa is excessive destruction of bone by osteoclasts, with replacement by fibrous tissue; osteoporosis is deficiency of both bone matrix and calcification; and osteosclerosis is abnormally dense bone. The term renal osteodystrophy spans the totality of these various bone diseases in the uremic patient.

Metastatic calcification results when the product of serum calcium times phosphorus (measured in milligrams per deciliter) is 75 or greater. One should therefore keep this calcium and phosphorus product below 70.

What symptoms does osteodystrophy cause?

Many patients complain of sore, painful feet or back pain. Fractures, when they occur, are painful and heal poorly. Metastatic calcification causes precipitates in soft tissue around joints. Less apparent, but more dangerous, are diffuse deposits of calcium in the heart muscle and in the lung. Itching may be intensified in the presence of a high calcium-phosphorus ratio. Skin ulcerations and gangrene of the tips of toes and fingers have occurred. Aggravation of hypertension is frequent.

How is osteodystrophy treated?

A priority system is necessary in the management of uremic osteodystrophy. The first objective is to maintain a low serum phosphorus to prevent metastatic calcification and hyperparathyroidism. The serum phosphorus level depends on intake, removal by dialysis, and binding of phosphate within the gastrointestinal tract. Restriction of dietary protein intake also limits phosphate intake. A variety of agents are available to bind phosphate to prevent absorption from the gastrointestinal tract. Those containing aluminum should be avoided and calcium-containing compounds should be used instead. Their activity depends on the surface area available for binding. The problem is to find the dose of phosphate binder that provides sufficient surface area throughout the day and is palatable enough for patient compliance. A change in medication periodically may make it more acceptable. Failure to bind phosphate adequately usually represents failure of the patient to take the phosphate binder.

Once serum phosphate is lowered to about 4 mg/dL, elevation of serum calcium to greater than 10 mg/dL reduces the parathyroid stimulation of osteoclasts that causes osteitis fibrosa. One must be cautious, however, not to reduce the PTH too much. Adynamic bone disease will occur if the PTH is decreased to normal. The goal should be a PTH between 1.5 and 3 times the upper limit of normal. Elevation of serum calcium can be achieved in several ways. The usual concentration of diffusible calcium in dialysis fluid is well above that of the serum, so each dialysis provides a surge of calcium. The administration of 1 to 2 g of calcium orally will often lead to an improved serum calcium level even in the absence of normal quantities of potent vitamin D compounds. If the desired level of serum calcium does not result from these efforts, 1,25-dihydroxycholecalciferol may be administered either orally or intravenously. Vitamin D may also be helpful in maintaining bone formation, apart from its role in the gastrointestinal absorption of calcium. Finally, don't forget that alleviation of chronic acidosis of uremia is another objective of treatment. Some patients will develop hypercalcemia on this regimen and will require a lower calcium in the dialysis bath.

Even if the treatment is successful in maintaining a low serum phosphorus and a high serum calcium, some patients may persist with the problems of renal osteodystrophy. Those with bone pain are likely to have a component of adynamic bone or osteomalacia. Those with fractures and a high alkaline phosphatase may suffer to a large extent from osteitis fibrosa. Persistence of renal osteodystrophy, with x-ray film changes consistent with hyperparathyroidism, high PTH levels, and a high alkaline phosphatase, may warrant a parathyroidectomy: either a four-gland removal or a subtotal parathyroidectomy. A bone biopsy is advisable before parathyroidectomy.

What is calciphylaxis?

Calciphylaxis is a rare but potentially life-threatening complication that may occur in ESRD patients. The causes of calciphylaxis are poorly understood but are usually the result of several comorbid factors. Hypercalcemia, hyperphosphatemia, and hyperparathyroidism all seem to be contributing factors in this condition.

When the serum phosphorus and the serum calcium levels become elevated together, insoluble calcium phosphate crystals develop. You will see this occur when the calcium phosphorus product exceeds 70 mg/100 mL. These calcium phosphorus crystals deposit in the soft tissues of the body including lungs, joints, heart valves, cornea, and skin. Soft tissue calcifications usually affect the trunk and lower extremities, but can occur in the breast, shoulder, or buttocks. Calciphylaxis usually begins as painful, purplish skin lesions that later form nodules. These nodules ulcerate and finally form eschar with underlying tissue necrosis. Blood flow is diminished to the tissue and the area eventually becomes necrotic. These lesions are difficult to heal and often become infected. Calciphylaxis is associated with a high mortality rate, with death occurring usually from sepsis from infected wounds or skin lesions. Prompt identification and treatment of this condition may help to diminish the morbidity and mortality associated with this disease.

Joint Disorders

Uric acid is frequently elevated in ESRD patients. The hyperuricemia may be associated with a goutlike involvement of one or more joints. Occasionally there is a true gouty attack, but most episodes are of pseudogout. Dialysis amyloidosis may also be seen in long-term dialysis patients.

What is pseudogout?

Pseudogout is an acute inflammation, usually involving a single area at or near a joint. The back of the hand or wrist, finger joints, and shoulders are common locations. Pain comes on abruptly, followed rapidly by tenderness, swelling, and limitation of motion. This lasts 3 to 5 days or longer unless treated.

How can pseudogout be treated?

Colchicine or one of the nonsteroidal antiinflammatory agents often relieves distress in 24 to 36 hours.

Are there residual effects of pseudogout?

Soft tissue swelling may persist for several weeks. Areas of metastatic calcification at the site sometimes are seen on an x-ray examination.

Is there any preventive treatment for pseudogout?

Frequent dialyses usually keep the uric acid below serious levels. If a very high level of uric acid persists, use of allopurinol may be considered.

What is dialysis amyloidosis (DA)?

Amyloid is a peculiar form of protein that precipitates in various body tissues. There are many different kinds of amyloid, including amyloid composed of β_2-microglobulin that is unique to dialysis patients. This protein is normally excreted by the kidneys, but is poorly dialyzed and therefore accumulates in the blood of patients with ESRD. This protein then deposits in joints and periarticular structures of the shoulders, hands, wrist, neck, and elsewhere, causing pain and limitation of motion. If progressive, this can be extremely debilitating.

Who gets dialysis amyloidosis?

Patients on dialysis for long periods (more than 3 years) are prone to this complication. Of patients on dialysis more than 10 years, the majority will have DA. Patients dialyzed with high-flux synthetic membranes are less likely to get this complication.

What is carpal tunnel syndrome (CTS)?

CTS in dialysis patients is compression of the median nerve at the wrist by the carpal tunnel sheath, which has been thickened by deposition of amyloid. CTS causes pain, numbness, and tingling of the thumb and first two digits. Pain medications, nonsteroidal antiinflammatory drugs (NSAIDs), and deep therapeutic ultrasound may ease joint symptoms. Renal transplantation usually causes a rapid disappearance of symptoms.

NEUROLOGIC SYSTEM
What neurologic changes occur with uremia?

Fatigue, slow mental processes, anxiety, depression, and agitation are common. Seizures occur if azotemia increases rapidly. Sleep disturbances in the form of insomnia, restless leg movements, and sleep apnea are major concerns. Restless leg syndrome causes the individual to have an uncontrollable urge to move the extremities in response to unpleasant sensations. The lower extremities are most often affected and the discomfort occurs usually when the patient is at rest. Movement helps to alleviate the symptoms. Symptoms occur most often in the evening and begin to diminish in the early morning. The causes of restless leg syndrome are not definitively defined but might be associated with anemia. Electroencephalographic (EEG) changes (increased slow wave activity)

occur and are related to increased PTH level. Calcium content of brain tissue is increased, and brain aluminum is elevated.

Describe the potential for insomnia in this patient population.

Inability to sleep or fitful sleeping during the usual hours of rest is a common problem in ESRD patients. Often the patient sleeps throughout the dialysis procedure, and it may be that the need for sleep at other times is reduced. Other patients seem to have a pathologic inability to rest soundly.

Response to sedatives and tranquilizers is usually poor and the risk of dependency is considerable. We have seen no adverse effects from the lack of sleep and suspect the problem is most often one of fitful or interrupted sleep, which is interpreted as "no sleep." Sleep apnea is more common in ESRD patients than in the general population. The reason for this is unclear, but formal sleep studies may be useful in selected patients.

What is dialysis dementia?

This is a rare syndrome, first described in 1972. It may appear after a few months or several years in patients who are seemingly well dialyzed and doing well. There is a peculiar complex of garbled speech (dyspraxia), asymmetric muscle jerking, mental deterioration, and seizures, along with characteristic EEG changes. A number of studies have implicated aluminum accumulation as a cause, primarily from administered aluminum hydroxide. With the use of calcium-containing phosphate binders in place of aluminum hydroxide, this syndrome has largely disappeared.

What is uremic neuropathy?

Neuropathy indicates deterioration of nerve function. It may develop gradually as renal failure progresses, or it may appear suddenly after an intercurrent infection or an episode of fluid overload. Peripheral neuropathy may present as burning feet, twitching, restless legs, reduced vibratory sensation, and decreased reflexes. The latter relate to slowed nerve conduction velocity, present in most ESRD patients. A motor neuropathy or myopathy may present as weakness of proximal muscles of arms and legs. Changes usually begin at the toes and progress upward. The upper extremities may be involved, but less often than the lower ones.

Is neuropathy common?

Neuropathy, in subclinical or clinical form, has been reported in up to 80% of people with ESRD. It is often seen at the time dialysis begins, possibly because that is when a careful search is done. Clinically significant neuropathy is less common with earlier institution of dialysis.

Can neuropathy be detected before symptoms appear?

Nerve conduction velocity measurements are used to detect and to quantitate progression or improvement of neuropathy. Most patients with moderately advanced azotemia have some delay in nerve conduction, often long before symptoms appear.

The test, although not difficult, is subject to many variables that make its reproducibility questionable and small changes difficult to evaluate.

Is neuropathy relieved by dialysis?

If dialysis is begun early, when only prolongation of conduction time is demonstrable, frequent dialysis may prevent worsening. More severe nerve damage responds very slowly to dialysis. If the amount and frequency of dialysis are not adequate, neuropathy may develop or, if already present, will worsen.

How does the dialysis prescription relate to neuropathy?

When adequate dialysis is prescribed and delivered (kt/V_{urea}* $\geq$ 1.2, with PCR 1 g/kg/day), neuropathy is rarely seen. If it does develop, it strongly suggests that underdialysis and urea kinetic modeling should be performed to assess this. Even if the modeling parameters fall within an acceptable range, worsening neuropathy requires intensification of the dialysis procedure (larger dialyzer, more time, higher blood flow).

What is the cause of neuropathy?

This is not known. The pathologic changes in the nerves are similar to those seen in some cases of diabetes mellitus, in certain vitamin deficiency states, and in chronic alcoholism. A number of authorities believe it results from accumulated medium-size to large toxic metabolites in the body. However, specific toxic agents have not been identified.

Is there involvement of other than the peripheral nerves?

A few patients develop deafness, for which no other cause can be demonstrated. Other patients on dialysis have developed gastric atony or bowel dysfunction resembling the autonomic disturbances seen in some diabetic individuals. Impotence may also be related to uremic toxin accumulation.

RESPIRATORY SYSTEM
What respiratory problems do the patient with ESRD exhibit?

Pulmonary edema from excess fluid accumulation and left ventricular dysfunction may occur and is seen more frequently in the patient with acute renal failure. The incidence of tuberculosis is estimated to be as much as tenfold higher in the hemodialysis population as compared with the general population (Daugirdas, Blake, and Ing, 2001). Kussmaul respirations may be seen in the patient with metabolic acidosis. The body will compensate by increasing the rate and depth of respirations in an effort to excrete excess carbon dioxide.

---

*Kt/V_{urea} is a way to measure the dialysis dose. The measurement takes into account the dialyzer efficiency (K), the treatment time (t), and the total volume of urea in the body (V_{urea}).

What is metabolic acidosis?

Metabolic acidosis is a condition that occurs when excess hydrogen ions build up in the blood. Initially, buffers in the blood combine with the excess hydrogen ions and there are no symptoms. As the number of hydrogen ions increase, fewer buffers are available to bind with these ions. The pH of the blood then lowers and the patient will respond physically to help eliminate the excess hydrogen ions. Under normal conditions the kidneys would eliminate more hydrogen ions in the urine to compensate.

REPRODUCTIVE SYSTEM
Does chronic dialysis contribute to menstrual dysfunction?

Women commonly have cessation of menstruation as a part of the uremic syndrome. A few pregnancies in women on maintenance dialysis have been reported. Other reports suggest that less than 20% of such women of childbearing age ovulate at all. Most are amenorrheic or have oligomenorrhea of an anovulatory nature. A significant proportion are troubled by galactorrhea. Endocrine studies suggest a defect at the hypothalamic-pituitary level, such that the hormonal feedback mechanisms do not function normally. To prevent unnecessary (undesirable) blood loss, patients should be instructed to report any abnormal or excessive menstrual flow. Early detection of the problem may eliminate the need for surgical intervention.

What about infertility?

Infertility, in both the male and female, is very common. Research studies indicate poor sperm formation in most men. The exact mechanism is less clear in women, but as indicated before is presumed to be endocrine in nature.

What other sexual problems have been associated with chronic dialysis?

Sexual dysfunction is a very real problem for most maintenance dialysis patients. Reduction of libido and impotence in men is common as uremia develops. Various sociologic and psychologic studies, largely depending on questionnaire responses, have suggested that total or partial impotence is a problem in 60% of men receiving maintenance dialysis. However, another study suggests that 50% to 70% of the impotence of male dialysis patients has an organic basis—whether neuropathic, endocrine, or vascular is unknown. In addition, medication (particularly antihypertensive agents) must always be considered a potential cause of impotence.

The reproductive problems described above are often relieved after correction of anemia with Epogen. The mechanism for this is unclear, but several successful pregnancies in women receiving EPO have now been reported.

METABOLIC DISTURBANCES

Uremia is associated with abnormal metabolism of glucose, lipids, and protein.

Glucose metabolism

Nondiabetics with ESRD have abnormal glucose metabolism. Cellular sensitivity to insulin is reduced. After a glucose load, peak blood sugar is near normal, but the rate of decline is slow.

When ESRD is the result of type 1 diabetes mellitus (onset before age 35), peripheral cellular resistance to insulin is especially severe. Violent swings between hypo- and hyperglycemia are frequent. Total insulin needs decrease somewhat after the patient begins dialysis, but wide swings of blood glucose and problems with insulin dosage continue because of the decreased ability of the kidney to metabolize insulin and consequent increase in the half-life of insulin.

Most diabetic ESRD in the United States is type 2 diabetes. Such patients are usually obese and have a resistance to insulin. Most are improved by weight reduction and increased activity. Many patients respond to oral hypoglycemic agents.

Lipid metabolism

Type 4 hyperlipoproteinemia is common. The elevated very low-density lipoproteins (VLDLs) are somewhat different from the usual VLDLs, which may be a result of reduced hepatic lipoprotein lipase activity, possibly related to insulin resistance. Carnitine deficiency has also been suggested to have a role.

Protein metabolism

Protein calorie malnutrition is common. Loss of lean tissue mass is masked by an increase in body water with occult edema. Serum albumin tends to be low because of poor protein intake, although impaired hepatic synthesis may play a part. Several nonessential amino acids are elevated, and certain essential polypeptides are decreased.

What other endocrine abnormalities occur with uremia?

Changes in insulin production and effect, and parathyroid hormone perturbations have been mentioned. Most other endocrine systems are also affected by uremia. These include the following:

- Plasma norepinephrine levels are increased; epinephrine values are inconsistent.
- Cortisol levels are near normal, with a normal response to adrenocorticotropic hormone (ACTH). Aldosterone is increased.
- Both glucagon and gastrin values are elevated. This results from loss of renal metabolic clearance.
- Hypothyroidism is more frequent in ESRD patients than in the general population. Euthyroid individuals on dialysis have low total thyroxine (T_4) and T_3 values and reduced free T_3, whereas free T_4 is normal. Conversion of T_4 to T_3 in peripheral tissue is reduced. Thyroid-binding globulin is low. Thyroid-stimulating hormone (TSH) is mostly normal, but the response to thyroid-releasing hormone (TRH) is reduced.

- Besides ACTH and TSH, the anterior pituitary produces four other hormones that are affected by uremia. Growth hormone and prolactin are increased. There is both increased production and decreased elimination. No systemic effect has been attributed to the elevation of either hormone.

Follicle-stimulating hormone (FSH) and luteinizing hormone (LH) each have critical roles in the pituitary-gonadal axis in both sexes. Production of abnormal estrogen and progesterone, or testosterone, by the gonads in uremia adversely influences the feedback mechanisms to the pituitary gland. LH levels are elevated in both men and women. FSH values are normal or minimally increased in both. End effects include testicular atrophy, low sperm count, and impotence in men, and dysmenorrhea or amenorrhea in women. Infertility is usual for both men and women. There is accumulating evidence that patients receiving recombinant human erythropoietin have fewer sexual problems of this sort. Much of the data is subjective. A number of objective studies support reductions of prolactin and growth hormone after administration of erythropoietin, but the mechanism is not clear. It is also unclear whether the effects that have been noted are the result of correction of anemia or are due to some specific effect of erythropoietin.

5

Laboratory Data: Analysis and Interpretation

IMPORTANT LABORATORY DATA FOR DIALYSIS PATIENTS

Important laboratory tests used to monitor dialysis patients include the following:

- Electrolytes (sodium, potassium, chloride, carbon dioxide)
- Blood urea nitrogen (BUN)
- Creatinine
- Hemoglobin
- Hematocrit
- White blood cell count
- Reticulocytes
- Platelets
- Iron and iron-binding capacity
- Ferritin
- Calcium
- Phosphorus
- Magnesium
- Albumin
- Total protein
- Glucose
- Alanine transaminase and aspartate transaminase (ALT, AST)
- Cholesterol
- Parathyroid hormone (PTH)
- Aluminum
- Hepatitis panel

What are normal laboratory values and how are they interpreted in the end-stage renal disease (ESRD) patient?

Review of the laboratory reports is included in the overall patient assessment. Any deviations from normal should be further evaluated for what is an acceptable value for a dialysis patient. For example, creatinine and BUN values may not fall within the range of normal because of ESRD. However, dialysis personnel should follow a protocol that defines when the BUN and creatinine values exceed the acceptable range for a person on dialysis and take appropriate action. Deviations from the acceptable range of laboratory values should be reported to the dialysis physician for appropriate intervention. Interventions may include a change in the dialysis prescription and/or medication(s).

What is albumin?

Albumin is a form of protein, which is a good measure of the nutritional status of an individual. It is also the protein of highest concentration in the plasma. Albumin carries smaller molecules in the blood such as medications, bilirubin, and calcium. Albumin helps to hold fluid in the blood vessels and is a good reflection of the patient's protein stores. It is well known that albumin is a powerful predictor of morbidity and mortality in the ESRD patient. The normal value ranges from 3.5 to 5.4 g/dL. A serum albumin greater than 4.0 g/dL is desired for the ESRD patient.

What are the symptoms of a low albumin?

A low albumin will cause edema as fluid shifts from the blood vessels into the tissues. Other symptoms of hypoalbuminemia include weight loss, fatigue, muscle wasting, and hypotension.

Why are dialysis patients at risk for low albumin levels?

Albumin levels are greatly influenced by diet. Dialysis patients are well known for having poor nutrition because uremia causes a loss of appetite. Lack of knowledge regarding adequate protein intake, difficulties with cooking or shopping for food, nausea, and loss of appetite for protein-rich food are all barriers supporting good nutrition in the dialysis patient. Some patients lose albumin into the urine, and peritoneal dialysis patients are at a high risk of lowering their levels as albumin is transported across the peritoneal membrane.

Why *do we* monitor albumin levels so closely?

A low albumin level (hypoalbuminemia) is linked to higher hospitalization rates and is one of the greatest predictors of death in the dialysis patient. In most studies, the risk for morbidity and mortality increases with a serum albumin level less than 3.5 g/dL (Ahmad, 1999).

What is the relationship between albumin levels and C-reactive protein (CRP)?

CRP is a protein produced in response to infection, inflammation, and tissue trauma. An elevated level of serum CRP is associated with a low serum albumin level in dialysis patients. A combination of the two factors has been identified as placing the dialysis patient at a higher risk for developing heart disease and inflammation of the blood vessels. CRP is present in the serum of normal individuals at levels between 0 and 5 mg/L. Serum CRP levels increase dramatically during infection or injury. Levels may increase 100 times or more during bacterial or viral infection. The CRP level will peak

2 to 3 days after an acute infection and begin to decrease 1 to 2 weeks after the infection subsides. This is why CRP is useful as an early marker for infection, inflammation, or injury. CRP measurements may help predict low serum albumin levels, evaluate for resistance to epoetin alfa (Epogen) therapy, assess the course of acute bacterial infections and their response to treatment, and detect occult infections or chronic inflammation (Spectra Renal Management, 2000).

Are dialysis patients at risk for aluminum toxicity?

Aluminum is a light metal found in cookware, soft drink and other beverage cans, antacids, cosmetics, antiperspirants, aluminum-containing phosphate binders—antacids, and contaminated water. The kidneys are the main organs for the filtration and excretion of aluminum in the body. The majority of aluminum is protein bound so it is not easily diffused through the glomerulus. Deposition of aluminum in the bone, tissues, and brain will be seen with elevated levels.

Aluminum toxicity was once prevalent among dialysis patients because they were exposed to aluminum from the water used in the dialysis treatment and from the oral intake of aluminum-based binders. The use of aluminum-based phosphate binders is now generally avoided due to the harmful effects of aluminum accumulation on the patient. The clinical consequences of aluminum toxicity involve symptoms to the brain, bone, and blood. These may or may not occur concurrently. High serum aluminum levels are associated with progressive neurologic symptoms that occur very subtly over time such as behavioral changes, slurred speech, and memory loss. Gastrointestinal irritation, loss of energy and appetite, anemia, and constipation also are associated with elevated aluminum levels. Dementia may be seen with advanced toxicity. Elevated aluminum levels may also cause epoetin alfa–resistant anemia and aluminum-induced bone disease. Normal serum levels are 0 to 10 mcg/L.

What is the treatment for aluminum toxicity?

Aside from removing the sources of exposure, the chelating agent deferoxamine mesylate (Desferal) may be used to remove the excess aluminum. To chelate means to remove a heavy metal, such as lead, mercury, or aluminum from the bloodstream. When administered, deferoxamine will form complexes with the aluminum, which can then be removed from the blood.

How does potassium work inside the body?

Potassium is the major intracellular cation and the second most abundant cation in the body. All but 2% of the total body potassium is within the cells of the body. Potassium is necessary for many cellular functions, neuromuscular control, skeletal, cardiac, and smooth muscle activity, and intracellular enzyme reactions. Potassium is influenced by acid-base balance as potassium ions are shifted out of the cell and replaced with hydrogen ions with acidosis. The majority of excess potassium in the body is excreted by the kidneys in the urine.

What causes hypokalemia?

Hypokalemia is a serum potassium level less than 3.5 mEq and may be caused by excessive gastrointestinal (GI) losses such as vomiting and diarrhea, diuretic use, excessive sweating, poor diet, and burns. Symptoms of low serum potassium include weakness and fatigue, and abnormal heart rhythms.

How is low potassium treated?

Dietary intake of potassium may need to be increased and intravenous potassium may be given if a rapid rise in the serum potassium level is needed. Dialyzing the patient on a higher potassium bath will minimize diffusion of potassium and help to maintain the serum level.

What is hyperkalemia?

Hyperkalemia is a serum potassium level greater than 5.5 mEq/L and usually the result of excessive dietary intake of high-potassium foods. Other causes of increased serum potassium are catabolic states, tissue or crush injury, blood transfusions, GI bleeding, hemolysis, missed dialysis treatments, and acidosis. Symptoms include abdominal cramps, shortness of breath, dizziness, diarrhea, muscle weakness, hypotension, electrocardiogram (ECG) changes, arrhythmias, and cardiac arrest. The rapidity of the change in potassium level rather than the actual serum measurement is a greater influence of the degree of symptoms produced.

What is the treatment for hyperkalemia?

A variety of treatment options exist for hyperkalemia. Sodium bicarbonate or glucose and insulin may be given intravenously to help drive the excess potassium into the cell. Sodium polystyrene sulfonate (Kayexalate) is a cation exchange resin that may be given orally or by retention enema. It works by exchanging two sodium ions for one potassium ion and allowing the potassium to be eliminated in the stool. Oral Kayexalate is more effective than retention enema.

The fastest and most efficient way to lower the total body potassium is hemodialysis. The dialysate potassium may be lowered to allow greater diffusion of potassium from the blood into the dialysate. Use with caution in the patient on digoxin therapy because toxicity may develop as the serum potassium is lowered. Potassium levels should always be monitored more frequently on the patient running on a lower potassium dialysate.

Is magnesium ever a problem for the patient with ESRD?

Magnesium is a mineral and the second most abundant cation in intracellular fluid. Most magnesium is eliminated in the stool, but the kidney is responsible for some of the excretion. Magnesium is responsible for neuromuscular activity and activates various enzymes for carbohydrate and protein metabolism. Magnesium is found in foods and medications such as antacids, laxatives, and phosphate binders.

Low magnesium levels (hypomagnesemia) may be caused by malnutrition, chronic diarrhea, certain diuretics, and antibiotics such as amphotericin B and neomycin. Symptoms of low magnesium include twitching, tremors, spasms, confusion, restlessness, and dysrrhythmias. Elevated magnesium levels (hypermagnesemia) may occur with dehydration and use of magnesium-based antacids or laxatives. Elevated levels of magnesium will cause excessive perspiration, hypotension, muscle weakness, and sedation. The normal magnesium level is 1.4 to 2.1 mEq/L.

How are calcium levels affected in the patient with kidney disease?

Calcium is the most abundant mineral in the body, with 99% located in the bones and the teeth. Calcium is necessary for blood clotting, bone growth and health, and conduction of neuromuscular impulses. Calcium may be ionized or nonionized. Only ionized calcium is free to be used by the body, and this represents 50% of the calcium in the body. The remaining calcium is bound to proteins.

The ESRD patient will normally have a lower serum calcium because calcium absorption is hindered by the suppression of 1,25-dihydroxycholecalciferol (vitamin D) production, decreased phosphorus excretion, and increased phosphorus retention. Normal calcium levels range from 9 to 11 mg/dL.

Why do we monitor the ESRD patient's phosphorus levels?

Phosphorus is normally excreted by the kidneys and accumulates in the patient with ESRD. As renal failure progresses, the ability of the kidneys to filter phosphorus decreases. High phosphorus levels are usually the result of decreased glomerular filtration coupled with excessive dietary intake. The normal phosphorus range is 2.6 to 4.5 mg/dL. The treatment for hyperphosphatemia is phosphate binders, which bind with the phosphorus in the GI tract, allowing it to be excreted through the intestines. Patients with high phosphorus levels would also benefit from dietary counseling.

What role does parathyroid hormone (PTH) play in maintaining calcium levels?

PTH is secreted by the parathyroid gland and helps to regulate calcium and phosphorus levels. PTH helps the body to absorb calcium and eliminate phosphorus. Low serum calcium levels stimulate PTH secretion. PTH secretion stimulates the movement of calcium out of the bone, increases calcium absorption from the small intestine, and minimizes calcium loss in the urine. Untreated hyperphosphatemia and hypocalcemia may lead to persistent and prolonged secretion of PTH in an attempt to raise calcium levels in the blood. Chronically elevated phosphorus levels will cause secondary hyperparathyroidism and the resultant renal osteodystrophy and calcium phosphorus deposits in the soft tissues of the body. Elevated phosphorus levels need to be controlled with the use of phosphate binders and nutritional education regarding phosphorus restrictions.

What is the relationship between calcium and phosphorus?

Phosphorus is a major intracellular anion. Eighty percent of the body's phosphorus is present in the bone. Phosphorus acts as a urinary buffer in maintaining acid-base balance, helps to maintain cell wall integrity, and is involved with transferring energy to cells in cellular metabolism. Calcium and phosphorus have an inverse relationship. When the phosphorus level is high, the calcium level is lowered. The normal phosphorus level is 2.5 to 4.5 mg/dL.

What is the importance of the calcium-phosphorus product?

Maintaining the calcium-phosphorus product between 40 and 60 is essential in avoiding bone disease. The calcium-phosphorus product is determined by multiplying the value of the calcium level by the value of the phosphorus level. For example, if your patient's calcium level were 10 mg and phosphorus level 9 mg, he or she would have a calcium phosphorus product of 90. A high product places the patient at risk for developing calcifications in the soft tissues, and coronary arteries.

Why do we monitor the ESRD patient's hematocrit and hemoglobin so closely?

A hemoglobin and hematocrit test is the most commonly monitored laboratory study used to evaluate anemia, and to prescribe a therapeutic dose of epoetin alfa. Both the hematocrit and hemoglobin are typically low in the ESRD patient due to decreased erythropoietin production. Hematocrit is the percentage of red blood cells in whole blood, and hemoglobin measures the oxygen-carrying capacity of red blood cells. Low levels of hematocrit are caused by decreased production of red blood cells, blood loss from the dialysis treatment, and shortened survival time of red blood cells. Low hematocrit values are associated with fatigue, shortness of breath, chest pain, palpitations, and feeling of cold. The normal hematocrit value for the kidney disease patient is approximately 30% to 36%.

Hemoglobin is a protein that contains the iron that carries oxygen from the lungs to all of the body's tissues. The target hemoglobin for the ESRD patient is approximately 11 to 12 g/dL. Two additional blood tests help determine iron availability: Ferritin is a protein that stores the iron until it is needed. The Kidney Disease Outcomes Quality Initiative (K/DOQI) guidelines for anemia of chronic kidney disease (2000) recommend a ferritin level of greater than 100 ng/mL and less than 800 ng/mL. Transferrin saturation measures the amount of iron immediately available for red blood cell (RBC) production. K/DOQI guidelines recommend a transferrin saturation level between 20% and 50%.

What is CHR and why is it measured?

Reticulocyte hemoglobin content (CHr) is a sensitive indicator of iron deficiency and a diagnostic tool that can monitor the efficacy of intravenous iron therapy. Reticulocytes are the most recent RBCs released into the bloodstream and circulate for only 1 to 2 days. CHr provides an assessment of the availability of iron to the red blood cells most recently produced by the bone marrow. Because the CHr is a more sensitive and specific marker of iron status at the reticulocyte level, determining the dose of intravenous (IV) iron therapy based on this index should improve hemoglobin levels in the ESRD patient.

BLOOD UREA NITROGEN (BUN)
What is urea?

Urea is the waste product of protein metabolism.

Why do dialysis patients have elevated BUN levels?

An increased BUN results from renal insufficiency, eating a diet high in protein, digesting blood from GI bleeding, dehydration, infection, injury, or elevated temperature, and could also indicate the need for a longer dialysis time, higher blood flow rate, or larger dialyzer. High levels of BUN will produce symptoms of fatigue, insomnia, irritability, dry and itchy skin, nausea, and an altered sense of taste and smell. The normal BUN level is 7 to 18 mg/dL but the normal level for a dialysis patient (pretreatment) is 60 to 100 mg/dL.

DIALYSIS ADEQUACY

Optimal dialysis can be defined as the dialysis treatment that makes patients feel almost as good and live almost as long as if they did not have end-stage renal disease. The amount of dialysis delivered during a single treatment is measured by the computed Kt/V and urea reduction ratio (URR). The higher the delivered dose of dialysis, the better the patient outcome. The National Kidney Foundation sets guidelines for recommended acceptable adequacy levels; however, many dialysis clinics set more stringent goals.

What is the Kt/V$_{urea}$?

Kt/V$_{urea}$ measures the effectiveness of the dialysis treatment in removing waste products, specifically, the ratio of urea clearance and time on dialysis to the volume of urea distribution (total body water). The National Kidney Foundation (NKF) K/DOQI clinical practice guidelines, hemodialysis adequacy (2000) suggest that the delivered Kt/V$_{urea}$ be at least 1.2. Urea is a good small molecule marker because its level correlates well with the nutritional state of the individual and with protein catabolism. The urea Kt/V$_{urea}$ index is the result of complex mathematical modeling of urea kinetics. K is the dialyzer clearance of urea (mL/min), t represents dialysis time (in minutes), and V indicates the volume of distribution of urea in body fluid. V$_{urea}$ is not a real volume that can be measured. It is derived from pharmacokinetic modeling and involves more than one fluid pool and rates of transfer between them. These cannot be directly measured.

What is the URR?

The URR measures the reduction of urea in the dialyzed patient from predialysis to postdialysis. The URR reflects the delivered dose of dialysis. The K/DOQI clinical practice guidelines, hemodialysis adequacy (2000) suggest a delivered dose of 65%.

What factors affect dialysis adequacy?

The NKF identifies the following factors as instrumental in adversely affecting the prescribed dose of dialysis:

Compromised urea clearance caused by

- Access recirculation
- Inadequate blood flow from vascular access
- Inaccurate estimation of dialyzer performance
- Inadequate dialyzer reprocessing
- Clotted dialyzer fibers
- Errors in blood and dialysate flow rates caused by miscalibrated equipment
- Inadequate blood and dialysate flow rate
- Dialyzer leaks

Reduced treatment time

- Premature discontinuation of treatment
- Time on dialysis incorrectly calculated
- Failure to account for interruption in treatment

Laboratory or blood sampling errors

- Dilution of BUN sample with saline
- Drawing predialysis BUN after initiation of dialysis
- Laboratory error
- Drawing postdialysis BUN before the end of dialysis treatment
- Drawing postdialysis BUN more than 5 minutes after the end of dialysis

When should serum glucose be monitored in the diabetic patient?

A serum glucose (Chemstick or Accucheck) assessment should be performed at the beginning of the dialysis. Unstable diabetics need more frequent checks. A serum glucose value less than 50 mg/dL may require a bolus of 50 mL of 50% dextrose to prevent hypoglycemic shock. An elevated glucose may require a dose of regular insulin to prevent diabetic coma (see Chapter 18).

What is creatinine?

Creatinine is a protein produced by muscle and is measured to determine kidney function. The amount produced by any person is relatively constant and the serum volume is determined by the rate it is being removed by the kidney. The amount of creatinine produced is relative to the muscle mass. The elderly will demonstrate lower creatinine levels due to decreased muscle mass. With declining renal function, the serum creatinine will rise. Normal creatinine values are 0.5 to 1.5 mg/dL. The serum creatinine value is a more sensitive marker of renal function because it is not influenced by diet or fluid volume.

What does it mean to measure the creatinine clearance?

Creatinine clearance is the amount of blood cleared of creatinine per unit of time and is normally expressed in milliliters per minute. The normal creatinine clearance is approximately 85 to 135 mL/min. With chronic kidney disease there is a decline in creatinine clearance. Normal values may vary slightly from laboratory to laboratory or textbook to textbook.

6

Principles of Hemodialysis

HISTORICAL BACKGROUND

Thomas Graham, a London chemist, reported the principles of the semipermeable membrane in 1861 and gave the process of selective diffusion the name dialysis. Then, in 1913, Abel, Rowntree, and Turner devised an apparatus for the dialysis of blood, using a number of collodion tubes, through which blood was flowed while a saline solution bathed the outside of the tubes (Fig. 6-1). This device was used successfully to treat animals with uremia. Later, Kolff and Berk developed the first clinically successful artificial kidney, after the development of heparin for anticoagulation and the ready availability of cellulose in the form of cellophane tubing. They employed a rotating drum of wood slats around which a spiral of cellophane tubing was wrapped. The lower portion of the drum was immersed in a bath of dialysis fluid, while the blood was propelled along the tubing by rotating of the drum. In 1948, Skeggs and Leonards first developed a parallel plate dialyzer; the first disposable dialyzer was the Travenol twin-coil unit, marketed in 1956. About 1965, Gambro began production of disposable parallel plate devices, while at the same time hollow-fiber artificial kidneys were developed in the United States.

SOLUTE TRANSFER
What does hemodialysis mean?

Hemo, of course, means blood. *Dialysis* connotes a separation or filtration process. Metabolic wastes or toxins are filtered from the blood by a semipermeable membrane and carried away by the dialysis fluid. The goals of hemodialysis are to manage the uremia, fluid overload, and electrolyte imbalances that occur as a result of chronic kidney disease.

What waste products are removed by dialysis?

A large number of substances accumulate in uremia (see Chapter 3). The molecular size of many of these is less than 500 daltons (Da). They diffuse readily across cellulosic membranes. Particles in the range of 500 to 2000 Da, sometimes called middle molecules, diffuse poorly across such membranes. Polypeptides in this size range have been suspected of causing some uremic symptoms, although this has never been

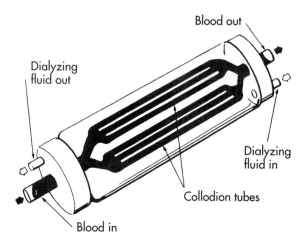

Fig. 6-1 Vividiffusion apparatus of Abel, Rowntree, and Turner. *(Adapted from Nosé Y: Manual on Artificial Organs. Vol 1. The Artificial Kidney, St Louis, 1969, Mosby.)*

proven. Molecules larger than 3000 Da are not generally regarded as toxic, with the exception of β_2-microglobulin (11,800 Da) and its relation to amyloid, bone disease, and anemia.

What factors affect the diffusion or removal of toxins in dialysis?

- Dialysate temperature: The higher the temperature, the greater the solute removal.
- Dialysate flow rate: The greater the dialysate flow rate, the greater the removal of solutes.
- Blood flow rate: The greater the blood flow rate, the greater the removal of solutes.
- Molecular weight of solutes: The smaller the molecular weight, the greater the removal of solutes.
- Concentration gradient: The greater the concentration gradient, the greater the amount of diffusion.
- Membrane permeability: The more permeable the membrane, the greater the removal of solutes.

What is a semipermeable membrane?

The semipermeable membrane is a selective membrane and acts as a sieve. The semipermeable membrane used in dialysis allows passage of some substances and fluid, but not all. It may be thought of as having submicroscopic openings or pores. Solute particles larger than these openings cannot pass through and are retained. Those particles small enough to pass do so at a rate inverse to their size: very small particles traverse more rapidly than those somewhat larger.

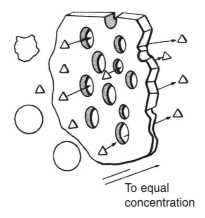

To equal
concentration

Fig. 6-2 Semipermeable membrane.

How does the semipermeable membrane function in hemodialysis?

The patient's blood is passed through a compartment formed by the membrane. Dialyzing fluid surrounds this compartment. Red cells, white cells, platelets, and most plasma proteins are too large to pass through the pores of the membrane. Water and small particles such as electrolytes cross by diffusion (Fig. 6-2), as do urea (60 Da), creatinine (113 Da), and glucose (184 Da).

What is diffusion?

Diffusion or, conductive transport, may be defined as the movement of solutes from an area of greater concentration of solutes to an area of lesser concentration of solutes. Molecules in solution are in constant motion and seek to spread uniformly throughout the solution. The rate of spread depends on the concentration, size, and electric charge of the particles. Diffusion of particles across a semipermeable membrane is the basis of dialysis. Diffusion will occur until equilibrium is reached (Fig. 6-3).

Why are all the solutes and water in blood not removed by the dialyzer?

The dialysis fluid is an electrolyte solution similar in composition to normal plasma water. Water molecules cross the membrane in both directions, as do electrolytes and other small particles. Only if the concentration of a particular kind of particle is greater on one side than on the other will there be a net flow from the side of high concentration to the side of lower concentration. Solutes and waste products of a small molecular size diffuse from the blood side concentration (high) to the dialysate concentration (low). This is the concentration gradient. A concentration gradient is necessary to accomplish solute removal in dialysis. A concentration gradient simply means a difference in concentration.

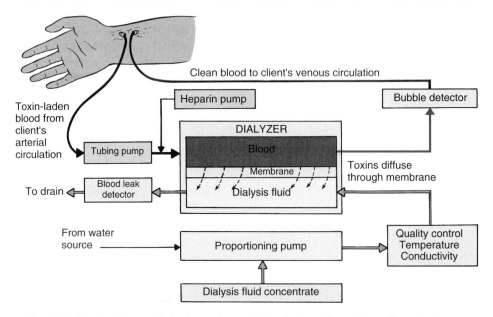

Fig. 6-3 Typical hemodialysis system. Toxin-laden blood from the client difuses across the membrane within the dialyzer into the dialysis fluid. Clean blood is returned to the client. *(From Black JM, Hawks JH, Keene AM: Medical-Surgical Nursing: Clinical Management for Positive Outcomes, ed. 7, Philadelphia, 2005, Saunders.)*

Are membranes permeable to middle and large molecules?

Several synthetic materials are used for high-flux dialysis. These include polyacrylonitrile (PAN), polycarbonate, polysulfone, polyamide, polymethyl-methacrylate (PMMA), and other membrane materials.

What is mass transfer rate, or solute flux?

Artificial kidneys, or dialyzers, are designed to remove metabolic wastes from the body, restore water and electrolyte balance, and correct acid-base disturbances. The dialysis process involves transport of unwanted or excess solute and excess water from the blood across a semipermeable membrane. The engineering term for such transport is mass transfer, and the rate of movement is the mass transfer rate, or solute flux.

What factors affect mass transfer rate?

Flux, at a constant temperature, is governed by the solute concentration gradient and the physical characteristics of the dialyzer. The latter include effective membrane surface area, membrane permeability, blood and fluid flow rates, and flow geometry. The mass transfer rate varies continually throughout the course of a clinical dialysis procedure.

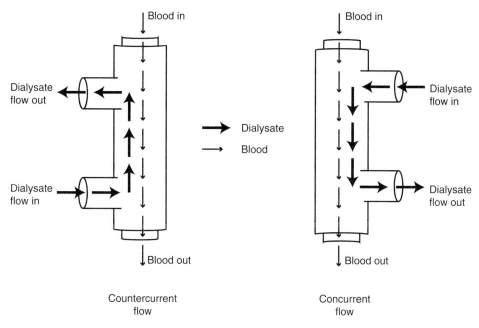

Fig. 6-4 Examples of blood and dialysate flow in the hollow-fiber dialyzer.

What is meant by flow geometry?

Flow geometry refers to the direction of flow of the blood and dialysate. Countercurrent flow is when the blood and dialysate flow in opposite directions, creating an optimal concentration gradient. Concurrent flow is when the blood and dialysate are both flowing in the same direction, creating a much smaller concentration gradient (Fig. 6-4).

TRANSPORT
What is meant by diffusive transport?

As noted, solute particles diffuse through the dialysis membrane from the side of higher concentration to the lower. This movement is termed diffusive transport or, less commonly, conductive transport.

What determines the rate of diffusive transport?

The rate of transfer depends on the following:
- The concentration gradient across the membrane for each solute
- The surface area of the membrane; the greater the area, the more solute moved per unit time.
- The mass transfer coefficient for the solute of interest for the particular membrane. The mass transfer coefficient increases for thinner or more porous membranes. It also is affected by the flow rates of both blood and dialysis fluid.

What is the sieving coefficient?

The amount of solute convected across a membrane in proportion to the quantity of fluid ultrafiltrated depends on particle size relative to pore size. If the pore-to-particle ratio is high, there is no restriction of solute transfer and the sieving coefficient is said to be 1. If none of the particles can be squeezed through, the sieving coefficient is zero.

What is convective transport?

When water moves across a membrane because of a pressure gradient (ultrafiltration), there is a friction effect on solute molecules, called solvent drag. This associated solute movement is termed convective transport (Latin *convectus*, "carried together").

What is the importance of convective transport?

Solute particles larger than 500 Da may have a low sieving coefficient, but because of their low diffusive transport, the convective component becomes a major fraction of their total transfer. Convective transport is of prime importance in high-flux hemodialysis and in the techniques of continuous arteriovenous hemofiltration, hemodialysis, and diafiltration.

What is meant by clearance?

Clearance is an empirical measure indicating a calculated volume of blood completely cleared of a substance in a given time. Clearance is expressed in mL/min. It is a theoretic, not a real, volume.

Controlled fluid removal at dialysis is essential. Ultrafiltration occurs in hemodialysis when fluid is removed under pressure. Most current dialyzers utilize elements of both positive blood compartment pressure and negative fluid compartment pressure (Fig. 6-5).

How does ultrafiltration occur?

Hydrostatic pressure is the pressure that forces plasma fluid out of the blood compartment and into the dialysate compartment of the dialyzer. The rate of fluid removal is influenced by the difference in hydrostatic pressure of the blood and dialysate compartments. The difference in the hydrostatic pressure of the blood and fluid represents the transmembrane pressure (TMP). The TMP reflects both positive and negative pressures in the dialyzer. Positive pressure is applied to the blood side of the dialyzer, which pushes the plasma fluid out. Negative pressure is applied to the dialysate side of the dialyzer to pull the plasma fluid out of the blood compartment to the dialysate compartment. It is very important that the dialysate compartment never exerts a pressure more positive than the blood compartment. This is referred to as reverse filtration.

What is reverse filtration?

During high-flux dialysis the ultrafiltration control system prevents excessive net fluid removal. The process generates a blood/dialysis fluid profile within the dialyzer that is

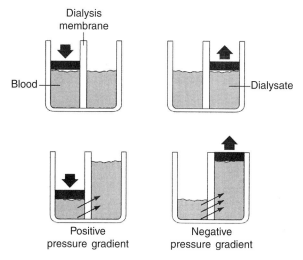

Fig. 6-5 Ultrafiltration.

positive (blood-to-fluid) near the blood inlet but that may, under some circumstances, become negative (fluid-to-blood) toward the outlet. The movement of dialysis fluid into the blood is termed *reverse filtration.*

What is the significance of reverse filtration?

The water used in preparation of dialysis fluid is not sterile. Addition of bicarbonate concentrate encourages and supports bacterial proliferation. Endotoxin and breakdown products form and may be carried across the high-flux membrane into the bloodstream when reverse filtration occurs. Pyrogen reactions as well as other adverse effects may occur.

How can the effects of reverse filtration be countered?

A molecular filter (ultrafilter) can be placed in the fluid delivery line just ahead of the dialyzer. These devices use ultrafiltration membranes to remove suspended particles of molecular size, but not dissolved solutes. Bacteria and pyrogen or pyrogen fragments are rejected by the ultrafilter (see Chapter 7).

What is the relationship between the hydrostatic pressure and the ultrafiltration rate?

For a particular dialyzer, at any given TMP, a certain amount of fluid will be removed per unit time at specific blood and fluid flow rates. During the investigational phase of a new dialyzer, an average ultrafiltration rate per mm Hg TMP is calculated. This is the ultrafiltration coefficient (k_{UF}) and is unique to each dialyzer. The k_{UF} is expressed as mL/hr of fluid removed for each mm Hg. The higher the k_{UF}, the greater the amount of fluid that can be removed with less pressure being applied to the semipermeable membrane. (See Chapter 11 for information on how to calculate the TMP for a patient treatment.)

What affects the resistance in the blood circuit?

The two major components are (1) the viscosity of the blood and (2) the geometry of the blood pathway.

1. Viscosity is largely a matter of hematocrit. The viscosity of blood of 30% hematocrit is approximately 2.3 to 2.5 centipose, about 2 to 2.5 times that of water.
2. Several aspects are important to the geometry of the blood pathway:
   - Length of the pathway. Hollow-fiber dialyzers have low resistance because of the short (15 to 50 cm) pathway.
   - Number of pathways. With a large number of pathways, the divided resistance is lower. Hollow-fiber dialyzers have several thousand pathways and have low resistance.
   - Cross-sectional area of the pathway. A large cross-sectional pathway has low resistance; a small one has high resistance. For hollow-fiber dialyzers, the control factor is the internal radius of the fiber.

How is the amount of ultrafiltration controlled during hemodialysis?

In the past, control of ultrafiltration was sought by manipulating the TMP. Blood outlet and fluid inlet pressures, critical variables in the calculation, are often inexact. The k_{UF} information provided by manufacturers is most often based on in vitro studies and may differ from actual patient experience by as much as plus or minus 30%. Even with conventional cellulosic membranes and blood flow rates of 200 to 300 mL/min, wide discrepancies between planned and actual fluid removal may occur. With use of high-efficiency or high-flux dialysis, precision in ultrafiltration management became crucial, leading to development of equipment to directly control ultrafiltration on a minute-to-minute basis.

How do ultrafiltration controls function?

There are two basic systems: (1) volumetric or balancing type and (2) servo-feedback or flow sensor type (see Chapter 7).

In the volumetric system, inflow and outflow through the fluid compartment are exactly balanced by special pumps. A separate pump removes fluid from this closed loop at a rate set by the operator. This creates negative pressure in the fluid loop, causing ultrafiltration across the membrane to match the rate of fluid removal.

The servo-feedback system uses very sensitive flowmeters to constantly monitor dialysis fluid inflow and outflow. This information feeds into a microprocessor that subtracts dialysate inflow (Q_{di}) from dialysate outflow (Q_{do}) to determine rate of ultrafiltration

(Q_{uf}) continuously. The desired ultrafiltration rate is programmed by the operator; the microprocessor adjusts TMP so that measured Q_{uf} matches desired Q_{uf}.

Direct ultrafiltration control systems, when operating correctly, achieve a plus or minus 10% accuracy in volume of fluid removal.

What is ultrafiltration profiling?

Ultrafiltration (UF) profiling is a technology available on some dialysis machines to vary the volume of fluid removal during the course of the dialysis treatment. Normally the dialysis nurse or technician will enter the volume of fluid to be removed or the patient's goal for that dialysis treatment. The machine will automatically divide the total volume to be removed by the length of the treatment. With UF profile, fluid removal is varied based on what profile is chosen. For example, the machine may be set to remove the greatest volume of fluid in the first half of the treatment, when most of the fluid is available to be removed. The rate of removal will then be decreased for the remainder of the treatment when there is less fluid available to refill the vascular space. Other profiles are available and can be selected based on the types of symptoms the patient's experience predialysis, intradialytically, and postdialysis. All of the profiles will remove the required total volume during the patient's treatment, but at different intervals and rates.

What shifts occur between intracellular and extracellular fluid compartments during hemodialysis?

Ultrafiltration can rapidly remove fluid from the vascular compartment. If the rate of removal exceeds the repletion rate from interstitial space, hypovolemia and hypotension occur. Infusion of hypertonic saline will increase osmolality in both the vascular and extravascular spaces. This in turn attracts fluid from the much longer intracellular pool and avoids the hypovolemia that causes the low blood pressure.

What is sodium modeling?

Sodium modeling or sodium variation is a tool that may be used to minimize some of the complications associated with the hemodialysis treatment. The specific treatment complications that can be prevented with the use of this therapy are dialysis-associated hypotension and cramping. An understanding of how these complications occur is essential in order to understand this technology. As the hemodialysis patient is ultra-filtrated, the plasma fluid is being removed from the intravascular space. With rapid dialysis, the intravascular space is depleted of fluid and the "refill" from the extravascular space does not occur quickly enough. When the plasma volume is depleted or decreased, hypotension results. Cramping in the extremities may occur because their perfusion is also compromised with a decreased vascular volume. Hypoalbuminemia and right-sided heart failure may also contribute to the vascular refilling being delayed.

The sodium variation system (SVS) helps maximize the refilling of the vascular space during ultrafiltration. This procedure involves the development of a computer model of sodium and water movement between compartments during dialysis. Sodium content of the dialysis fluid is varied during the procedure according to the preprogrammed plan. The sodium concentration of the dialysate being delivered to the dialyzer is increased. This may be done in either of two ways: (1) addition of a special NaCl concentrate to the dialysis fluid by an infusion pump, or more commonly (2) varying the proportion of the usual concentrate as the treatment progresses, thus changing the final sodium concentration. For example, a commonly used proportioning yields a dialysis fluid sodium of 140 mEq/L; a 10% increase in the amount of concentrate as it is mixed increases the final fluid sodium to 154 mEq/L, with only minor quantitative changes in other electrolyte concentrations such as potassium and calcium. The sodium level can be raised to as much as 160 mEq/L. The sodium level is slowly returned to normal by the end of the dialysis treatment with no adverse effects on the patient such as hypertension or increased thirst.

How is acid-base balance achieved during hemodialysis?

When continuous fluid proportioning systems were introduced in 1963, bicarbonate could not be used in the concentrate because the calcium and magnesium precipitated. Sodium acetate, which the body metabolizes to bicarbonate, was substituted, avoiding the precipitation problem. Acetate-based concentrate became standard for many years. It had several disadvantages, particularly the production of cardiovascular instability.

Introduction of short, rapid dialysis and high-flux dialysis made the return to bicarbonate-based fluid mandatory for these procedures. Bicarbonate dialysate is now the standard of practice at most facilities. One of the goals of hemodialysis is to correct the acidosis associated with renal failure. During the dialysis treatment, there is a transfer of bicarbonate from the dialysate to the blood. The diffusion of bicarbonate helps the patient to achieve acid-base balance by buffering the hydrogen ions.

How is bicarbonate used in dialysis fluid production?

The concentrate to be used is packaged in two parts. The "acid concentrate" contains chemicals other than sodium bicarbonate, plus a small amount of acid. The "bicarbonate concentrate" has the sodium bicarbonate and some sodium chloride (necessary to increase conductivity for monitoring purposes). Three streams of fluid are blended by the proportioning equipment: (1) water (34 parts); (2) acid concentrate (1 part); and (3) bicarbonate concentrate (1.8 parts).

Different types of equipment utilize concentrates of different composition and different mixing proportions. Accidental use of mismatched concentrate is a potentially fatal error.

7 Dialyzers, Dialysate, and Delivery Systems

The dialyzer is a selective filter for removing toxic or unwanted solutes from the blood. The filtration process uses a semipermeable membrane between blood flowing on one side and dialysis fluid, called dialysate, flowing on the opposite side. The delivery system prepares dialysate of correct chemical composition, and then delivers it at proper temperature and other parameters to the dialyzer.

All dialyzers consist of a series of parallel flow paths designed to provide a large surface area between blood and membrane, and membrane and dialysate. There are two basic flow path geometries: (1) rectangular cross section, seen in parallel plate dialyzers; and (2) circular cross section, seen in hollow fiber dialyzers.

PARALLEL PLATE DIALYZERS
What are characteristics of plate dialyzers?

They are assembled in layers, like a sandwich. Sheets of membrane are placed between supporting plates, which have ridges, grooves, or cross hatches to support the membrane and allow the flow of dialysate along it. The blood flows through the sheets of the membrane. The contained volume of blood is small, and heparin requirements are also usually small. A disadvantage of plate dialyzers is that they are compliant. This means that the volume of blood that they hold increases as the TMP increases. The main disadvantage of plate dialyzers is that they are not well suited for reuse.

HOLLOW-FIBER DIALYZERS

The hollow-fiber artificial kidney (HFAK) is by far the most commonly used dialyzer. HFAKs are available in a wide variety of sizes and membranes.

What serves as the semipermeable membrane in the HFAK?

Tiny hollow fibers of about 150 to 250 μm in diameter are used. Blood flows through these tens of thousands of hollow fibers. They are formed from a variety of materials, cellulosic and synthetic. Wall thickness may be as little as 7 μm, although some synthetics have walls of 50 μm or more (Fig. 7-1).

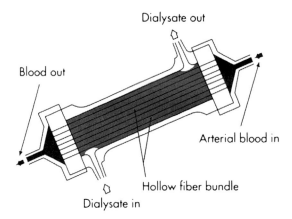

Fig. 7-1 Hollow-fiber dialyzer.

What are advantages of hollow-fiber dialyzers?

The contained blood volume is very low in relation to the dialyzer's surface area because of the dialyzer's flow geometry. Resistance to blood flow is low because of the large number of blood passages. Hollow-fiber dialyzers are not compliant; therefore, they do not increase in shape or in the volume of which they hold under high transmembrane pressure. Ultrafiltration can be precisely controlled. They are well adapted to reuse.

What are disadvantages of the HFAK?

- Meticulous deaeration of the fiber bundle is required before beginning a dialysis procedure. Otherwise, fibers may air lock and not admit blood.
- There may be uneven distribution of blood at the inflow header space, with reduced perfusion of some of the center fibers.
- Hollow-fiber dialyzers are most commonly sterilized with ethylene oxide (ETo). Residual toxic products of ETo sterilization retained in the potting material of the headers can cause adverse patient reactions.

Are there other ways to sterilize hollow-fiber dialyzers?

Yes. Some producers use gamma irradiation. Other manufacturers employ steam sterilization. Both methods are effective. Electron beam, or e-beam, is a newer method of factory sterilization of hollow-fiber dialyzers. Electron beam sterilization inactivates microorganisms or destroys the microorganisms by a chemical reaction. The electron beam does not use chemicals or radioactive materials for its sterilization process and may be a good alternative for the patient who is sensitive to ETo.

MEMBRANES FOR HEMODIALYSIS

Membranes used in hemodialysis are of two basic types: (1) organic cellulose derivatives and (2) synthetic membranes.

Willem Kolff used cellulose sausage casings for the first successful clinical dialysis. Cellulosic membranes continue to be basic for many dialyzers. Synthetic membranes were developed in the search for efficient, large-volume seawater desalinization by reverse osmosis. The development of volume-controlled ultrafiltration equipment for hemodialysis made the use of these high-hydraulic permeability membranes practical. They in turn have made high-flux hemodialysis, hemofiltration, and continuous renal replacement therapy (CRRT) viable options in renal treatment.

What is the nature of a cellulosic membrane?

Cellulose $(C_6H_{10}O_5)$ is a complex carbohydrate polymer that is the structural material of plants. Commercial cellulose is obtained from wood products and cotton. Treatment with heat and chemicals produces a liquid slurry, which is coagulated and formed into sheets or extruded through dies as hollow fibers. Different kinds of processing result in membranes of various thicknesses, water-absorptive qualities, and permeabilities.

What accounts for the permeability of cellulosic membranes?

Electron microscopy shows that the fibers of cellulose membranes swell when wet, forming a tortuous maze. The "pores" are actually twisting, irregular tunnels that force water or a solute molecule to travel a distance several times the thickness of the membrane to get through it.

What are some cellulose membranes now used in hemodialysis?

Cuprophan has been widely used. The cellulose is treated with ammonia and copper oxide during manufacture; Cuprammonium rayon and Hemophan are modifications. Saponified cellulose ester, cellulose acetate, and triacetate are other widely used cellulose materials.

What are the advantages and disadvantages of cellulose membranes?

One distinct advantage is the fact that they have been used for many years, and their transport characteristics are well known. They are also relatively inexpensive. However, all the cellulosic membranes have some degree of bioincompatibility with blood. This poses a number of problems, which will be discussed later in this chapter.

What are features of synthetic membranes?

These synthetics are thermoplastics. They have a thin, smooth luminal surface supported by a spongelike wall structure. Those used for hemodialysis include polyacrylonitrile (PAN), polysulfone (PS), polyamide, polymethyl-methacrylate (PMMA), and others. Convective transfer accounts for their overall mass transport. All have ultrafiltration coefficients of 20 to 70 mL/hr/mm Hg or more. They are well adapted to reuse. Synthetics have much fewer bioincompatibility problems than cellulose membranes.

What are negative aspects of synthetic membranes?

There are several negative aspects, including the following:
- They are expensive in comparison with cellulosics
- Automated ultrafiltration control is required because of the very high water permeability
- Adsorption of proteins to the membrane surface can be a problem
- The high permeability creates a risk of backfiltration from dialysate to blood

MEMBRANE BIOCOMPATIBILITY

Each time blood comes in contact with a foreign surface, an inflammatory response is elicited. This response is used to gauge the biocompatibility of a hemodialysis membrane. When there is an intense reaction and a high level of inflammation, the membrane is said to be bioincompatible. When the response and inflammation are mild, the membrane is classified as biocompatible. The level of membrane biocompatibility may be associated with both short- and long-term consequences.

How does one measure the level of inflammatory response resulting from blood/membrane interaction during hemodialysis?

The intensity of the reaction is measured by the level of complement generation following initiation of hemodialysis. Markers used to evaluate complement activation are C3a, C5a, and the "membrane attack complex"—C5b through C9—in the patient's blood.

What is complement activation?

The complement system is a series of plasma proteins that react sequentially to cause a variety of biologic events. This system works with the immune system to defend the body from substances that the body determines to be "nonself." When blood encounters a hemodialysis membrane, the response elicited is similar to that occurring when the body's immune system is challenged by bacteria.

What are some of the intradialytic manifestations of complement activation?

The first clinical manifestation to be associated with complement activation is leukopenia. Immediately after starting hemodialysis using cellulosic membrane, patients' white cell counts drop sharply. This begins to correct after about 15 minutes. By the end of a 4-hour dialysis, the white cell count will be back to the initial level or perhaps slightly higher, due to a compensatory response by the bone marrow. This leukopenia is transient, but it may be important to patients with compromised cardiac or pulmonary systems. C5a, an end product of the complement cascade, activates white cells. When white cells are activated, they become "sticky." These cells aggregate, or clump, and are sequestered in the first capillary bed they encounter, usually the lungs. The clumps of white cells reduce pulmonary capillary perfusion, and reduce the patient's ability to efficiently exchange oxygen and CO_2 between blood and alveolar air. This may be manifested as an intradialytic hypoxemia. Other intradialytic problems likely associated with complement activation include chest pain, back pain, coagulation abnormalities, and in severe cases, anaphylaxis. Activation of complement peaks at 15 minutes and can last as long as 90 minutes. The amount of complement generated relates to the type and surface area of the membrane being used.

Which membranes induce the highest levels of complement activation?

Cellulose and cellulose-based membranes induce more complement activation than do synthetic membranes (Table 7-1). The chemical composition of the cellulosic surface is similar to that of the cell wall of bacteria: both are chains of polysaccharide structures. The body responds to blood-cellulose contact much the same as it does to invasion by bacteria. Free hydroxyl groups on the membrane surface are likely the primary source of the intense complement activation. Chemical alterations to buffer the free hydroxyl groups are used to create "modified cellulosic membranes" like cellulose acetate and Hemophan. Membranes of cellulose acetate have some of the surface hydroxyl linked with acetyl groups. Hemophan membranes have amino groups attached to the reactive sites to buffer them. Both of these modifications reduce the amount of complement

Table 7-1	Types of Dialyzer		
Membrane type	Hydraulic permeability	Examples	Biocompatibility profile
Regenerated cellulose	Low flux	Cuprophan	Poor
Modified cellulose	Low/high flux	Cellulose acetate Cellulose diacetate Saponified cellulose ester	Intermediate
Synthetic	High/low flux	Polyacrylonitrile Polysulfone Polyamide Polycarbonate Polymethyl- methacrylate	Good

From Johnson RJ, Feehally MA: *Comprehensive clinical nephrology*, ed 2, St Louis, 2003, Mosby.

generated; however, these membranes are still less effective than synthetics in minimizing complement production.

Why do synthetic membranes induce less complement than cellulosic membranes?

Being synthetic, they lack the reactive sites found on cellulose-based membranes; thus the amount of complement generated during hemodialysis is less than with cellulosic membrane.

What are some of the long-term considerations when selecting a membrane for hemodialysis?

Long-term use of bioincompatible membranes may be associated with an increased incidence of infection and malignancy, and impaired nutritional status. Patients dialyzed on cellulose membranes have a higher incidence of β_2-amyloid disease than those on synthetics. The increased risk of infection and malignancy is thought to be due to repeated attacks on the patient's immune system. When patient blood is repeatedly exposed to bioincompatible surfaces, the body responds as though under attack. The immune system kicks in, complement is generated, and the inflammatory response is triggered. There can be tissue damage, and future stimuli may elicit only a limited response, thus predisposing the individual to infection and potential malignancy.

Malnutrition is a major contributor to morbidity and mortality of patients on hemodialysis. Even with adequate protein intake, malnutrition is a problem and seems to relate to an accelerated catabolic process, most evident on dialysis days. A catabolic effect associated with bioincompatible membrane is well documented. However, recent studies have demonstrated an increase in protein catabolism during hemodialysis with synthetic membranes as well (Ikizler et al, 2002). β_2-amyloid disease (β_2AD) is important in long-term morbidity. Clinical manifestations include arthropathies, bone lesions and pathologic fractures, soft tissue swelling, and carpal tunnel syndrome. Patients being dialyzed with cellulosic bioincompatible membranes exhibit more pronounced clinical symptoms of amyloidosis (Schiffl et al, 2000). Possible reasons for the difference include the following:

- Cellulose membranes do not have the capability to remove molecules as large as β_2-microglobulin.
- Cellulose membranes induce high levels of complement generation, and some products of complement activation may be responsible for the release of β_2-microglobulin from monocytes.

How does membrane biocompatibility affect patients with some residual renal function?

In one study, patients dialyzed on cellulose acetate membranes appeared to lose residual renal function more rapidly than those dialyzed with polysulfone membrane.

Does biocompatibility of the membrane affect patients in acute renal failure?

This is not clear. There is a consensus that the more compatible membranes do contribute to better recovery and survival. Less complement activation, less white cell activation, and less inflammation associated with more biocompatible membranes are believed responsible.

DIALYZER REUSE

Dialyzer reuse is the cleaning, processing, and sterilizing of a dialyzer once used, to be used again on that same patient. Dialyzer reuse has been done for many years in many dialysis clinics and is a safe and effective way to keep the cost of the dialysis treatment within reason.

What are the advantages of reuse?

Fundamentally, the average cost per dialysis is substantially reduced. The "first-use syndrome," an infrequent phenomenon of chest or back pain, nausea, and malaise occurring in the first half hour of a run with a new cellulose dialyzer, is absent or rare with reused dialyzers.

What are disadvantages of reuse?

Processing, testing, identification, and storage of reused units require space and personnel time. Consumption of high-quality water is greatly increased. Sterilizing agents, particularly formaldehyde, are a hazard to personnel and to patients. Quality control of manual processing is difficult to ensure. Automated systems minimize these problems, but at high initial cost.

Are there guidelines for reuse procedures?

Yes. Guidelines were defined by the Association for the Advancement of Medical Instrumentation (AAMI) and subsequently given the force of law by the US Food and Drug Administration (FDA). (See Chapter 9 for more on reuse of dialyzers.)

DELIVERY SYSTEMS

The delivery system prepares and delivers dialysate to the dialyzer unit. Most systems provide dialysate for a single patient; others have the capacity to supply several dialyzer stations simultaneously.

What is the Solution Delivery System (SDS)?

The SDS is a method of delivering the solutions used to make dialysate to the machine. Bicarbonate from a mixing tank and acid from a storage tank are transferred to an overhead holding tank called a "head" tank. The solutions are then gravity fed to a solution distribution system and then fed out to the patient care area to be delivered through a series of pipes to the machines.

What are the functions of dialysate?

Dialysate carries away the waste materials and fluid removed from the blood by the dialysis procedure, prevents the removal of essential electrolytes, and averts excess water removal during the procedure. These functions are achieved by making the chemical composition of the dialysate correspond as nearly as possible to that of normal plasma water.

What chemicals are used?

There are usually five compounds involved: sodium chloride, sodium bicarbonate or sodium acetate, calcium chloride, potassium chloride, and magnesium chloride. Glucose may be included in some formulations.

How are the chemicals made into dialysate?

Manufacturers provide dialysis concentrate in various sized containers. The sodium chloride content is near saturation, and the other constituents are in proportion to their final concentration in the dialysate. There is some equipment for making concentrate on site from dry chemicals, reducing transportation costs.

How is bicarbonate-based dialysate prepared?

Calcium and magnesium will not remain in a solution with bicarbonate because of the low hydrogen ion content. To solve this, two separate concentrates are used. The proportioning (delivery) system is more complex because it must mix and monitor three liquids instead of only two.

What chemicals are in the bicarbonate concentrates?

The "A" (indicating acidified) concentrate contains most of the sodium, all of the calcium, magnesium and potassium, chloride, and a small amount of acetic acid to maintain pH low enough to keep the calcium and magnesium in solution when mixed into dialysate.

The "B" (bicarbonate) concentrate contains the sodium bicarbonate. Some systems include part of the sodium chloride as well as the B concentrate; this raises the total conductivity, making it easier to monitor the concentrate. Table 7-2 shows the tabular formula used with one volume-volume type dilution.

Table 7-2	Tabular Formula for One Volume-Volume Type Dilution						
	mEq/L IN FINAL DILUTION						
Component	Na^+	K^+	Ca^{++}	Mg^{++}	Cl^-	HCO_3^-	CH_3COO^-
Concentrate B	59				20	39	
Concentrate A	81	2	3.5	0.7	87.2		4
Final	140	2	3.5	0.7	107.2	35	

In the proportioning system, the B concentrate is usually diluted partially with water; the A concentrate is then proportioned into the mixture just before it goes to the dialyzer. In the closed system, CO_2 cannot bubble off, the reaction between sodium bicarbonate and acetic acid cannot proceed to completion, and the hydrogen ion content keeps the calcium in solution.

What are the potential problems with bicarbonate dialysate?

Liquid B concentrate is not stable; some manufacturers add a small amount of special polymer as a stabilizer. Others provide dry $NaHCO_4$ as the powder, to be mixed at the facility. The mixing process requires care so that much of the CO_2 formed during the procedure is not lost from solution; it must be used within 24 hours of mixing.

Bicarbonate concentrate is very susceptible to bacterial contamination and proliferation. Even the stabilized solution should not be used if the container has been opened more than 72 hours. All containers for mixing, holding, or dispensing B concentrate must be scrupulously sanitized at regular intervals. Contamination must be avoided.

One manufacturer utilizes a delivery system that accepts a closed container of dry bicarbonate onto a special holder. Warm water passes through the column, producing a saturated solution of bicarbonate that is proportioned with water and then with the A concentrate by a conductivity-controlled feedback system.

There are many formulations of A concentrate to tailor the final dialysate sodium, potassium, calcium, and magnesium to the dialysis prescription. Each brand of delivery system has its unique proportioning and mixing ratios. Extreme care must be exercised to ensure that the concentrates selected are correct for the delivery system being used.

What kind of water is used to prepare dialysate?

The water must meet AAMI standards for chemical content and for bacterial and pyrogen content. In most instances, this involves complex and expensive treatment of feed water. Chapter 8 gives the various processes involved to achieve "dialysis-quality water."

Current AAMI standards for product water used to prepare dialysate states the microbial count has to be lower than 200 CFU/mL and an endotoxin concentration lower than 2 EU/mL.

What is the LAL test?

LAL is the abbreviation for limulus amebocyte lysate. It is an assay for endotoxin that uses a protein extract from the *Limulus,* or horseshoe crab. It is reported in nanograms per milliliter or in endotoxin units (EU) (1 ng/mL = 5 EU/mL).

Why is dialysate verification and monitoring so important?

Serious patient reactions and deaths have resulted from dialysate preparation errors or equipment malfunction. Dialysate must be verified for each dialysis. Each delivery system should have a function check daily.

What methods are used to check the dialysate composition?

There are two general methods, primary and secondary. A primary method specifically measures the concentration of one solute by a laboratory method of known reliability. Usually two solutes are determined, such as sodium by flame photometry and chloride by titration. This is particularly important for bicarbonate dialysis to ensure proper ratio of acid to bicarbonate, as well as the ratio of concentrate to water.

What secondary tests are used?

The most common test of dialysate is the total conductivity. This does not measure specific ions, but the overall conductivity contributed by all the ions (hence it is a secondary test). Conductivity meters must be calibrated carefully to the "normal" or "safe" range for each type of concentrate used. If two or more dialysate formulas are used, the safe range for each must be clearly identified since each has a different ionic concentration. Most manufacturers indicate on the label of the concentrate containers the conductivity of their dialysate when it is properly mixed.

An alternative secondary check of dialysate is the measurement of total osmolality by either freezing-point depression or vapor pressure. These measure total solute in the dialysate.

How do proportioning systems correctly mix dialysate?

Liquid concentrate is required. Several systems for mixing the correct proportions of concentrate and water have been used, but those in most widespread use employ microprocessor circuitry to control the speed of proportioning pumps, based on continuous conductivity and other parameter monitoring downstream of the mixing area (Fig. 7-2). The speed of the pumps and thus the volumes of the concentrates added are precisely controlled by the electronic feedback circuit to ensure that the dialysis fluid is properly mixed.

What are disadvantages of proportioning systems?

These very complex, highly sophisticated, microprocessor-controlled electronic and hydraulic devices are quite expensive. Many functions are preprogrammed and may not be readily changed. Sensors and monitoring devices must be fail-safe and redundant. Troubleshooting is often difficult, and factory-based service personnel may be needed for repairs.

How does a sorbent regenerative supply system work?

In this system, a small volume of dialysate is recirculated through a cartridge of adsorbent materials and chemically regenerated. Metabolic waste products transferred from the dialyzer to the dialysate are removed and the electrolyte content and pH are restored (Fig. 7-3).

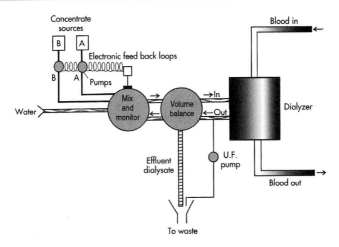

Fig. 7-2 Prototype of electronic proportioning system for bicarbonate dialysate, with volumetric ultrafiltration control.

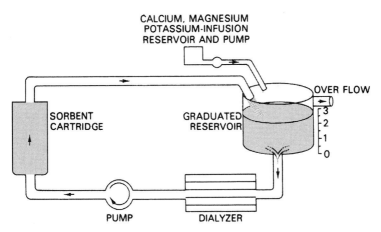

Fig. 7-3 Sorbent regenerative supply system.

How does a sorbent system function?

Three actions are involved: (1) conversion of urea to ammonium carbonate, (2) adsorption of creatinine and other nonionized solutes, and (3) ion exchange resins (sodium zirconium phosphate and zirconium oxide).

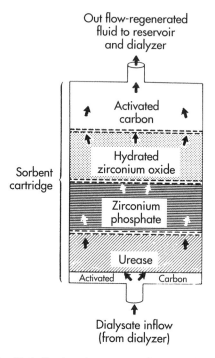

Fig. 7-4 Sorbent regenerative cartridge.

What is the process of urea conversion?

As dialysate enters the regenerative cartridge (Fig. 7-4), it first passes a carbon layer, which removes heavy metals and oxidants; it then contacts a bed containing urease. Urease is an enzyme that converts urea to ammonium and carbonate.

How are ammonium ions handled?

The next segment of the cartridge contains sodium zirconium phosphate, which acts as an exchange resin, taking up the ammonium ions and releasing sodium and hydrogen ions at about 1 Na^+ to 9 H^+. The carbonate ions equilibrate with hydrogen ions to yield bicarbonate ions (as $NaHCO_3$) and carbon dioxide.

Are other ions exchanged in the column?

Yes. Calcium, magnesium, and potassium ions are also exchanged for sodium ions by the sodium zirconium phosphate. In addition, the third portion of the cartridge contains hydrated zirconium oxide, which removes phosphate ions and fluoride.

How are creatinine and nitrogenous materials removed?

The final layer of the sorbent column contains activated carbon (charcoal) that binds by adsorption of creatinine, uric acid, guanidines, and other organic metabolites.

Is it necessary to replace calcium, magnesium, or potassium?

Yes. An infusion of calcium and magnesium is made just before the dialysate returns to the dialyzer to keep the desired concentration of these ions. Potassium is added, or omitted, according to the physician's desire.

What are advantages and disadvantages of the sorbent system?

Advantages include its portability and the absence of need for a special water supply or drain connections; it can be used wherever electricity is available.

Disadvantages include the somewhat expensive sorbent cartridge. There is a limit to the capacity to digest urea and to the absorption of ammonia. Ammonia may accumulate in the system and in the patient. Very large patients or those with very high serum urea values may require more than one cartridge per dialysis.

ADDITIONAL EQUIPMENT AND FUNCTIONS

Along with the dialysate mixing function, heaters, deaerators, pH and concentration monitors, dialysis delivery systems include a number of complementary functions essential to the hemodialysis procedure. These include the blood pump with an indicator for an estimate of blood flow rate, heparin infusion pump, air/foam detector, and inflow and outflow pressure sensors. On the dialysate side are temperature controls and monitors, conductivity monitors, flow rate controls, pressure sensors, and ultrafiltration volume controls. An online urea sensor in the effluent dialysate line has potential for truly accurate quantification of urea removal. These functions are controlled by several electronic microcontrollers and programmable microprocessors with appropriate parameters displayed on video screen(s).

How is dialysate temperature controlled?

The heater and/or heat exchanger is controlled by one or more sensors and a microcontroller circuit. Fluid temperature should hold within 0.5° C of the set point. There should be a separate sensor, independent of the heat control, for online monitoring with visual and audible alarms for any out-of-limits state. Accuracy should be checked regularly with a certified glass thermometer. Many end-stage renal disease (ESRD) patients have a body core temperature of 36° to 36.5° C. Added heat in excess of replacement causes a vasodilatory response, which may be detrimental at a time when the normal vasoconstrictive response to reduced volemia from ultrafiltration is acting to minimize hypotension. Fluid temperature greater than 41° C causes hemolysis of red blood cells, which can continue for several hours.

Why are deaeration devices necessary?

Water contains considerable dissolved air and microbubbles. When it is warmed, the dissolved air comes out of solution as expanding microbubbles. These have a negative effect on temperature and conductivity sensors, and flowmeters. Bubbles can reduce dialysate/membrane contact in hollow-fiber dialyzers.

Most deaeration devices use warmers along with negative pressure to bring the dissolved gases out of solution. An air trap or coalescing filter then captures the gases and vents them to the outside.

What problems are associated with dialysate flowmeters?

Solute film tends to build up with time and reduce accuracy. Calibration of the flowmeter or flow controller should be part of the routine servicing of the machine. At the bedside, actual flow can be quickly determined by a timed, measured outflow collection from the drain hose. Ultrafiltration control should be set to zero temporarily, during the measurement.

What is the importance of the dialysate pressure monitors?

If ultrafiltration is regulated by adjusting dialysate negative pressure, both inflow and outflow monitors must have high and low alarm set points, and must be accurate within ±20 mm Hg, or 10% of reading. Manufacturer's directions must be followed carefully in adjusting and calibrating these monitors.

If ultrafiltration is controlled volumetrically or flowmetrically, the dialysate pressure monitors serve as a check on the ultrafiltration control and the transmembrane pressure.

How is dialysate concentration controlled and monitored?

The most suitable apparatus for this is the conductivity monitor (Fig. 7-5), which must be temperature compensated. Normal accuracy is ±1% to 3%. The conductivity sensor is basically an electrolytic cell, as described in Chapter 2. The electrodes of continually

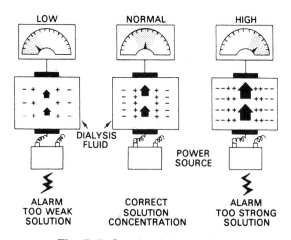

Fig. 7-5 Conductivity monitor.

operating monitors are eroded by electrolytic action with a gradual loss of sensitivity over time. Most delivery systems use at least dual conductivity sensors, the readings of which must match. A confirmation test with a handheld conductivity meter should be routine each day. Before any adjustment of the conductivity monitors, a primary test, such as the laboratory measurement of sodium or of chloride, should be done to verify the actual composition of the dialysate at the time.

Is dialysate pH monitored?

There should be some type of pH verification. The usual limits are pH 6.8 to 7.6. There should be audible and visual alarms for any out-of-limits state. Sensors for pH drift with passage of time and must be recalibrated by the manufacturer's personnel.

What kinds of blood pumps are used?

A pump with internal components exposed directly to blood can present major problems in cleaning and sterilization. Peristaltic roller pumps, which work by progressively compressing special segments of blood tubing against the semicircular housing, are used almost universally.

How is blood flow rate measured?

Most blood pumps have speed indicators calibrated to show flow according to the speed of rotation. The internal diameter of the pumping segments of the tubing in use must match that for which the pump indicator was calibrated. Variations in tubing, pressure conditions in the blood circuit, and lack of linearity across the indicator scale cause discrepancies of $\pm 10\%$ to 15% between indicated and actual blood flow.

The calibration of each pump should be verified regularly, under standard conditions, with the same brand and lot of tubing used clinically. Water at 37° C should be pumped from a container, through the tubing, which is partially clamped to approximately the negative pressure between the needle and the inflow side of the pump during dialysis. The outflow should be collected in a graduated cylinder for 3 to 5 minutes. Volume (milliliters) divided by time (minutes) gives the flow rate. A record of each calibration should be kept on the machine, and in the central file.

How do blood leak detectors work?

Blood leak detectors are situated in the effluent dialysate line (Fig. 7-6). A beam of light is directed through a column of dialysate onto a photoelectric cell. A change in translucence and light scatter in dialysate reduces the light received by the photocell, stopping the blood pump and activating visual and audible alarms.

AAMI standards require detection of less than 0.45 mL/min of blood at hematocrit 45 over a range of dialysate flows. Particulate matter or air bubbles are frequent sources of false alarms. If a blood leak is not easily confirmed visually, the dialysate should be checked with a Hemostix. If standard maintenance procedures do not eliminate the problem, the manufacturer's representative should correct or replace the unit.

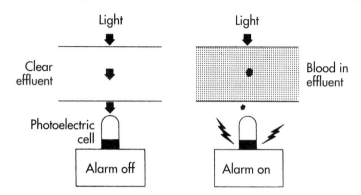

Fig. 7-6 Blood leak detector. *(Adapted from Nosé Y: Manual on Artificial Organs. Vol 1. The Artificial Kidney, St Louis, 1969, Mosby.)*

How do air bubbles in blood detectors behave?

Whenever a pump is used to propel blood through the extracorporeal circuit, some degree of negative pressure is created at the intake side. Air may be sucked into the line at connections that are not absolutely tight (as at the needle hub), through needle punctures or breaks in the tubing, or from empty fluid containers attached at the infusion sidearm. These potential air sources are especially important as pumping speed is increased in the efforts to achieve high blood flow rates. Air in blood can obstruct fibers of hollow-fiber kidneys, and if the quantity is sufficient, air may pass the venous bubble trap and go on to cause massive air embolism to the patient.

A commonly used detector employs an ultrasonic beam to identify air, foam, and microbubbles in blood (Fig. 7-7). Sound travels more quickly through fluid than through air, thus even minuscule bubbles slow the sonic beam and result in an alarm. Sonic detectors may be armed while the bloodlines contain only saline; they do not respond to light or light changes in the surrounding environment.

Most air/foam detectors have no external sensitivity adjustment. The dialysis delivery system can be operated with the detector disarmed for priming and rinsing. There should be a low-level alarm, clearly discernible from a distance, to indicate the disarmed status. No patient should be permitted to dialyze with the air/foam detector in the disarmed state.

How do ultrafiltration controls work?

These devices exactly match the outflow dialysate volume with the inflow volume, plus a precisely measured extra effluent volume representing the desired (programmed) ultrafiltrate. There are two basic types of ultrafiltration controllers: (1) volumetric and (2) flowmetric (Figs. 7-8 and 7-9).

How do volumetric ultrafiltration devices operate?

The most common system employs two diaphragm chambers to balance the inflow and outflow dialysate (Fig. 7-10). While one side of the first chamber is filling with fresh

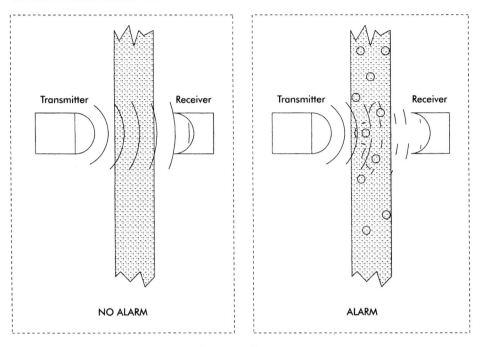

Fig. 7-7 Sonic air/foam detector.

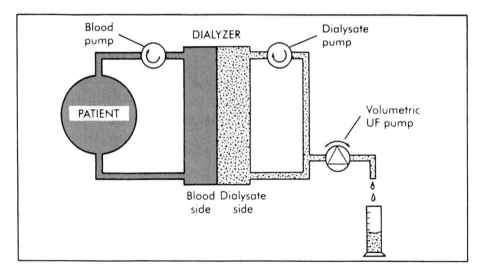

Fig. 7-8 Volumetric ultrafiltration control. *(Redrawn from Vlchek DL: Staying tuned in to the high-tech world—part 2: dialysis delivery systems,* Dial Trans, *Aug 18, 1989.)*

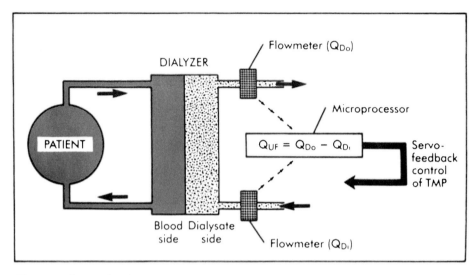

Fig. 7-9 Servo-feedback ultrafiltration control. *(Redrawn from Vlchek DL: Staying tuned in to the high-tech world. Part 2: Dialysis delivery systems,* Dial Trans, *Aug 18, 1989.)*

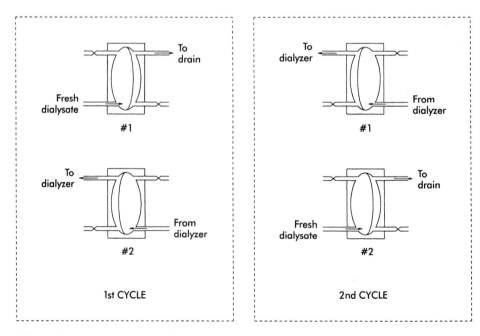

Fig. 7-10 Volumetric ultrafiltration. Matched double diaphragm chambers.

dialysate, its diaphragm is forcing out an equal volume of used fluid from the other side. Simultaneously in the second chamber, one side is filling with spent fluid from the dialyzer while the opposite side is ejecting an equal volume of fresh dialysate to the dialyzer. When the diaphragms have deflected across the width of the chambers, valves are reversed so that the side that was emptying now fills, and vice versa. The volume for ultrafiltrate is removed from the outflow dialysate channel by a metering pump before the outflow volume is matched to inflow, thus removing the desired amount of ultra-filtrate from the patient. Because the volumes in and out of the controller are precisely equalized, whatever pressure (negative or positive) is necessary will be created for the removal of the measured ultrafiltrate volume by the dialyzer.

How does the flowmetric ultrafiltrate control system work?

In a flowmetric system there are one or two very accurate flowmeters in both the in-flow and the outflow dialysate pathways to measure the flow of fluid passing through these pathways. The speed of the dialysate pump in the outflow path is varied by the electronic control module so that the volume through the outflow meter is exactly equal to the volume through the inflow meter, plus the programmed amount of ultrafiltrate.

HIGH-EFFICIENCY AND HIGH-FLUX DIALYSIS
What are equipment needs for high-efficiency dialysis?

There are the following four requirements:
- A highly permeable cellulose membrane (ultrathin Cuprophan, Hemophan, cellulose acetate ester, etc.) with surface area 1.5 m^2 or more
- Reliable blood flow of 350 mL/min or more; dialysate flow of 750 mL/min or more
- Bicarbonate dialysate delivery system
- An ultrafiltration control system

The combination of a large area of membrane of high mass transfer capability and high Q_b and Q_d produces increased small molecule transfer. Intermediate-sized and large solute transfer rates are enhanced by the area and permeability increases.

What are the system requirements for high-flux dialysis?

As with high-efficiency dialysis, in the high-flux system it is important to maintain high blood flow rate, high dialysate flow rate, and precision control of ultrafiltration volume. High-flux dialyzers use synthetic membranes of very high permeability, with convective transfer providing a major share of solute transport (see page 66). These dialyzers have ultrafiltration coefficients of 20 to 70 mL/hr/mm Hg or more.

The ultrafiltration controller precisely manages net fluid removal, but in so doing generates a dialysate pressure profile that creates reverse filtration from dialysate to blood in the distal portion of the dialyzer (Fig. 7-11). A problem of contamination of blood by pyrogenic material and endotoxin fragments is created because high-flux

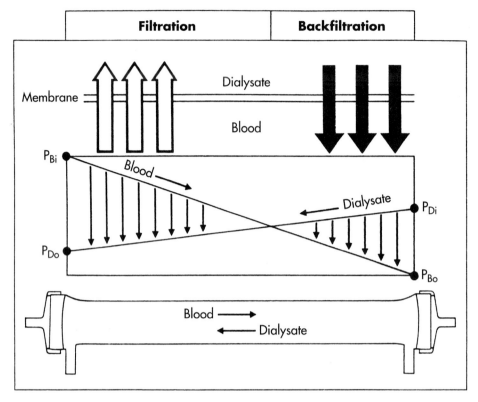

Fig. 7-11 Backfiltration and pressure distribution. *(From Baurmeister U, et al: Dialysate contamination and back filtration may limit the use of high-flux dialysis membranes,* Transact ASAIO *35:21, 1989.)*

membranes readily pass particles of 2000 to 10,000 Da. The LAL test (see Glossary and page 79) is used to monitor dialysate for endotoxin.

How might the problem of reverse filtration be countered?

AAMI standards require not more than 200 colony-forming units (CFU) of bacteria per milliliter in water for dialysate, and not more than 200 CFU bacteria or 2 EU by LAL test for endotoxin in dialysate leaving the delivery system. Bacterial multiplication continues as the dialysis fluid courses through the dialyzer; pyrogenic materials increase and cross the high-flux membrane during backfiltration.

Addition of a molecular filter or ultrafilter (see Chapter 8) to the dialysate path immediately ahead of the dialyzer may be necessary for high-flux dialysis. A 50,000- to 100,000-Da ultrafilter will reject intact endotoxins; the 1000- to 10,000-Da ultrafilter will be necessary if endotoxin fragments are the problem. Some manufacturers have a provision for ultrafilters in their delivery systems.

8 Water Treatment

Water is a complex and incompletely understood chemical compound. The purest form of water is freshly formed rain as it leaves the cloud. It is also a very high-energy form of water. In the journey from rain cloud to final delivery tap, much of this energy is expended in acquiring various impurities as solute or suspension.

Improved dialysis technology has made high-purity water critical for dialysis fluid preparation. Fortunately the science of water purification has made parallel advances. Enhanced membranes for reverse osmosis, ultrafiltration (UF) devices to screen out endotoxins as well as bacteria, and improved monitoring systems are being applied in the renal community.

What impurities may be present in tap water?

Three categories of contaminating substances can cause patient injury or equipment malfunction: (1) chemical solutes, (2) bacteria or bacterial products, and (3) particulate matter. Of these, the chemical and bacterial contaminants may be directly harmful to patients receiving dialysis.

How do impurities get into water?

Falling rainwater passing through the air contacts carbon dioxide and sulfur dioxide, forming carbonic and sulfuric acid in weak solution. Upon hitting the ground, this water encounters limestone and other minerals to form calcium bicarbonate and sulfate, magnesium carbonate, and other salts. Calcium carbonate is the more prevalent impurity in tap water and accounts for most of its hardness.

What other inorganic chemicals may be present in tap water?

Sodium, chloride, iron, aluminum, nitrates, manganese, copper, zinc, iodide, and fluoride are common ionic constituents. The types of mineral present in the geographic area and the time the water is in contact with them determine the content.

Trace elements that may be present include arsenic, silver, strontium, selenium, chromium, lead, cadmium, cyanide, barium, tin, and others.

Are these chemicals harmful?

Nitrates and chloramines may cause methemoglobinemia, in which red cell hemoglobin cannot transport oxygen. Copper in excess may cause hemolysis. Manganese can be toxic, and iron may possibly be toxic. Fluoride is believed to aggravate uremic bone disease; it does accumulate in bone, and it is toxic to enzyme systems. Tin has been found in significantly higher quantity in tissues of dialyzed uremic patients than in nonuremic individuals. Aluminum accumulates and is related to dialysis-dementia syndrome, as well as to a form of anemia and osteodystrophy. Zinc causes gastrointestinal upset and may produce anemia. In areas of radioactivity, the presence of 90Sr may pose a danger.

Are there other materials in tap water?

Nonionic organic compounds, particularly nitrogenous matter such as proteins and polypeptides, phenols, indoles, and aldehydes, may be present. Solid particles of iron, sand, and silica are frequent. Suspended material, including mud, algae, plankton, bacteria, viruses, pyrogenic matter, and dissolved gases (ammonia, carbon dioxide, chlorine) are often present. The most common soluble organic compounds are chloramines from urban water treatment systems. The content of these materials as well as ionic impurities vary with the water source, season, and distribution system.

Some water supplies have identifiable amounts of pesticides or herbicides, such as chlordane, DDT, aldrin, lindane, 2,4,4-T, and others.

Most water supplies contain various kinds of bacteria. Many are not detected by routine testing for coliform organisms. Such organisms include *Flavobacterium*, *Achromobacter*, *Serratia*, *Pseudomonas*, and several atypical mycobacteria.

If a water supply meets the requirements of the Safe Drinking Water Act and Environmental Protection Agency standards, is it safe for dialysis?

No. Contaminants in the water used to make dialysis fluid may enter the patient's bloodstream through the dialysis membrane. In addition, most dialysis procedures use bicarbonate as the buffer. Some delivery systems, in bicarbonate mode, will not function properly if the pH is outside the range of 6.5 to 7.8. The pH of untreated tap water may be extremely acidic or extremely alkaline.

Why is special water treatment necessary to make dialyzing fluid?

During hemodialysis the amount of water that contacts the patient's blood is more than 25 times the amount taken in by drinking. A substance present in water to only one quarter of its upper limit of safety for drinking purposes may enter the body during hemodialysis in amounts 10 to 25 times that much. Ingested water is processed by the gastrointestinal tract before reaching the bloodstream. This selective membrane can alter the rate at which foreign substances are absorbed from ingested water. In a dialyzer system the dialyzer membrane cannot select ions to be absorbed or rejected, and they pass by diffusion. Substances that are harmless in drinking water may be toxic in dialysis water.

What methods are used to treat water for use in hemodialysis?

- Filtration
- Activated carbon filters (adsorption)
- Water softeners
- Reverse osmosis (RO)
- Deionization (DI)
- Ultraviolet light exposure

What is accomplished by filtration?

Suspended particles (mud, sand, rust, algae) are removed by mechanical filtration through a wound filament or membrane cartridge or by tanks containing granular material that can be backflushed. These effectively filter particles down to about 5 mm in size. Submicron filters are available that screen out particles as small as 0.2 mm. The smaller the number of the filter, the more efficient it is at filtering substances. The number of the filter represents the size of the particle that it is capable of filtering.

What types of filters are used?

The use of multimedia depth filters (i.e., sand filters) is a very economical and efficient way to remove suspended particles by filtering the water through sand. Cartridge filters remove particulate matter by filtering the water through a very stiff or rigid device. An ultrafilter is a very thin and delicate filter that removes much smaller solutes such as endotoxins. Ultrafilters are highly effective for the removal of fine particles, bacteria, endotoxins, and other pyrogenic matter, as well as high-molecular-weight organic molecules.

What is the silt density index?

The silt density index (SDI) is an indicator of the colloid and suspended particulate matter present in tap water. The measuring device indicates the pressure drop over time as the tap water crosses a 0.45-mm membrane filter. The more suspended material present, the slower the water passes. An SDI of less than 5 is required of feed water for most reverse osmosis systems.

What is the action of the carbon tank?

The carbon tank contains granular activated carbon, which removes chlorines and chloramines from the water by adsorption. Carbon filters or tanks also remove organic matter and odor-producing materials by the same method. Adsorption is a physical process that does not require a chemical reaction and is simply the process in which liquids, gases, or suspended materials cling to a surface such as the activated carbon. The carbon tank will not remove electrolytes, such as calcium or sodium. Most water treatment systems have two carbon tanks. The first tank removes virtually all of the chlorine, and the second tank acts as a standby or backup in the event the first tank did not effectively remove all of the chlorines and chloramines. These tanks are sometimes referred to as the working tank and the polishing tank. The tanks must be backwashed nightly to redistribute the carbon for more effective adsorption. The polishing tank has a low flow through it and little chlorine present, making it a good source for bacterial growth. Rotating the polishing and the working tanks will help minimize the growth of organisms and extend the life of the tanks. Commonly, there are two types of carbon tanks: (1) portable exchange or (2) "permanent" portable exchange. Portable exchange tanks are "changed out" on a cycle that is developed by the facility. The vendor then replaces them with "new charcoal"–filled tanks. Permanent tanks are equipped with a control unit that allows them to be backwashed at the facility's discretion. At intervals the carbon is replaced by the vendor. Backwashing does not regenerate the carbon beds. It actually "fluffs" the carbon particles so that channels are removed and the total bed is once again available to contact water passing through it.

What is the action of the water softener?

A water softener is a device located after the carbon tanks that exchanges ions in the water. Water hardness is caused primarily by calcium and magnesium ions. A water softener exchanges calcium and magnesium ions for sodium ions on a milliequivalent-for-milliequivalent basis. Other positively charged ions such as aluminum are also removed by the water softener. For each calcium ion removed, two sodium ions are added. The sodium is later removed by the reverse osmosis (RO) system. Permanent softeners have a concentrated brine tank that holds the sodium chloride and controls for onsite regeneration of the softener.

If the feed water is very hard, a softener will remove most of the calcium and magnesium before further treatment. If a deionizer is used downstream, the softener will reduce the divalent ion load presented to the deionizer resin bed and prolong its life. If the subsequent treatment is RO, the removal of calcium and magnesium by the softener may result in higher quality product water and longer RO membrane life.

What problems occur with the use of water softeners?

If the raw water is very hard, considerable sodium is substituted in the exchange for calcium and magnesium. Municipal water supplies often vary seasonally or even during a single day if multiple sources are used.

There are two types of softeners, portable exchange and permanent. Portable exchange units are provided ready for use by the vendor. Regeneration of the media resin is performed by the vendor at a central facility.

There are no online monitors that will indicate "hard" or "soft" water, but commercial test kits for total hardness are available and are quite reliable. The degree of hardness of both source water and product water should be determined each day. This will indicate the need for the regeneration cycle, as well as any softener malfunction.

What is RO?

RO represents the ultimate in ultrafiltration and is the most effective method of treating water used in dialysis. The RO process removes most contaminants left in the water by the pre-RO treatment systems including bacterial endotoxins and other contaminants. The RO process involves the movement of water under high pressure across a semipermeable membrane. The dissolved solutes or contaminants will form on the feed side of the membrane and the pure water will form on the product side of the membrane. It is expected that the percent rejection of the water going through the membranes will have a rejection rate of at least 80%. The product or purified water will then be sent to a holding tank, where it will be stored before use.

How are organic compounds processed by the membrane?

Organic compounds have no net charge and are not electrically repelled but are physically screened by the membrane. Almost all particles of molecular weight greater than 200 Da are rejected. This includes bacteria, viruses, and pyrogens.

What types of membranes are used for RO?

Membranes for RO use must be (1) freely permeable to water, (2) highly impermeable to solutes, and (3) able to tolerate very high operating pressures. Desirable characteristics include tolerance to a wide range of pH and temperature and resistance to attack by bacteria and by chemicals such as chlorine.

Membranes in general use include (1) cellulose, (2) aromatic polyamide, (3) thin-film composites, and (4) high-flux, chlorine-resistant polysulfone.

- Cellulose acetate membranes have high water permeability but poor rejection of low-molecular-weight contaminants. Range of pH tolerance is limited; they degrade at temperatures greater than 35° C (95° F) and are vulnerable to bacteria. They are relatively inexpensive.
- Polyamide membranes have wide pH tolerance and are more resistant to bacterial action and to hydrolysis than are cellulose membranes. They are very susceptible to degradation by free chlorine.
- Thin film composites are expensive. The supporting layer is usually a porous polysulfone. Fixed to this is a thin, dense, solute-rejecting surface film such as polyfurane cyanurate or a polyamide. Composite membranes have better water flux and better solute rejection than cellulose acetate. They are less subject to compaction and bacterial action.
- Chlorine-resistant polysulfone membranes have a very long service life. They tolerate a wide span of pH and temperatures. Water flux is high. They differ from other membranes in that if divalent ions are present in the feed water, rejection of monovalent ions is sharply reduced. Therefore it is essential that the feed water be softened or deionized before entering the RO unit.

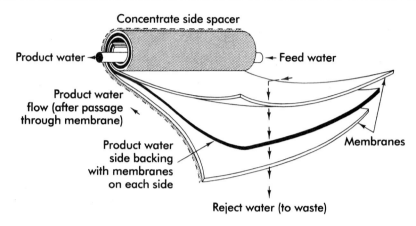

Fig. 8-1 Spiral-wrap reverse osmosis module.

What configuration of RO modules is used?

Module design must include such features as a large membrane surface area, a tolerance for very high pressure (up to 500 psi), good flow characteristics, and a low pressure drop. Configurations in use for hemodialysis water are (1) the spiral-wound or spiral-wrap (Fig. 8-1) and (2) hollow-fiber modules.

Spiral-wound units consist of two layers of membrane with a fabric material fastened between, sandwich fashion. The fabric material is the product carrier. The membrane-sandwich sheet, along with a plastic mesh separator, is wrapped in a spiral around a central perforated tube in a manner somewhat similar to that of an old-style coil dialyzer. Feed water under high pressure enters one end of the unit and flows along the channels provided by the plastic mesh; some water is forced by the hydraulic pressure through the membrane. The central fabric conducts this filtered water to the central tube, from which it emerges as product water.

In hollow-fiber units the membrane is formed as capillary fibers of 80 to 250 mm inside diameter. Several thousand of these fibers are bundled inside a high-pressure cylinder. Pressurized feed water surrounds and permeates the hollow fibers, forming the product water inside the capillary lumina. The small internal diameter of the hollow fibers can contribute to plugging and reduced permeate flow.

What are special advantages of RO over other types of water treatment?

There are several advantages:

- Bacteria, viruses, and pyrogen materials are rejected by the intact membrane. In this respect RO water approaches distilled water in quality.
- Available units are relatively compact and require little space. They are well suited to home dialysis.
- In average use, the membrane has a life of a little more than 1 to 2 years before replacement is necessary.

- Periodic complete sterilization of the RO system with formalin or other sterilant is practical.

What are disadvantages of RO systems?

Disadvantages include the following:

- The membranes have a limited service life. For instance:
  - Cellulose acetate membranes have limited pH tolerance. They degrade at temperatures greater than 35° C. They are vulnerable to bacteria. They eventually hydrolyze.
  - Polyamide membranes are intolerant of temperature greater than 35° C. They have poor tolerance for free chlorine.
  - Thin-film composites are intolerant of chlorine.
  - High-flux polysulfones require softening or deionization of feed water to function properly.
- As with hemodialysis membranes, leaks are possible. Continual monitoring of product water flow rate and conductivity is necessary.
- Product water is 25% to 50% of feed water. The remaining 50% to 75% goes to waste, a matter of economic and environmental concern.
- The membrane must be kept continually wet throughout its entire life. The flow cannot simply be stopped and the unit maintained filled with water; bacterial growth, hydrolysis of the membrane, and pyrogen production are likely to result. When not in operation, the unit should be held in a sterilant-filled state.
- Chloramines (oxidant compounds formed from the reaction between chlorine and ammonia used as bactericidal agents in some city water supplies) are nonionic and freely cross the RO membrane. Anemia resulting from chloramine has occurred in some dialysis patients. A carbon filter should always be used ahead of an RO system to remove any chloramine.
- To meet peak flow needs in large hemodialysis facilities, a reservoir or holding tanks for processed water from the RO unit may be necessary. The water is recirculated in a continuous loop from RO unit to tanks and back to prevent stagnation. The tanks and plumbing are sites for potential microbial growth and endotoxin formation. Tank design is important in minimizing contamination. A steeply rounded or conical tank bottom with the drain port at the extreme low point ensures complete emptying. The reentry port should be near the top and use a special nozzle to spray the underside of the cover. This prevents water droplets from forming on the cover, and the cascade of water down the sides prevents the collection of stagnant water. The top should have a microbial filter in the air vent. This design also provides excellent sterilant contact during chemical disinfection, and complete flushing away of sterilant at "rinse-out." Chlorine or iodine may also be metered into the system between the RO unit and the tanks to control the growth of organisms (Fig. 8-2).

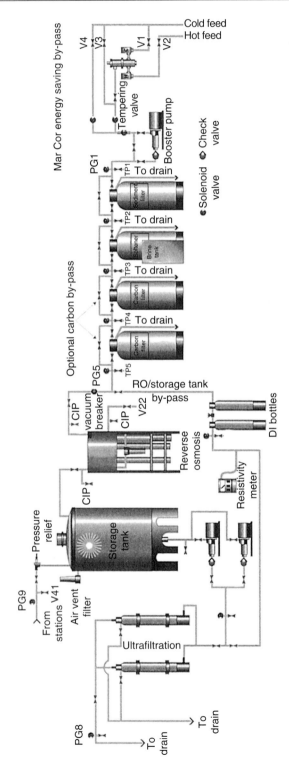

Fig. 8-2 Recirculating loop water treatment system with holding tank. *(Courtesy Mar Cor Services, Harleysville, Pa.)*

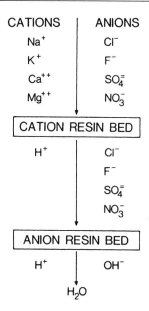

Fig. 8-3 Schematic diagram of two-bed deionizing system.

What is deionization?

Deionization (DI) refers to the removal of ionized minerals and salts from a solution, in this case, the feed water. Positively charged ions are exchanged by the resin beads for hydrogen ions and the negatively charged ions are exchanged to form hydroxide ions. (Fig. 8-3). The hydrogen and hydroxide ions formed as a result combine to create water molecules. Deionizers produce water of high ionic purity, but they do not remove bacteria or pyrogens. Indeed, deionizers often make the quality of water worse in terms of bacteria and endotoxin content; the resin bed provides an environment conducive to bacterial proliferation. It is prudent to follow deionization equipment with submicron filtration or an ultrafiltration unit (Fig. 8-4).

How is water quality monitored with the use of a deionizer?

It is imperative that some type of monitor be installed to ensure the chemical quality of the product water. Deionizer water quality values are expressed in resistivity units. The Association for the Advancement of Medical Instrumentation (AAMI) guidelines state that product water should not be allowed to go below 1 MΩ resistance; at that point the tanks should be exchanged.

What problems occur with deionizers?

The following are several problems to watch out for:
- An initial problem is obtaining the maximum flow rate needed. As with softeners, proper size of the DI set is critical. Peak and normal operating

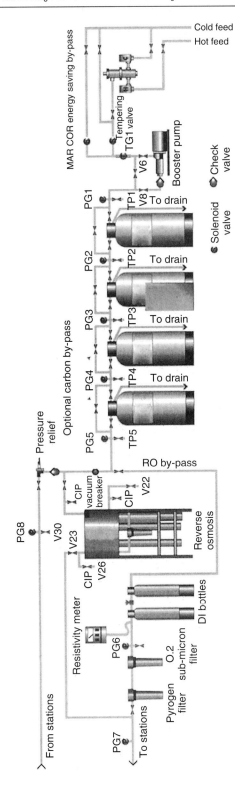

Fig. 8-4 Direct feed water treatment system to produce ultrapure water. (*Courtesy Mar Cor Services, Harleysville, Pa.*)

flow rates and operating line pressures should be determined. The user then should look at the operating specifications for a variety of tank sizes and select the size that best meets the facility's needs, taking account of the pressure drop across the DI set. Pressure indicators before and after this subsystem are advisable so that the difference in pressure can be easily determined.

- Total ion content of the feed water is a problem; only a finite quantity of ions can be removed by a resin bed of given size. Service life of the deionizer depends on water composition and volume. If a DI unit is positioned ahead of an RO unit, its service life will be short. It will be processing water of high ionic content while the RO unit will serve primarily as a bacterial and endotoxin screen. If the DI unit is located downstream from the RO device, the DI then becomes a "polisher." It also increases chances of microbiologic contamination. It is recommended that a submicron filter or an ultrafilter be placed downstream.

- Resin beds tend to exhaust suddenly. A parallel bypass installation is necessary so that switchover can be made while the exhausted tanks are replaced. The water in tanks that are standing idle will be stagnant. Provision for flushing a reasonable volume to the drain should be part of the system. The volumetric capacity of deionizers (gallons of water passing through the tanks) is rated in grains per gallon (GPG) of total dissolved solids (TDS), expressed as calcium carbonate. (Note: 1 GPG approximates 17.1 mg/L $CaCO_3$.) Rated capacity of the deionizer divided by the TDS of the feed water will give an approximation of the volume of water that may be treated before the unit exhausts. Online, continuous readout resistivity meters should be positioned to monitor the effluent water. When the resistance degrades to 1 MΩ/cm, the tanks should be exchanged (an AAMI standard).

- Usually the anion and cation resins exhaust at different times. If the tanks are used to exhaustion, ions previously removed may be released, possibly in a concentration greater than that of the feed water. The water may become extremely acidic or extremely alkaline, depending on which resin exhausted first. This situation may be hazardous to patients or equipment.

How is ultraviolet light used in treating water?

Ultraviolet (UV) light is a form of radiation that penetrates the cell walls of microorganisms and destroys them by altering their deoxyribonucleic acid (DNA). In the dialysis water treatment system, the UV light source is housed in a clear protective quartz sleeve. It is placed so that water can pass through a flow chamber, where it is exposed to intense UV radiation. It is important that the water flow not be too turbulent and that the water is free of suspended particles. UV light passes more easily through clear translucent fluids. Cloudy liquids make the UV light more difficult to penetrate and could potentially allow microbes to hide behind the suspended particles and not be eliminated. The UV light does not destroy endotoxins.

What degree of water purity is required for hemodialysis?

The AAMI developed a set of water quality guidelines that is recognized as the US national standard. The standard now applies not only to chemical or inorganic contaminants but to microbiologic contaminants as well. These requirements are shown in Table 8-1 as well as the adverse effects of exposure.

Table 8-1	AAMI Water Quality Guidelines*	
Water contaminant	**AAMI suggested maximum level (mg/L)**	**Adverse effects from exposure†**
Aluminum	0.01	Anemia, bone disease, neurologic changes
Antimony	0.006	*Nausea/vomiting*
Arsenic, lead, silver	0.005 each	
Bacteria		Hypotension, nausea/vomiting
Beryllium	0.004	Bone damage
Cadmium	0.001	*Nausea/vomiting, diarrhea, salivation, sensory disturbances,* kidney/liver/bone damage
Calcium	2 (0.1 mEq/L)	*Nausea/vomiting, headache, muscle weakness, tachycardia, hypertension,* abnormal bone mineralization, soft tissue calcifications, pancreatitis
Chloramines	0.1	*Hemolysis, chest pain, arrhythmias, nausea/vomiting*

From Vlchek DL, Burrows-Hudson S: *Quality assurance guidelines for hemodialysis devices,* Washington, DC, February 1991, U.S. Department of Health and Human Services, Food and Drug Administration; Potential Drinking Water Contaminant Index, www.epa.gov/safewater/mcl.html; Association for the Advancement of Medical Instrumentation, 2001, Arlington, Virginia.
*The physician has ultimate responsibility for determining the quality of water used for dialysis.
†Acute symptoms in italics.

Table 8-1	AAMI Water Quality Guidelines*—Cont'd	
Water contaminant	AAMI suggested maximum level (mg/L)	Adverse effects from exposure†
Chlorine	0.5	
Chromium	0.014	Liver damage
Copper, barium, zinc	0.1 each	*Chills, flushing, headaches, projectile vomiting, hypotension,* anemia, liver damage, pancreatitis
Endotoxin	2 EU/mL	Hypotension, nausea/vomiting
Fluoride	0.2	*Chest pain, nausea/vomiting, hypotension,* headache, bone disease
Magnesium	4 (0.3 mEq/L)	Nausea/vomiting
Mercury	0.0002	Kidney damage
Nitrate (N)	2	*Hemolysis, hypotension, nausea/vomiting, weakness, confusion*
Potassium	8 (0.2 mEq/L)	
Selenium	0.09	*Fatigue, irritability,* hair/nail loss, kidney/liver damage
Sodium	70 (3 mEq/L)	*Increased thirst, nausea, headache, hypertension, pulmonary edema, seizures, coma*
Sulfate	100	Metabolic acidosis, nausea/vomiting
Thallium	0.002 mg/L	Liver/kidney damage

What problems are there in handling very pure water?

As water is treated increasingly near its pure state, its energy level also increases. Such pure water very quickly reacts chemically with materials it contacts. Only pipe or tubing of medical-grade stainless steel, polyvinyl chloride (PVC), or one of the new inert materials may be used to carry the product water. Tanks must be of such material. If exposed to air, ultrapure water will quickly absorb and react with carbon dioxide.

What problems are there with bacteria and pyrogens in water treatment?

The original AAMI standard was based on dialysis fluid made with acetate concentrate and dialyzer membranes of Cuprophan. The microbial standard of 200 CFU/mL in water for preparing dialysis fluid, and 2000 CFU/mL in the proportioned dialysate exiting the dialyzer, was appropriate for such hemodialysis. Because dialyzer membranes have changed significantly (see Chapter 7), the standards for proportioned dialysate exiting the dialyzer have been changed from 2000 CFU/mL to 200 CFU/mL. New membranes are much more porous to water, solutes, and suspended matter. Transmembrane movement is bidirectional, relative to pressure and solute concentration gradients. Proper prefilters with an RO unit, or DI with submicron postfiltration, will in most instances meet the standard. Bacteria proliferate on filter surfaces, carbon tanks, softener and DI resin beds, and the feed water surface of the RO membrane. A regular schedule of backflushing with an approved sterilant must be used to minimize bacterial growth in all components of the water treatment system. The sterilant must, of course, be thoroughly rinsed from the system before water is used for patients. Chemical sterilization kills bacteria but does not destroy them, and actually fixes some of the protein and polysaccharide components and endotoxins. Copious backflushing is needed to wash this debris away from the collecting surfaces.

A majority of facilities use bicarbonate-containing concentrate in their fluid-proportioning systems. Many facilities use dialyzers with high-flux membranes, along with controlled ultrafiltration devices.

Bicarbonate concentrate, when stored, supports proliferation of endotoxin-forming microorganisms. Whether these originate from the water used to prepare the concentrate or from the bicarbonate powder, it is likely that more strict microbial and endotoxin limits will be necessary. For high-flux dialysis where backfiltration poses a problem, delivery of sterile, pyrogen-free fluid from the proportioning system to the dialyzer may become necessary.

How may microbiologic contaminants be further reduced?

The following four means are most commonly used:

- Chlorine may be metered into RO product water. This is sometimes utilized in facilities that recirculate RO water through a holding tank system. However, the chlorine produces problems also.

- Submicron (0.05 mm) filters will stop passage of bacteria and viruses. Such filters must be replaced frequently and are expensive. They do not exclude all pyrogenic matter.
- UF will reject bacteria and endotoxins effectively. Initial installation is relatively expensive, but operation is economical. Sanitization is simple, and service life is good.

How is ultrafiltration used to remove bacteria and endotoxin?

UF membranes have an effective pore size of more than 0.001 mm. Pores of this size do not retard the movement of osmotically active solutes; hence less hydraulic pressure is needed for the transmembrane movement of water than is needed with RO membranes.

UF membranes are often called molecular filters; they filter suspended particles of molecular size rather than dissolved substances. The larger particles do not have the osmotic effect of dissolved solutes. There is little osmotic backpressure, compared with RO membranes, hence less need for high hydraulic pressure. However, these molecular filters reject bacteria, endotoxin, and endotoxin fragments that are thousands of daltons in size. Ultrafilters are available that exclude particles of 50,000 to 100,000 Da; in fact, an even tighter membrane of 1000 to 10,000 Da is available.

UF devices may be placed ahead of RO units to prevent bacterial growth or accumulation of particulate material on the feed water surface of the RO membrane. When used as the final step before delivery of product water to the proportioning system, UF will ensure its microbiologic quality.

What tests are done to maintain the water treatment systems?

Bacteria culturing. Bacteria culturing is performed to detect the presence of bacteria in the water. A colony count is typically read in 24 and 48 hours. Bacterial cultures are also performed on the dialysate.

Conductivity. Conductivity is verified on the feed and product water to make certain it contains the proper amount of ions. It can be measured with a Phoenix meter (which also measures pH and temperature). Conductivity may also be measured with a handheld meter such as the Myron-L.

Resistivity. Resistivity determines the efficiency of removal of ions from water processed in a deionizer. Water with a high resistivity will have a low conductivity due to the low amount of ions in the solution.

Hardness test. This test detects the presence of calcium and magnesium in the water.

Total dissolved solids (TDS). TDS determines the total dissolved solids in water. TDS is the sum of all the ions in a solution and verifies the effectiveness of the RO membranes. This can be checked with a handheld meter. The results are expressed in parts per million (ppm).

What microbiologic standards apply to dialyzer reuse?

This is defined in the *AAMI Recommended Practice for Reuse of Dialyzers (RD47)*. The water used in reprocessing should have a bacterial count of no more than 200 cfu/mL, or an endotoxin level of 1 ng/mL (5 endotoxin units [EU]) limulus amebocyte lysate (LAL). This also may be made stricter because of the problems with bicarbonate and with high-flux dialyzers.

What kind of water processing is best for the individual dialysis unit?

This depends on the quality of available tap water and its solute content. Feed water should be analyzed on a regular basis for chemical and bacteriologic content and should meet the EPA Drinking Water Standard. Product water—the final purified water used to prepare dialysis fluid should meet the AAMI and other applicable standards. Components of a system to meet these requirements may include the following:

- Initial sediment filter(s)
- Resin-type softener (water hardness checked twice daily)
- Activated carbon filter (two in series)
- RO unit (with continuous conductivity/resistivity monitoring of inflow and outflow water)
- DI unit (continuous conductivity monitoring of outflow, plus monthly bacteriologic, limulus test, and chemical analysis)

A complete system of this type will provide maximum purity water, approaching 18 MΩ/cm resistance. Thorough investigation is necessary to reach the desired purity of water in the most economic manner. Ongoing monitoring is essential to ensure its maintenance.

Where may information about available tap water quality be obtained?

State departments of health conduct regular and detailed analyses of public water supplies, except for Indiana and Wyoming, where the Environmental Protection Agency (EPA) has responsibility. The reports are available upon request, and often, upon request, any periodic reports will be sent to the facility. The department of health may do an analysis of a specific water supply on request. Manufacturers of water treatment equipment and supplies seek to tailor their equipment to each individual dialysis facility's needs. They may provide a detailed water analysis as part of their service.

Information on chemical content is usually given in parts per million (ppm). This is equal to milligrams per liter. To convert to mEq/L, multiply milligrams per liter times valence and divide by molecular weight. For example, for calcium:

$$60 \text{ ppm} = 60 \text{ mg/L}$$

$$\text{mEq/L Ca}^{++} = 60 \times 2 \text{ (valence)} = 120 \div 40 \text{ (molecular weight)} = 3$$

$$\text{Thus 60 ppm Ca}^{++} \text{ represents 3 mEq/L}$$

What cost factors are involved in establishing an adequate water treatment system?

Before setting a dollar figure on how much to spend, the facility should consult with a knowledgeable designer of dialysis facility water treatment systems and reliable supplier/installer. Facility needs, current and future, should be determined. Consideration should be given to each of the following factors:

- Peak volume needs
- Desired quality of product water (minimum should exceed AAMI standards)
- Expertise of the technical staff
- Cost of feed water
- Compliance with standards
- Type(s) of therapy to be delivered
- Ease of operation
- Maintenance requirements

Components listed above should be included only to achieve a particular goal, with the final objective of meeting or exceeding AAMI standards. If the source water is of very low mineral content, it may be possible to achieve 1 $M\Omega$/cm product water by RO alone, or by DI alone, after appropriate filtration. Only the minimum number of components necessary should be used to meet or exceed AAMI standards.

Preparation of bicarbonate dialysate and high-flux dialysis may necessitate more stringent microbial control than is required by current AAMI standards and the 1991 Quality Assurance Guidelines.

What are the FDA's Guidelines for Water Treatment Equipment?

According to the FDA guidelines, each premarket notification for a water purification component or system should include the information listed in Box 8-1. This helps the FDA

Box 8-1

FACTORS INCLUDED IN PREMARKET NOTIFICATION FOR WATER PURIFICATION PRODUCTS

- Device name, including both the trade or propriety name and the classification name
- Establishment registration number, if applicable, of the owner or operator submitting the premarket notification
- The generic class (class 2) in which the device has been placed under Section 513 of the Federal Food, Drug, and Cosmetic Act and the appropriate panel
- A statement of the action taken by the registered manufacturer for special controls

---

Modified from FDA guidelines, U.S. Department of Health and Human Services Food and Drug Administration, May 30, 1997.

(Continued)

Box 8-1

FACTORS INCLUDED IN PREMARKET NOTIFICATION FOR WATER PURIFICATION PRODUCTS—cont'd

- The Safe Medical Devices Act of 1990 (SMDA) requires all persons preparing a premarket notification submission to include (a) a summary of the safety and effectiveness information in the premarket information notification submission upon which an equivalence determination could be based, or (b) a statement that safety and effectiveness information will be made available to interested persons upon request
- Proposed labels, labeling, and advertisements sufficient to describe the water purification component or system, its intended use, and the directions for use (including maintenance, operation, cleaning, and troubleshooting), accompanied by a specific intended use statement and any warnings, contraindications, or limitations clearly displayed
- Statement comparing the water purification component or system to a legally marketed predicate device (one which was in commercial distribution prior to May 28, 1976, or one that has been cleared for marketing in the United States under Section 510[K] of the act)
- For a device or device labeling that has undergone a change or modification that could significantly affect the safety or effectiveness of the device, the 510(K) must include any additional supporting data to show that the manufacturer has considered the effects that the change or modification might have on the safety and effectiveness of the device
- Requirements are listed for these water purification components:
  - Reverse osmosis (RO)
  - Water softeners
  - Carbon absorption beds
  - Deionization (DI)
  - Sediment and cartridge filters
  - Ultraviolet (UV) disinfection unit
  - Ultrafilters
  - Auxiliary components
  - Water storage tanks
- Additional requirements for water purification systems applications:
  - Provide a description of the decision-making process utilized to meet the needs of the user.
  - Describe the consequences of failure for each component and the required corrective action.
  - Provide user's manuals for each component of the system, as well as guidance for the installation, start-up, and maintenance of the system.

Box 8-1

FACTORS INCLUDED IN PREMARKET NOTIFICATION FOR WATER PURIFICATION PRODUCTS—cont'd

- Label each component in the system with the name and address of the supplier.
- Provide the results of leech testing and identify the chemical composition of any material that leeches from the system.
- Certify that the water produced by each purification system will meet or exceed current standards and regulations.

---

determine whether the application has "substantial equivalence" to a water purification system already on the market. A copy of the guidelines can be obtained from the Center for Devices and Radiological Health's Division of Small Manufacturers Assistance (DSMA).

9 Dialyzer Preparation and Reprocessing

DIALYZER PREPARATION

Each dialyzer has its own specific characteristics and procedure for preparation for patient use. Manufacturers' instructions are updated frequently as alterations are made or as improved techniques are developed. It is very important to read package inserts frequently to ensure adherence to current recommendations.

What are the essential parameters when a dialyzer is prepared for patient use?

- All air in the dialyzer must be removed. Any air left in the dialyzer could be dialyzed across the membrane and into the patient's vascular system. Air trapped in the wall of the hollow fibers will reduce the dialyzer clearance by preventing diffusion between the blood and dialysate compartments. Also, air will promote clotting in the hollow fibers of a dialyzer.
- Any particulate matter left in the dialyzer from the manufacturing process must be flushed out with the saline prime.
- Dialyzers must have all disinfectant used in the reprocessing procedures removed, and be free of residual disinfectant.
- Dialyzers must always be flushed and primed with a physiologic saline solution (0.9 g NaCl/100 mL water) compatible with patient blood.

How is air removed from a dialyzer?

To remove the air from a dialyzer, prime normal saline into the dialyzer from the bottom. This is accomplished by attaching the bloodlines to the dialyzer, and then turning the dialyzer so that the venous end is up. Then run the saline in through the arterial bloodline, through the dialyzer into the venous bloodline, and into a basin. As the dialyzer is filled, the air will be forced out the top of the dialyzer. Tap the dialyzer lightly, and turn it from side to side to ensure that all of the air is removed from the header.

How much saline should be used to prime the dialyzer?

It will take from 500 to 1000 mL. The amount depends on the type of dialyzer and whether it has been reprocessed. A new dialyzer should have 1000 mL of prime to remove the glycerin and particulate matter remaining from the manufacturing process. A reprocessed dialyzer requires approximately 500 mL because the prime will be recirculated with the dialysate flowing counterclockwise to remove any residual disinfectant.

Should anything be different when priming a reprocessed dialyzer?

Yes. Reprocessed dialyzers are filled with a disinfectant, and it is important that all disinfectant be removed and no air be introduced into the dialyzer. Once air is introduced, it is very difficult to remove. All air must be removed from the arterial bloodline before attaching it to the dialyzer. This is accomplished by priming the arterial bloodline with saline, making sure all the air is removed before attaching the line to the dialyzer. After this is done, turn the dialyzer venous end up and continue the priming procedure.

Do manufacturers make any recommendations regarding the priming of their dialyzers?

Yes, all of them do. Some dialyzers should have the blood compartment filled first, and for others the dialysate compartment is filled first. Most hollow fiber dialyzers require that you "wet" the membranes first before attaching the dialysate lines. This ensures that the dialyzer fibers will not collapse when exposed to dialysate. Dialysis personnel should read and follow the instructions that come with the dialyzers used in the particular facility.

DIALYZER REPROCESSING

Cleaning and disinfecting a dialyzer to be used again for that same patient's treatment is dialyzer reprocessing or dialyzer reuse. Reuse of dialyzers is safe and cost effective. The guidelines in the Association for the Advancement of Medical Instrumentation's [AAMI] Recommended Practice for the Reuse of Hemodialyzers (RD47) must be followed because the Centers for Medicare and Medicaid Services (CMS) has adopted them as standards governing the practice. Dialyzer manufacturers are now required by the US Food and Drug Administration (FDA) to label their dialyzers so that users know that they are appropriate for reprocessing. The manufacturer must also recommend appropriate reprocessing techniques.

Bloodlines and other disposable items have been reused, but are regulated and restricted by the FDA and are rarely reused in the United States. The Department of Health and Human Services' CMS has taken an official end-stage renal disease (ESRD) program position on reuse and has published specific written requirements. Some chemicals used to reprocess dialyzers are considered hazardous and are regulated by the Occupational Safety and Health Administration (OSHA).

What are some advantages to dialyzer reuse?

There are purported clinical advantages to the reuse of dialyzers. With each dialysis treatment, the patient's blood leaves proteins on the wall of the membrane. These protein deposits create a secondary membrane that reduces the amount of exposure of the patient's blood to the artificial membrane on subsequent treatments. Bleach, however, when used in the disinfection process, will decrease this protection as it strips the protein layers from the dialyzer.

On rare occasions a patient may react to a new dialyzer. These reactions are believed to be caused by either bioincompatible membranes or ethylene oxide residue left in the sterilized dialyzer. A reaction may occur shortly after initiation of dialysis, and could be life-threatening. Once the dialyzer has been reprocessed for reuse, such reactions are not observed during subsequent treatments.

Reused dialyzers also help to contain the cost of each patient treatment, and with reuse there is a significant reduction of medical waste products and biohazardous trash.

How many times can a dialyzer be reused?

Some centers arbitrarily settle on three or five reuses per dialyzer, whereas other centers use a dialyzer until it has been determined that its effectiveness is no longer adequate to deliver the recommended dose of dialysis for the patient. Even these small numbers represent a significant savings. To determine cost effectiveness of reuse, divide the original cost of the dialyzer by the total cost of reprocessing. To qualify for reuse, a dialyzer must meet defined criteria: residual volume must be 80% or greater of original volume, it must pass a pressure-holding test, and the appearance evaluation should show no more than a few clotted fibers. After each clinical use, the dialyzer is evaluated using these criteria and must meet them to be used again for a patient.

What are the basic steps for reuse?

The basic steps in most reprocessing programs are as follows: (1) flushing the dialyzer to remove most of the blood residuals; (2) cleaning, usually done with chemicals (bleach or Renalin) and reverse ultrafiltration; (3) testing to verify that the membrane is intact and that the dialyzer will remove waste products as expected; and (4) disinfection with either a chemical or heat.

What are specific criteria used to determine if a dialyzer may be reused?

The four main criteria for reuse are as follows:
- Total cell volume (TCV) measurement is the most widely used method to determine whether a reused dialyzer maintains adequate solute removal capability. In this test, the dialyzer is filled with water, pumped dry, and the contained volume is measured in a graduated cylinder. This volume is the standard for that dialyzer and the value against which it will be compared after each use. If less than 80% of initial volume remains, the dialyzer is rejected for further patient use. A dialyzer with 80% of its initial volume still has 90% of its initial solute removal capability.
- Pressure testing of the dialyzer is performed to determine whether there are broken fibers that would lead to a blood leak during dialysis. Pressure is applied to the dialyzer and then held. If the pressure drop is too great, the dialyzer is discarded. This is sometimes referred to as leak testing.

- Some reuse machines test the dialyzer's k_{UF} (ultrafiltration coefficient). Though this is not a test to predict dialyzer clearance, it is an indication of how "open" the dialyzer membrane may be to large molecules.
- Finally, appearance or visual inspection is an important criterion. A dialyzer with larger streaks of residual blood, indicating a large number of clotted fibers, is cause for immediate rejection.

To be used again, a dialyzer must meet minimum requirements of TCV and pressure tests.

Is large solute clearance affected by reprocessing?

Yes. The extent of this effect depends on the dialyzer membrane and reprocessing technique; some membranes tend to become more open when exposed to bleach cleaning. Most membrane clearance of large solutes such as β_2-microglobulin is decreased when Renalin is used. It is very important to understand how particular dialyzers are affected by the reprocessing technique used.

How are reprocessed dialyzers disinfected?

Renalin is the most commonly used chemical disinfectant, used by about 70% of dialysis units; formaldehyde (formalin) is the second most common disinfectant used. Glutaraldehyde and heat are used by some facilities to disinfect dialyzers.

What types of labeling are required for the reprocessed dialyzer?

Meticulous care must be taken to ensure that each dialyzer is used on only one patient. The dialyzer must be labeled with the patient's name, the number of previous uses, and the date of the last reprocessing. Careful attention must be given to patients with the same or similar names. Additional means of identification, such as the use of a social security number or birthdate, is recommended as an additional check to verify the correct dialyzer is being used on the patient. Some facilities will place a warning on the dialyzer to alert the staff member to exercise extra caution when placing the patient on that dialyzer.

What exposure time is required for Renalin and formaldehyde?

Renalin, a mixture of hydrogen peroxide, peracetic acid, and acetic acid, is a sterilant and requires a 0.5% solution for an 11-hour contact time. In contrast, aqueous formaldehyde, a high-level disinfectant, kills all microorganisms, including spores and viruses, with a minimum exposure of 24 hours and a 4% concentration of formalin at room temperature. A lower concentration, 1.5% formalin, is effective at 100° F for a 24-hour exposure.

What happens if a dialyzer is not adequately disinfected?

If there is not sufficient exposure (concentration and time), bacteria in the dialyzer will not be killed and may even multiply. This could result in a patient becoming bacteremic when the blood is exposed to the dialyzer during a subsequent treatment.

What information should be verified before using a reprocessed dialyzer for a patient?

Several checks must be completed. The most important is to verify that the dialyzer is being used for the correct patient. Other requirements include ensuring that the dialyzer contained an adequate level of disinfectant before it was rinsed, and that all of the disinfectant was removed during the rinsing process. Finally, the dialyzer must pass all reuse testing such as TCV and pressure tests.

What precautions are necessary when using chemical disinfectants?

The use of protective gear—including eye shield, gloves, and a waterproof gown—is necessary. Adequate ventilation (in adherence to OSHA guidelines) is also required. Any splashes on skin or eyes should be flushed with copious amounts of water and appropriate medical care should be sought.

Note: OSHA requires that personnel be well informed about these hazardous chemicals and their potential toxicity. Every dialysis facility must have printed OSHA requirements and regulations related to the use of disinfectants. Training records of staff education and health monitoring records must be maintained. Material safety data sheets (MSDS) must be available for each chemical housed in the facility and which the employee may have the potential for exposure to. The MSDS must be accessible to staff at all times.

What precautions should be taken when working with formaldehyde?

The OSHA standard, Title 29 of the Code of Federal Regulation (CFR) Part 1910.1048, protects workers who have the potential to be exposed to formaldehyde. Formaldehyde is a suspected carcinogen associated with nasal and lung cancer. Airborne concentrations as little as 0.1 parts per million (ppm) may cause irritation to the nose, eyes, and throat. Allergic reactions may occur with exposure causing wheezing, cough, or asthmalike symptoms.

Air quality monitoring and patient education are used to protect staff from potential dangerous exposure. OSHA has set permissible exposure limits (PELs) at 0.75 ppm measured as an 8-hour time-weighted average (TWA). The OSHA standard for short-term exposure limit (STEL) is 2 ppm during a 15-minute period. The action level is 0.5 ppm for an 8-hour TWA. OSHA mandates that all staff be educated on the hazards of and how to work safely with formaldehyde on an annual basis. An emergency shower and eyewash station must also be available to the staff in the event of an exposure. Mandatory respiratory training must also be done on reuse personnel as well as fit testing for a respirator.

Are these chemicals stable over time?

No. Renalin is broken down fairly rapidly by temperature greater than 80° F, exposure to light, and exposure to organic matter (such as blood). Time is another factor: once diluted, Renalin has a relatively short shelf life. It is very important to test each dialyzer for Renalin potency just prior to preparing it for patient use. Formaldehyde is quite stable for long periods.

How should the dialyzer be prepared before the next run?

After the dialyzer is filled with disinfectant at the end of the reprocessing procedure, it is necessary to document the presence of the disinfectant by an appropriate chemical test. This helps to confirm that the dialyzer is stored with the disinfecting chemical. Before the next clinical use, the disinfectant must be removed. The bloodlines are connected to the dialyzer, and sterile saline is rinsed through the blood side of the dialyzer. Usually 250 to 500 mL of saline is run through the dialyzer and discarded. The arterial and venous bloodlines are then connected to establish a closed loop. The blood pump is started, and the recirculation of saline, with ultrafiltration, should remove any residual chemical left in the system. Essentially, the disinfectant is simply dialyzed out of the system.

Just before use, the recirculating saline in the dialyzer is sampled using the test appropriate for the disinfectant used. After the test is performed, the absence of the disinfectant must be documented. Only after a negative test has been confirmed is the dialyzer considered safe for patient use. Many dialysis units and some state agencies require two people to verify that the dialyzer is correct for a specific patient and has a negative disinfectant test before using the reprocessed dialyzer.

When Renalin is the disinfectant used, is there a specific order in which the compartments are primed?

Yes. Renalin is a strong acid, so it is important to prime the blood compartment with normal saline before attaching the dialysate lines. If the dialysate compartment is primed first, reaction between the dialysate and Renalin will cause some of the CO_2 to come out of solution as a gas. These bubbles can be trapped in the fibers, creating an air gap between the blood and dialysate, with poor diffusion.

Are there circumstances in which reuse is inappropriate for a particular patient?

Yes, patients with systemic infections or with sepsis are generally excluded from reprocessing programs. Patients with hepatitis B cannot participate in reuse programs.

Are patients required to give their consent for reuse of dialyzers?

Yes, CMS requires that patients give consent in writing. The consent must be made part of the patient's clinical record. If the patient does not give this written consent, reuse is not permitted.

10 Access to the Bloodstream

HISTORICAL BACKGROUND

Effective hemodialysis became a reality in the 1940s. Each treatment required a surgical cutdown. Hollow tubes (cannulas) of glass or metal were inserted into an artery and a vein. The glass and metal tubes were later replaced with cannulas of polyvinyl chloride or other plastic materials. During the 1950s, attempts were made to leave the cannulas in place for more than one treatment. Different methods of maintaining patency were tried. These attempts, at best, lasted only a few treatments.

In 1960, Scribner, Quinton, and Dillard at the University of Washington, devised a cannula that could be left in place much longer. It consisted of Teflon tubes, one placed in an artery, and one in a vein. These tubes were connected externally, allowing for continuous rapid flow of blood through the device. This technique was improved in 1962 with the use of Silastic (silicone rubber) for the external shunt loop, and Teflon for the vessel tips. This allowed for greater flexibility of the tubing and increased comfort for the patient. This innovation was not only effective for a single hemodialysis but also offered a method for repeat treatments.

Another major development came in 1966 when Cimino, Brescia, and co-workers developed the forearm internal arteriovenous fistula. This was created by performing a surgical anastomosis between a forearm artery and vein. The subsequent flow of arterial blood into the vein permitted percutaneous puncture of this vessel that offered adequate flow for hemodialysis.

Use of internal synthetic graft materials began in 1974. Today the most common type of synthetic graft is polytetrafluroethylene (PTFE). A "button" needle-free form of vascular access was developed in 1980. The button needle-free worked, but not as well as the other internal synthetic graft material. These new synthetic grafts and devices offered new possibilities for patients who did not have adequate vessels for a Cimino fistula.

Shaldon described temporary access for hemodialysis via cannulation of the femoral vein in 1961. Uldall, in 1979, devised a special catheter for temporary access in the subclavian or internal jugular vein. When the dual lumen catheters were introduced, this further enhanced a means of temporary access, by allowing one catheter to function as both the inlet and outlet ports.

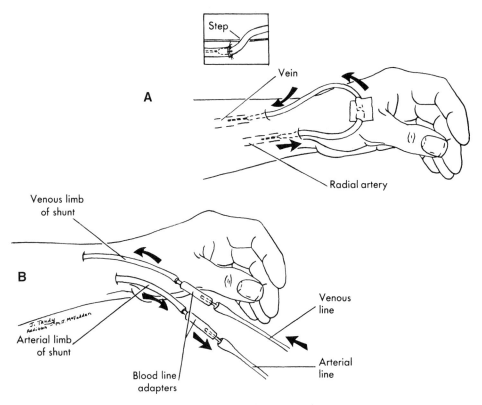

Fig. 10-1 A, Quinton-Scribner shunt with connector in place between dialysis runs. **B,** Shunt arms separated and connected to dialyzer bloodlines. *(From Larson E, Lindbloom I, Davis KB:* Development of the Clinical Nephrology Practitioner, *St Louis, 1982, Mosby.)*

Vascular access, as used for hemodialysis in the early 1960s, has evolved considerably during the past 30 years or more. However, maintaining patent access with adequate blood flow remains one of the major problems in the chronically hemodialyzed patient (Fig. 10-1).

INTERNAL ACCESSES

The National Kidney Foundation (NKF) has established guidelines for the selection of a permanent vascular access for chronic hemodialysis. Current guidelines recommend that 40% of all patients should have a native arteriovenous fistula as their permanent chronic access and that less than 10% of all patients have a central venous catheter as a permanent access. The order of preference for a vascular access for patients undergoing chronic hemodialysis is: a wrist (radial-cephalic) (Fig. 10-2, *A*) primary arteriovenous fistula, an elbow (brachiocephalic) primary arteriovenous fistula, an arteriovenous graft of synthetic material (Fig. 10-2, *B*) or a transposed brachiobasilic vein fistula, and lastly,

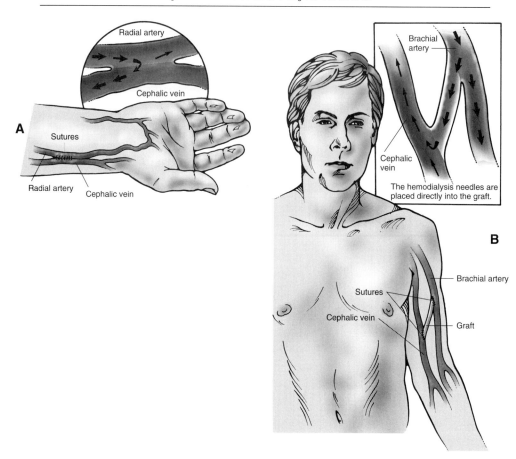

Fig. 10-2 Options for long-term vascular access for hemodialysis.
A, A surgically created venous fistula. The increased pressure from the artery forces blood into the vein. This process causes the vein to dilate enough for fistula needles to be placed for hemodialysis. When the vein dilates in this matter, the fistula is said to be "developed." **B,** A surgically placed straight vascular graft in the upper arm. The graft creates a shunt between arterial and venous blood. *(From Ignatavicius DD, Workman ML,* Medical-Surgical Nursing: Critical Thinking for Collaborative Care, *ed 4, St Louis, 2002, Saunders.)*

a cuffed tunneled central venous catheter, which should be discouraged as a permanent vascular access (NKF-Kidney Dialysis Outcomes Quality Initiative [K/DOQI] Vascular Access Clinical Practice Guidelines Update, 2000).

The time of vascular access placement should be well before the need for dialysis treatment. The 2002 National Kidney Foundation K/DOQI Clinical Practice Guidelines for chronic kidney disease recommend initiation of a vascular access when the glomerular filtration rate (GFR) is less than 30 mL/min/1.73 m^2.

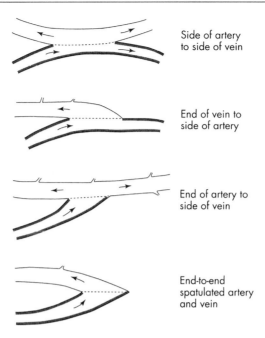

Side of artery
to side of vein

End of vein to
side of artery

End of artery to
side of vein

End-to-end
spatulated artery
and vein

Fig. 10-3 Four different anastomoses commonly constructed between the radial artery and cephalic vein. *(From Wilson SE:* Vascular Access: Principles and Practice, *ed 4, St Louis, 2002, Mosby.)*

ARTERIOVENOUS FISTULAS
What is an arteriovenous fistula?

An arteriovenous (AV) fistula is an internal access surgically created by a vascular surgeon using the patient's own blood vessels. In an internal AV fistula, a small (5 mm) opening is created surgically in an adjoining artery and vein, and the two vessels are joined at this opening, creating an AV fistula. The two blood vessels utilized are anastomosed in a side-to-side, end-to-side, or end-to-end connection (Fig. 10-3). The diversion of arterial blood into the vein causes the vein to become enlarged, distended, and prominent, allowing placement of large-gauge needles for the dialysis treatment.

Eventually the access will be able to deliver a blood flow of 300 to 500 mL/min. Maturation occurs when there is dilation and thickening of the venous segment of the fistula. This is due to the increase in blood flow and pressure of arterial blood. The vein used to create the AV access will sometimes develop additional branches, which will also enlarge and mature enough to be cannulated for dialysis. This is called collateral circulation and increases the available surface area for cannulation. However, if the collateral circulation prevents the development of the main vein, ligation would be necessary.

The AV fistula can be placed in either the upper or lower arm. The radial artery and cephalic vein (lower arm) (Fig. 10-4) and brachial artery and cephalic vein (upper arm) are commonly used. Proper evaluation of the patient's vasculature and physical

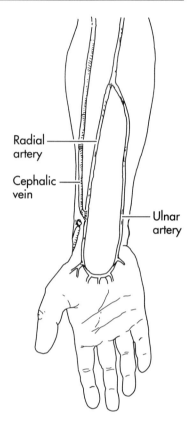

Fig. 10-4 Mid-forearm radiocephalic fistula is used if the distal radial artery is not suitable. *(From Wilson SE: Vascular Access: Principles and Practice, ed 4, St Louis, 2002, Mosby.)*

assessment play a role in determining the access of choice for that patient. A major cause of early AV fistula failure is the selection of suboptimal vessels. Venography allows for identification of appropriate veins and helps to rule out sites that are not suitable for use. Doppler flow studies may also be used if venography is not available.

Every attempt is made to use the patient's nondominant arm in order to help them to maintain their present standard of living and also to facilitate self-cannulation if they perform their own dialysis care. The patient must have sufficient arterial blood flow to maintain the access and to provide an adequate dialysis treatment. The AV fistula may take up to 4 months or longer to mature enough to allow for cannulation.

What is Basilic Vein Transposition?

Basilic vein transposition is a new technique used to create a vascular access in patients with inadequate vessels in the wrist. This transposed vessel technique involves dissecting the basilic vein and transposing it anteriorly and subcutaneously while anastomosing it to the brachial artery (Fig. 10-5). This transposed vessel provides a large surface area for cannulation and requires only one anastomosis. The incision for this access is rather large with the start of the incision being at the midantecubital

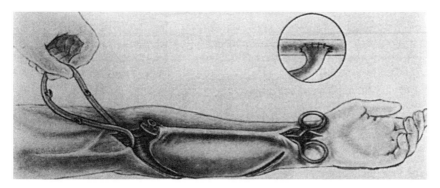

Fig. 10-5 Radial-basilic fistula in the forearm, with transposition of the vein to the anterolateral aspect. *(From Patrick W, May J: Basilic Vein Transposition,* Am J Surg *143:254, 1982.)*

fossa and extending to the medial aspect of the arm to the axilla. The main advantage to this type of access placement is the avoidance of using a synthetic graft. As with other autologous grafts, you will see a longer patency rate and fewer risks of infection.

What is an AV graft?

When a patient is not a candidate for a native AV fistula, a vascular graft is substituted. An AV graft can be of biologic or synthetic material; however, synthetic grafts are utilized most frequently. The graft material is implanted subcutaneously into either the forearm or upper arm. In some circumstances when the arm cannot be utilized, the chest or leg area may be used. The graft bridges an artery on one end and a vein on the other end. Blood flow direction is from the artery into the vein. With the AV graft, the needles for cannulation are placed directly into the graft material.

The synthetic graft is used most often in patients who do not have adequate vessels to create an internal AV fistula. The graft may be placed in several configurations: straight, looped, or curved. NKF-K/DOQI guidelines recommend the use of PTFE over biologic or other synthetic materials. The AV graft may be used as early as 2 to 6 weeks after placement, with the surgeon's approval. The tissue surrounding the graft will grow into and around the graft, helping to stabilize this vessel.

Why do you need to know the direction of blood flow in the arteriovenous graft?

The direction of blood flow in the access is necessary to know in order to properly place the needles for the hemodialysis treatment. The venous needle should always be placed in the direction of the blood flow (artery to vein). Placing the venous needle against the flow of blood will cause increased resistance to the blood returning to the patient. This will be signified by a high venous pressure reading on the machine.

How do you determine the flow of blood in a looped configuration AV graft?

In a looped or horseshoe AV graft, after gently depressing the graft at midpoint, you can listen for a bruit or feel for a thrill on each side of the graft. Because you have occluded the flow of blood at midpoint, you will still be able to fill a thrill or hear a bruit on the side where the blood is entering the access (arterial side). The side of the graft with little or no thrill or bruit would be the venous side. Other techniques used to determine the flow of blood is to palpate the graft at midpoint once the needles are placed. The arterial needle will continue to have a flashback of blood when the graft is compressed midpoint.

What types of grafts are available?

Synthetic grafts are the most common grafts currently in use. Many synthetic materials (Dacron, PTFE) are available in various diameters and lengths. A newer form of PTFE allows for needle insertion immediately after placement, although the manufacturer recommends waiting 5 to 7 days. Fig. 10-6 shows two types of placement for synthetic grafts.

What are the advantages of an AV graft?

AV graft can be used sooner than AV fistulas, usually after 2 weeks. Maturation time for the vessel to enlarge is not required. The larger vessel size allows for easier cannulation. Table 10-1 lists the advantages and disadvantages of internal accesses.

What are the special care needs and potential problems with use of the AV fistula for access to the bloodstream?

Needle insertions are necessary for each hemodialysis. With repetitive venipunctures, scar tissue forms over the fistula, making insertion of needles more difficult and painful. Furthermore, if a needle becomes accidentally dislodged and passes through a vessel wall (infiltration), bleeding into the tissues may result in formation of a painful hematoma. Use of the fistula may be difficult or impossible until swelling decreases. At the end of each hemodialysis treatment, after the needles are withdrawn, firm pressure must be applied over the puncture area for 10 to 20 minutes to prevent persistent bleeding.

Are there special problems with an internal AV fistula?

Size and location of arterialized veins are important. It is often a matter of weeks, and sometimes months, before the veins become sufficient in size that large-gauge needles may be inserted without difficulty. In women, this process takes longer than in men. The veins of the forearm vary in their pattern and distribution. The location of easily accessible vessels may be limited, so that a few sites must be repeatedly used for insertion.

Occasionally, the desired blood flow is difficult to obtain through the inlet needle. This problem may result from the size of the vein or from branches that divert the flow.

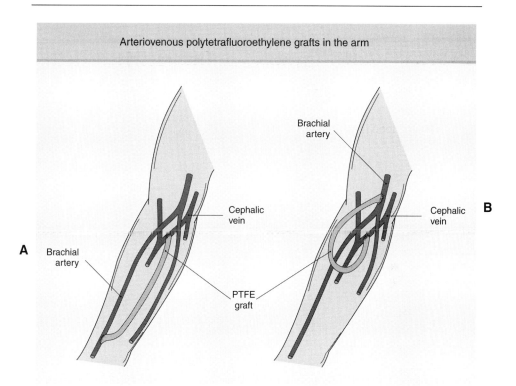

Arteriovenous polytetrafluoroethylene grafts in the arm

Fig. 10-6 Polytetrafluoroethylene (PTFE) grafts in the arm. **A,** Straight forearm PTFE graft. **B,** PTFE loop graft. *(From Johnson RJ, Feehally J: Comprehensive Clinical Nephrology, ed 2, St Louis, 2003, Mosby.)*

Occasionally the needle must be placed very near the anastomosis to obtain sufficient flow (the needle tip should never be closer than 3 cm from the anastomosis). Sometimes with side-to-side AV fistulas, most of the dilation of the veins occurs over the back of the hand, and the arm veins do not become prominent. Surgical revision may be required to correct the flow of the blood.

A third problem is spasm of the vessel, which is common. This usually occurs at the beginning of hemodialysis, causing decreased arterial blood flow. Spasms occur when attempting to maintain high blood flows in an immature fistula. The lumen of the needle sucking against the vessel wall can cause spasms. This is painful and is accompanied by a fluttering sensation at the needle. The use of back-eye needles may help.

On the return-flow side, resistance may be high secondary to venous stenosis in the outflow vessel above the anastomosis. Other mechanical causes of return flow resistance include position of the extremity and placement of the needle against the vessel wall. Repositioning of the needle may be necessary.

A fourth problem is accidental tearing of the vessel during venipuncture. This may result in formation of a large hematoma, making the vessel difficult or impossible to use

Table 10-1	Advantages and Disadvantages of Internal Accesses	
	Arteriovenous fistula	**Arteriovenous graft**
Advantages	Excellent patency rate	Large surface area for
	Can last for decades	cannulation
	Highest blood flow rates	Ability to span large areas of
	Lowest rate of complications	the body
	(infection, steal syndrome,	Easy to cannulate
	stenosis)	Little time required for
	Improved performance over	maturation
	time as access develops	Variety of shapes and
	Development of collateral	configurations
	circulation, which creates	Ease of surgical implantation
	additional branches for	
	cannulation	
Disadvantages	Failure of vein to enlarge	Higher rates of infection
	More difficult to cannulate	May reject graft material
	than graft	Higher rates of thrombosis
	Cosmetically unattractive	Stenosis at venous anastomosis
	Must find healthy veins that	from intimal hyperplasia
	are in proximity and not	No development of collateral
	too tortuous	circulation
	Requires time to mature	
	before use	

for many days. The same type of accident may occur if the patient suddenly moves or thrashes about during dialysis.

In addition, the "radial artery steal" syndrome may develop. A few patients develop ischemic changes of the fingers. This is manifested by coldness, poor function, and even gangrene and necrosis of tips of the fingers. The "steal" is caused by low arterial pressure at the fistula site, resulting from diversion of radial artery blood to the vein. Because the radial artery distal to the fistula normally connects with the ulnar artery, the pressure gradient causes ulnar blood to be diverted from the arteries to the fingers and flows instead toward the fistula. Hypoperfusion of the palm and fingers results causing pain and coldness, which worsens during the dialysis treatment. If recognized early, the syndrome may be corrected by surgically tying off the radial artery distal to the fistula.

Infections, thromboses, and aneurysms are three additional potential AV fistula problems. Infection of the fistula can occur secondary to poor personal hygiene or poor aseptic technique during cannulation. This local infection can lead to thrombosis or sepsis if not treated. Signs and symptoms include redness and swelling of the access and/or pain and fever. Diagnosis is confirmed by culturing the drainage and/or doing blood cultures. Antibiotic therapy is employed.

Thrombosis is the most common complication of AV fistulas. In addition to infection, it can be caused by hypotension or stenosis of the fistula. Thrombosis can also be secondary to compression of blood flow, either by the use of tight bandages or a fistula-needle-holding device, by the patient sleeping on the fistula arm, or from hematoma formation. The simultaneous use of two fistula-needle-holding devices is discouraged. The bruit should always be auscultated after placing a fistula-needle-holding device or clamp on a patient's access.

Finally, aneurysms (outpouchings of the vessel wall) can occur from repeated cannulation of the same site and from infection. Large aneurysms limit available cannulation sites.

How does one assess the internal access before needle insertion?

Assessment involves several steps:

- A thorough assessment is key to skillful cannulation and will help to increase the longevity of the access as well as minimize other complications. A complete assessment of the access must be done before cleaning the site or actual cannulation.
- Visibly observe the access, noting any signs of infection. Look for signs of redness or inflammation. The access extremity should have a normal skin temperature and not be too hot or too cold. The skin should be of a normal temperature for the patient. A hot feeling may indicate an infection and, an access, which is noticeably cool, might be thrombosed. Observe previous needle insertion sites for proper healing and scab formation. Make note of any open areas or drainage. The nurse should be informed of any unusual findings. A culture of drainage may be indicated, and the nurse must make the determination whether the access may be cannulated.
- The skin should not be discolored or bruised and the patient should not complain of any pain or numbness in the access or extremity. Swelling may be seen in the access, which has recently been placed. Some patients have poor venous drainage in the access limb, causing swelling. Finally, swelling may be present because of a previous needle infiltration. Elevation of the affected limb is helpful to increase the venous return and decrease the swelling. Swelling should be monitored from treatment to treatment for improvements or worsening conditions. The circumference of the arm may be measured with a tape measure and compared for any increases or improvements. The registered nurse should be informed of any unusual findings before cannulation of the patient is attempted.
- Check for circulation or patency. Palpate the internal access for a "thrill," which should be felt over the entire length and resembles a gentle vibration. A thrill is indicative of adequate blood flow throughout the vessel of 450 mL or greater. A pulse will indicate less than adequate blood flow through the access. Listen with the bell of a stethoscope for a bruit or a swooshing sound. This should be clearly

audible over the entire length of the access. The bruit should be heard with greater intensity over the anastomosis. Intensification in the normal sound of the bruit may indicate a stenotic area in the access. The absence of a bruit or thrill indicates the access is clotted or no longer patent. A clotted access should never be cannulated. The patient should be taught to assess the access daily by palpating for a thrill.

What is the proper aseptic preparation for cannulation of a graft?

An antiseptic solution, such as povidone-iodine, should be used to cleanse the skin over and around the fistula. Apply the antiseptic in a circular motion away from the puncture site until a circle of 2 inches in diameter has been covered. Be sure to follow the antiseptic manufacturer's directions for effective disinfection. The povidone-iodine must be allowed to dry on the epidermis before needle insertion. If the patient is allergic to povidone-iodine, isopropyl alcohol may be used, but needle insertion must be performed before the alcohol dries.

What types of needles are used for puncturing the AV fistula?

Large-gauge, thin-wall, back-eye needles are preferred. The larger gauge needle is used for the high blood flows necessary for high-flux or high-efficiency dialysis. Blood flows of 400 to 500 mL/min may be attained with 14-gauge needles. Smaller, 17-gauge needles are used with children or infants to accommodate their small vessel size and decreased blood flow rate requirements. It is generally recommended practice to use at least a 15-gauge needle with blood flow rates of 350 mL/min or greater. Dialyzing a patient at a high blood flow rate with a small-gauge needle may cause hemolysis of the red blood cells as the cells are passed through a small needle opening with such shear force.

Are there particular points to be observed in placing the needles?

The flow of blood through the access determines needle placement because the venous needle must always be placed in the direction of blood flow. Blood flow is sometimes identified as antegrade and retrograde with the former meaning in the direction of blood flow and the latter, against the flow of blood. The arterial needle should be placed nearest the anastomosis but at least 3 cm away from the site. A thorough assessment must be done to ensure that the needle is placed at least this far away from the anastomotic connection to avoid cannulating this site. The arterial needle may point toward the hand or the heart, or either antegrade or retrograde. The venous needle should be located so that the point is at least 5 cm proximal to the arterial needle. It should always be directed toward the heart or in the direction of blood flow (antegrade).

The AV fistula and AV graft are cannulated at different angles. Angle of entry depends on the depth of the access: the deeper the access, the steeper the angle required. Angle of insertion ranges from 20 to 45 degrees.

Cannulation of a new AV fistula must be approached with extreme care. The vessel is very fragile in its early stages and prone to infiltrations. Preferably, only the most seasoned employees will initially access the fistula. Many facilities have adopted cannulation protocols in which the AV fistula is initially only cannulated with one needle (arterial outflow) and the venous return is through the central venous catheter for the first few treatments. Smaller-gauge needles are also used for the first few treatments as well as lower blood flow rates. The temporary catheter is usually removed when cannulation with two needles has been successfully performed over consecutive treatments.

Why is this positioning of the needles important?

The manner in which needles are placed will affect the long-term patency rate of the access. Care must be taken to avoid placing the needles in the same general area each treatment. Over time, this will cause the wall of the vessels to thin and aneurysms will develop. Aneurysms are weakened areas of the vessel, which actually dilate, enlarge, and balloon out. These areas are generally avoided as sites for cannulation. Needle sites should be rotated each treatment and it is best to utilize the entire length of the access to get maximum surface area and development.

Placing the arterial needle near the anastomosis will achieve the best blood flow. The tip should not be closer than 3 cm from the anastomosis. Placement of the needle toward or away from the anastomosis depends on the optimal blood flow. Usual practice is to place the arterial needle point with the flow. Finally, spacing the needles at least 5 cm apart minimizes recirculation of blood that may result in an inadequate dialysis.

What conditions favor recirculation?

A fistula with a low blood flow rate leads to recirculation. The low flow can be caused by stenosis at the arterial end, or more commonly, by stenosis at the venous end. It is usually associated with an increase in venous pressure and, if the recirculation is sufficiently great, may result in the "black blood" syndrome.

What is the "black blood" syndrome?

When recirculation is severe, the blood becomes acidotic, and the red cells cannot carry oxygen. The pH of this blood is usually below 7, and the blood appears very dark.

How is occurrence of recirculation determined?

The concentration of any substance (urea or creatinine) should be the same in the arterial bloodline going into the dialyzer as in the patient's systemic circulation. If the arterial concentration is less, the substance may be diluted by venous blood returning from the dialyzer so that some blood is going through the dialyzer more than once without returning to the systemic circulation. To calculate the percentage recirculation, three blood samples are obtained simultaneously. One represents the systemic circulation (peripheral blood, or P). Also necessary is a specimen from the inflow line just before it enters the dialyzer (arterial blood, or A), and the outflow line just after it leaves the dialyzer (venous blood, or V). Calculate the estimated recirculation as follows:

$$\text{Percent recirculation} \ = \ \frac{P - A}{P - V}$$

Example: P = 100, A = 90, V = 25

$$
\begin{aligned}
\text{Percent recirculation} \ &= \ \frac{100 - 90}{100 - 25} &&= \ \frac{10}{75} \\
& \ 10 \div 75 &&= \ 0.13 \\
& \ 0.13 \times 100\% &&= \ 13\%
\end{aligned}
$$

Given a good fistula and use of two well-placed needles, the percentage of recirculation should be less than 10%. With double-lumen catheters, recirculation commonly may be as high as 15%. Recirculation greater than 15% is excessive and should be investigated and corrected.

How is the peripheral (P) blood sample obtained?

Peripheral veins are no longer used. The peripheral sample is obtained from the inflow line before the dialyzer, using the slow/stop flow technique for measuring access recirculation (see Box 10-1).

What other techniques are available to measure access recirculation?

Newer techniques allowing for real-time measurement of access recirculation include the HD01 hemodialysis monitoring system (Transonic Systems, Ithaca, New York) and the Crit-Line instrument (In-Line Diagnostics Corporation, Farmington, Utah).

How do these devices measure recirculation?

The Transonic Systems device uses flow dilution sensors placed on the arterial and venous bloodlines. Saline is injected through the venous drip chamber or a port in the venous

---

Box 10-1

REVISED SLOW/STOP FLOW TECHNIQUE FOR MEASURING ACCESS RECIRCULATION

1. Perform test after approximately 30 minutes; turn off ultrafiltration (UF) device
2. Draw arterial (A) and venous (V) line samples
3. Immediately reduce blood flow rate (BFR) to 120 mL/min
4. Turn blood pump off 10 seconds after reducing BFR
5. Clamp arterial line above sampling port
6. Draw systemic or peripheral blood sample from arterial line port
7. Unclamp line and resume dialysis

From Sherman R, et al: Recognition of the failing vascular access: a current perspective, *Sem Dial* 10(1):1-4, 1997.

tubing. A laptop computer preloaded with dilution measurement software measures the volume flow through the bloodlines and the changes in the ultrasound signal velocity and calculates the percentage of recirculation. The Transonic Systems device also measures cardiac output.

The In-Line Diagnostics device uses a disposable blood chamber placed between the end of the arterial blood tubing and the arterial port of the dialyzer. An optical sensor is placed on the blood chamber and is attached to the In-Line Diagnostics device. The In-Line Diagnostics device calculates the percentage of recirculation based on changes in hematocrit following microinfusions of saline. This instrument also measures hematocrit, oxygen saturation, and blood volume change (Fig. 10-7, *A* and *B*). (See Chapter 11 for a discussion of the Crit-Line instrument.)

May the venous needle be placed in another extremity?

Occasion may arise when two needles cannot be placed in the fistula extremity (usually because of hematoma formation or infiltration upon needle insertion). Often a vein in the opposite extremity can be found that will accommodate the outflow from the machine.

Does the patient require an anesthetic before needle placement?

Some patients experience discomfort with needle insertion, particularly patients with newer or never used accesses. An anesthetic such as lidocaine 1% (Xylocaine) may be used intradermally. The lidocaine is administered at a 15-degree angle just under the top tissue of the skin. You must always aspirate before giving lidocaine to make sure that you are not in a blood vessel. If you do withdraw blood with aspiration, you must discard that syringe and begin again. With repeated cannulations, scar tissue develops and the patient experiences less pain with cannulation. EMLA cream, a topical anesthetic, is another option for patients who require some type of anesthetic before needle insertion. The patient applies this cream before arriving for treatment. The cream must be removed before the patient is cannulated.

Can anything be done to cause the veins of an arm with an AV fistula to enlarge more quickly?

Nothing should be attempted for 4 or 5 days after the fistula is created. A tourniquet or blood pressure cuff may be placed around the upper arm, snug enough to cause distention of the veins; it may be left in place for a half hour and may be repeated several times each day. Hand exercises, such as squeezing a rubber ball while the tourniquet is in place, may help. Warm compresses or soaks several times a day may speed up the venous distention.

What care is required for the fistula arm between dialyses?

An arm with a new fistula should be elevated on a pillow between treatments to decrease swelling in the extremity. It is important to maintain adequate pressure, either by hand or with a light pressure dressing, over the puncture sites for 10 to 20 minutes after the

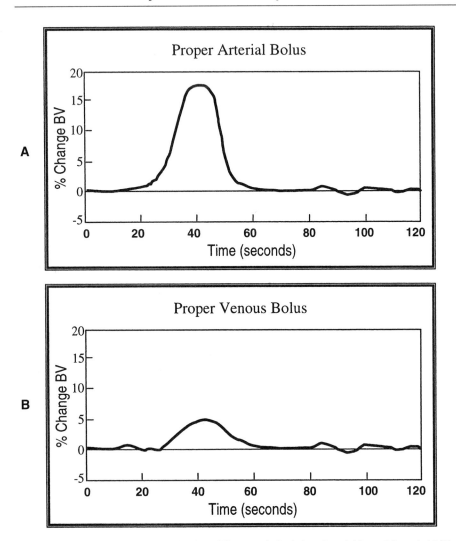

Fig. 10-7 A, Proper arterial bolus. The peak height should be at least 15%.
B, Proper venous bolus. The screen now displays a smaller bolus. If
recirculation occurs, Crit-Line will calculate the area under the curve.
*(Crit-Line manufactured by In-Line Diagnostics Corporation, Farmington,
Utah.)*

needles are removed. Most patients still have some heparin effect at the end of dialysis,
and bleeding can be a serious problem. Even oozing under the skin can cause hematoma
and scar formation, which eventually makes the vessel difficult to use. After the bleeding
has stopped, bandages are sufficient to protect the puncture sites. If bleeding continues from the puncture site more than 20 minutes after removal of needles, the heparin
dose should be evaluated and readjusted. Activated clotting times should be monitored

during dialysis to ascertain optimal heparin requirements for each patient. Daily cleaning with soap is advised. Some people like to use an ointment to keep the skin soft.

What is the LifeSite Hemodialysis Access System?

The LifeSite system is an implanted device used as a central venous blood access for hemodialysis. The LifeSite system consists of a round metal valve approximately 1.2 inches in diameter, a height of 0.5 inch, and a 25-inch cannula line (Fig. 10-8). The valve is implanted subcutaneously and the cannula is placed in a vein, the subclavian or jugular, which is tunneled to the LifeSite valve. The LifeSite system is made up of a mixture of titanium alloy, stainless steel, and silicone clastomers. Two LifeSite systems are implanted in the patient for both the draw and return of blood. A special 14-gauge needle is inserted through the skin into the LifeSite valve. An internal pinch clamp is opened with needle insertion, allowing the flow of blood. Removing the needle once again engages the pinch clamp, preventing the flow of blood. Repeated cannulations into the valve create a tract or buttonhole between the skin and the valve entrance. The buttonhole remains closed after needle removal by tissue interstitial pressure. An antimicrobial solution is irrigated into the pocket valve in between treatments with a 25-gauge, 1-inch needle that does not open the pinch clamp, and prevents the solution from becoming systemic. Not all patients are candidates for a LifeSite Access system. Contraindications include (1) recent infection associated with positive blood cultures, (2) a systemic or localized infection unresponsive to antibiotic therapy, (3) lack of adequate tissue to support the valve, and (4) known or suspected allergy to the device materials. The LifeSite system may be used as a temporary or long-term vascular access and only Vasca-approved needles are used to access the device. Complications may include the following: inadequate blood flow, bleeding/hematoma at injection site, difficulty with cannulation, thrombosis, site infections, valve pocket/cannula tunnel infections, bacteremia/septicemia. Dialysis staff are specially trained by nurse

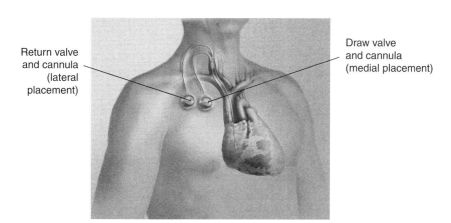

Fig. 10-8 The LifeSite system (Vasca, Inc.). Two implanted subcutaneous ports. *(Courtesy LifeSite/Vasca.)*

specialists to work with this type of access (LifeSite Hemodialysis Access System, Instructions for Implantation and Use for the LifeSite Hemodialysis Access System).

What is the buttonhole method of accessing the vascular access?

The buttonhole technique (constant-site technique) used to cannulate AV fistulas has been used on a limited basis for approximately 25 years. In the buttonhole technique of cannulation, the access is cannulated in exactly the same spot and angle of insertion, from treatment to treatment. A tunnel tract of scar tissue eventually develops, which then allows the needle to be easily inserted into the same channel with each cannulation. This type of cannulation is associated with less pain and fewer incidents of infiltrations. This method is a useful alternative for the patient who self-cannulates or the patient dialyzing at home. Medisystems offers a buttonhole needle set with antistick dull bevels. This blunt needle can be used once the buttonhole develops. The antistick dull bevel prevents cutting of the tissue surrounding the scar tissue tunnel track.

SINGLE-NEEDLE TECHNIQUE

Kopp developed the single-needle device in 1970 for use with the internal AV fistula and the single-lumen catheter. Single-needle dialysis has not been practiced in the United States for several years; however, it is popular in Europe.

What is the principle of operation of single-needle dialysis?

A Y-type hub is connected to a single needle or catheter. As blood is drawn into the dialyzer, a clamp simultaneously occludes the outflow line. Then the inflow line is occluded while the outflow is released to return blood from the dialyzer to the patient. In Europe, two blood pumps are used, one for the arterial bloodline and one for the venous bloodline. High-flux dialysis, with its need for high blood flow rates, and the popularity of dual-lumen catheters has minimized the use of single-needle devices outside of Europe.

Temporary Vascular Access

Dialysis catheters are used in the management of the hemodialysis patient in certain situations: (1) as an access for acute dialysis, (2) in the patient who is imminently awaiting a kidney transplant, (3) when allowing for maturation of the AV access, (4) as a permanent access when the availability of vessels is limited for a permanent internal access, (5) patients undergoing plasmapheresis, (6) patients receiving venovenous continuous renal replacement therapy, and (7) patients on peritoneal dialysis requiring temporary hemodialysis because of peritonitis. It should be noted that prolonged use of subclavian vein catheters would result in subclavian vein stenosis.

The NKF-K/DOQI guidelines suggest that only 10% of chronic maintenance hemodialysis patients should have catheters as their permanent vascular access. The use of central venous catheters as a permanent access for hemodialysis is not the best choice, but is an alternative in access selection.

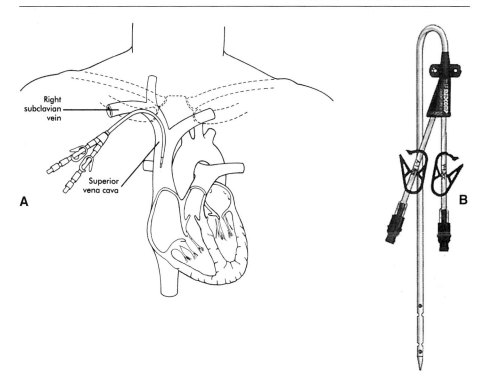

Fig. 10-9 A, Temporary vascular access using subclavian dual-lumen venous catheter. **B,** Dual-lumen temporary catheter. *(Courtesy MEDCOMP Corp., Harleysville, Pa.)*

Which veins are used for temporary access?

The subclavian, internal jugular, and femoral veins are used (Fig. 10-9, *A*). Vessels are accessed using double-lumen catheters (Fig. 10-9, *B*).

What are the contraindications for using subclavian or jugular catheters?

Subclavian or jugular catheters should not be used on the following patients:
- Patients with acute respiratory distress who cannot be positioned either supine or in the Trendelenburg position
- Patients with known subclavian vein stenosis

How is the subclavian or jugular catheter placed?

The physician uses strict aseptic technique. The patient lies supine in the Trendelenburg position with the head turned to the opposite side. The skin around the area is cleaned and covered with sterile drapes. With local anesthesia, the catheter is inserted and sutured into place. Verification of correct placement by chest x-ray examination is required before the catheter may be used.

What complications can occur?

Immediately after the insertion, pneumothorax, hemothorax, or air embolism may occur. Bleeding is another complication if the artery is inadvertently punctured during insertion.

What are indications for using a femoral catheter?

A femoral catheter is used in the following types of cases:
- The acutely ill patient confined to bed
- The end-stage renal disease (ESRD) patient whose access is clotted, but who requires urgent dialysis
- Continuous renal replacement therapy
- Patients who may have subclavian vein stenosis

What complications can occur?

- Retroperitoneal hemorrhage from puncture of the vein during insertion
- Bleeding at the insertion site

Is special nursing management necessary with these catheters?

Aseptic technique when initiating and when terminating dialysis is of utmost importance. All catheters are prone to infection. The caps and ports should be wrapped in a 4 × 4 dressing soaked in an approved disinfectant before initiating or ending dialysis. It is of the utmost importance that the caregiver is aware of the type of catheter the patient has placed in order to be able to provide the appropriate site care. The manufacturer's recommendations for disinfectant must be followed to maintain the integrity of the catheter. The exit site should be cleaned with the facility recommended disinfectant after every treatment, and a sterile dressing should be applied. The appearance of the exit site, especially if there is redness or drainage, must be documented.

Heparin is instilled into the port(s) of the catheter following dialysis. This heparin must be removed before the next dialysis to avoid the patient's receiving a bolus. Do not attempt to instill saline into a clotted catheter; this might force the clot into the vascular system.

What technical problems can occur with these catheters, and how are they best combated?

The main problem, poor blood flow, can be corrected with the following measures:
- Lowering the patient's head, or turning the patient's head to the opposite side from the catheter, if using a subclavian or jugular vein
- Keeping sterile dressing intact until the end of the treatment
- Applying external pressure to the exit site
- Rotating the catheter shaft 180 degrees if the catheter has wings
- Reversing the lines, using the arterial port for venous return (as a last resort)

The other difficulty that commonly occurs is clotting. Proper heparinization of the catheter after dialysis, according to the manufacturer's directions, will help to alleviate this problem. Fibrinolytic agents may be prescribed if the catheter is clotted or to prevent clotting.

Are dual-lumen catheters available for permanent use?

The permanent catheter is becoming more widely used. A silicone rubber catheter is inserted intraoperatively. The catheter has a subcutaneous Dacron graft that impedes infection. These catheters are usually placed in the internal jugular vein and a subcutaneous tunnel is created that allows the catheter to exit through the chest wall (Fig. 10-10, *A*). Permanent catheters are also placed in the subclavian, mammary, and femoral veins. Another type of PermCath is a Tesio catheter (Fig. 10-10, *B*), which uses two single-lumen catheters placed side by side in the same vein. This allows for customized catheter placement with increased blood flow rate. PermCaths are useful in pediatric patients whose small arteries and veins prohibit placement of an AV graft.

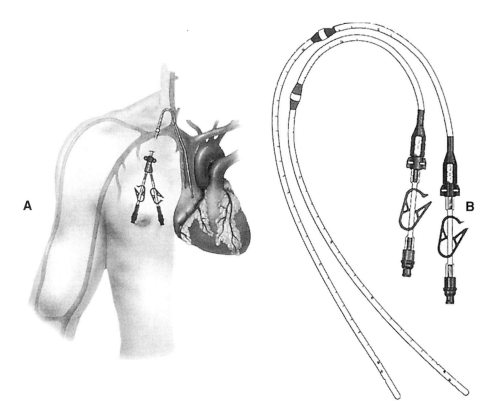

Fig. 10-10 A, Internal jugular permanent vascular access using the Tesio catheter. **B,** PermCath modified by Tesio. *(Courtesy MEDCOMP Corp., Harleysville, Pa.)*

What continuous quality improvement issues are important with vascular access?

Greatest concern surrounds issues of assessment, clotting, and venous pressure. In assessment, documentation on the treatment record should include absence or presence of a bruit and thrill with fistulas and grafts. A decrease in thrill may denote graft stenosis and impending graft clotting. Note the appearance of the access, including redness, swelling, and any drainage. It is important to document the ease or difficulty of cannulation.

Second, adequate blood flow is important to prevent clotting of the lines and dialyzer, resulting in unnecessary loss of blood. Clotting occurs most often with catheters. Increased bleeding from the needle sites after dialysis may indicate venous stenosis.

Finally, increasing venous pressure is often a sign of stenosis. Venous pressure is measured immediately after initiation of hemodialysis at a blood flow rate (BFR) of 200 mL/min. With 16-gauge needles, the venous pressure should be <150 mm Hg. With 15-gauge needles, the venous pressure should be <100 mm Hg.

What are the DOQI guidelines for vascular access?

The K/DOQI guidelines, formulated by the NKF in 1997, advocate both early placement of an AV fistula predialysis and avoidance of temporary catheters. The guidelines also emphasize that the AV fistula should be the first access attempt. K/DOQI guidelines also suggest that the percent of AV fistulas should be increased. To follow these guidelines, each dialysis unit should have an aggressive continuous quality improvement (CQI) access program. Copies of the K/DOQI vascular access guidelines can be obtained from the NKF. (See page 338 for additional information on NKF-K/DOQI.)

What are some of the newer trends in blood access?

Innovative locations are used for AV graft and PermCath placement when usual sites are no longer available. Examples include the axillofemoral or the mammary artery to mammary vein graft. Research continues, in hope of devising a graft that does not clot.

In summary, when the Scribner shunt was developed in 1960, the impact it would have on prolonging the life of the patient with ESRD was unforeseen. More than 326,000 patients in the United States are on maintenance hemodialysis, and there are many in acute renal failure whose care is facilitated by technologic advances in vascular access. Experimentation with new devices is ongoing. The future portends innovations that will enhance the care and the quality of life of the patient with renal failure.

11 Patient and Machine Monitoring and Assessment

Initial and ongoing assessment of the patient and continuous monitoring of dialysis equipment are among the most vital functions of dialysis personnel. Both registered nurses and patient care technicians (PCTs) have defined roles and responsibilities. State boards of nursing regulate the practice of nursing, including the direct supervision of nonprofessionals to whom specific tasks may be delegated. Readers are advised to review the regulations guiding practice in the states in which they practice.

In some states, only registered nurses are allowed to perform assessment as described by the Nurse Practice Acts. Several states, however, have special laws that allow the unlicensed dialysis PCTs to perform certain tasks. In many states, PCTs are certified by the state to infuse normal saline intravenously for priming and hypotension, inject intradermal lidocaine (Xylocaine) before insertion of dialysis needles into the vascular access and to administer IV heparin for anticoagulation per protocol or physicians' orders. These tasks are allowed under the direct supervision of a registered nurse.

In this chapter, assessment refers to the nurses' role. Monitoring or collection of data is the role of the PCT. After data are collected, the nurse and the PCT work together to initiate changes in the dialysis treatment per physicians' orders or protocols.

What is patient monitoring?

Patient monitoring is a series of repeated or continuous observations and documentation of the patient's physiologic state and response to dialysis. Machine monitoring is continuous and includes the following: arterial and venous pressures, blood flow rate, transmembrane pressure (TMP), ultrafiltrate removed, dialysate temperature, dialysate flow and conductivity, and remaining treatment time. Dialysis personnel are responsible for reading, documenting, and evaluating these parameters. Vital signs are measured at least every hour or more frequently in unstable patients. Assessments determine the appropriate dialysis intervention to attain the goals of treatment.

What are dialysis treatment outcome standards?

The National Kidney Foundation–Kidney Disease Outcomes Quality Initiative (NKF-K/DOQI) provides guidelines with indicators for outcomes. Four different clinical practices guidelines (hemodialysis adequacy, peritoneal dialysis adequacy, treatment of anemia, and vascular access) are used to assess and improve the outcome of each dialysis. Other guidelines have been developed, including nutrition, dyslipidemia, bone disease, and hypertension. An additional guideline for pediatrics is being developed (see Appendix A for additional information on NKF-K/DOQI).

What are the different types of hemodialysis assessment?

Types of assessment include the following: physical assessments, laboratory data analysis and interpretation, first dialysis assessment, intradialytic assessment (predialysis, post-dialysis, and monitoring of hemodialysis procedure), and the multidisciplinary team assessment using the NKF-K/DOQI clinical practice guidelines.

GENERAL ASSESSMENT PARAMETERS

Assessment involves collecting data through interviews, physical examination, performance of laboratory tests, and interpretation of patient observation. These data directly affect the patient's care.

What does physical assessment include?

Physical assessment consists of the following: assessing weight, blood pressure (BP), temperature, pulse, respiratory rate; evaluating respiratory effort, extent of edema; auscultating for quality of heart sounds and breath sounds; comparing apical and peripheral pulses; assessing skin integrity, skin color, jugular vein distention (JVD); and evaluating vascular access.

When are patients weighed?

Dialysis patients are weighed before and after each dialysis treatment. Some patients follow their weights at home to guide the adjustment of their fluid intake between dialyses.

Why is measurement of weight important?

Weight is a good indicator of how well the patient is controlling fluid balance between dialyses. Predialysis weight indicates how much ultrafiltration is required during the treatment. Postdialysis weight is the best indication of how much ultrafiltration occurred during the hemodialysis procedure.

What is meant by the patient's dry weight?

Dry weight is the ideal postdialysis weight after the removal of all or most excess body fluid. Patients who are at dry weight are usually normotensive. If the postdialysis weight suggests volume status is too high, the patient may be on the borderline for fluid overload and may be hypertensive. If postdialysis weight is too low, the patient may be hypovolemic and at risk for hypotension and clotting of the vascular access.

How much weight gain is permissible between dialysis treatments?

Weight gained between dialysis procedures is due to fluid retention. Most dialysis units encourage patients to limit their weight gain to 0.5 kg (or 1 lb) per day. (Refer to Chapter 14 for further discussion and calculation of fluid restrictions.)

Why is BP measurement important?

Blood pressure is often volume related. Hypertension may indicate volume overload. Hypotension may indicate dehydration. Blood pressure is measured while the patient is sitting and standing to evaluate orthostatic changes requiring intervention.

What is normal BP?

Normal BP is an individual matter. In the end-stage renal disease (ESRD) patient, blood pressure is analyzed for trends, rather than absolute values. A systolic value greater than 170 mm Hg or less than 90 mm Hg or a diastolic value greater than 100 mm Hg should be reported to the physician.

Where can the cuff be placed for BP measurement?

The upper arm is the most common cuff placement site but there are two alternative placements. (1) A large thigh cuff can be applied around the midthigh area. The pulse is audible via a stethoscope at the popliteal space. (2) A regular cuff may be applied above the ankle with auscultation over the posterior tibial or dorsalis pedis artery. This usually yields an audible BP, but the readings obtained will be 20 to 40 mm Hg higher than arm pressures. A notation should be made on the patient's chart whenever leg pressures are taken.

Why are temperature, pulse, and respiration (TPR) monitored?

TPR observations serve as a baseline at the start of dialysis. Temperature elevation suggests infection or complicating illness. An elevated temperature is often a sign of vascular access infection. Fever during dialysis may be caused by high dialysate temperature or by a pyrogen reaction. A rapid pulse may result from anemia or fluid overload. Irregular heart rate (arrhythmia) may indicate cardiac complications, including those associated with serum potassium levels. An increase in pulse rate during dialysis may be associated with falling blood volume (from ultrafiltration) and may occur just before a drop in BP. Increased respiratory rate may indicate excessive fluid gain. Any unexpected findings should be reported to the physician.

What is edema?

Edema is the excessive accumulation of fluid in the tissue spaces. Excessive weight gain between dialyses results in edema. Edema appears in different areas of the body in different patients. It may present at the ankle or sacrum, facial or periorbital areas, or peripherally. The jugular veins are often distended when the patient is fluid overloaded. Fluid status assessment determines the amount of ultrafiltration required during dialysis.

Are there other physical assessments?

The predialysis assessment includes a subjective analysis of the patient's health since the previous dialysis treatment. Ask whether he or she has experienced symptoms such as headaches, hypotension, bleeding, or diarrhea. Dialysis personnel can assess changes in mentation, speech, or thought processes while patients describe their health and any problems between dialysis sessions.

FIRST HEMODIALYSIS ASSESSMENT
Why is the first hemodialysis procedure so important?

The first hemodialysis is critical because it sets the atmosphere for all future treatment procedures. The first dialysis is usually performed in the hospital. The patient may be unstable and feel sick. The information the nurse gives the patient during this first dialysis is often forgotten or misunderstood. Therefore the nurse and dialysis personnel must reiterate teaching instructions regarding medications or access care again and again. Written manuals and instructions are helpful so patients have a reference as needed. Sometimes the first dialysis is performed in an outpatient dialysis facility. When this is the case, it is imperative that the dialysis personnel be cognizant of the emotional status of the new patient. The patient may be fearful because of the myths he or she has heard, or because of the equipment's appearance. These fears, combined with the fact that he or she is chronically ill, are strong reasons for the patient to be in emotional shock and to not recall instructions given during that first dialysis. The dialysis nurse and personnel must make the first dialysis as smooth and uneventful as possible.

What procedures take place before the first hemodialysis?

The physician evaluates and prescribes the dialysis orders for the new patient. The nurse reviews the orders, determines the proper dialyzer, and (after the fluid composition and machine settings are programmed) starts predialysis assessment. Before the first meeting with the patient, medical records should be reviewed. This information will be helpful during the physical assessment. After introductions, a brief tour around the facility should be conducted. The first visit should be as simple and as pleasant as possible. Remember that instructions will have to be repeated many times.

Make certain that a signed consent for the dialysis treatment is completed and retained in the patient's medical records. The physical assessment begins with the patient's weight, blood pressure, temperature, pulse, and respiratory rate. A general assessment of the patient's fluid status and overall well-being follows. Some questions that should be asked include the following: Is there edema? Is the patient in any respiratory distress or experiencing any pain? Any bleeding or bruising? Is there residual renal function? Are bowel movements regular? Are there sleep problems? Many units have assessment forms that offer guidelines to the caregiver.

During this first procedure some of the dialysis parameters will be set: for example, heparin requirements, tolerance of fluid removal, arterial and venous pressure readings, saline requirements, tolerance to the dialyzer, and the dialysate composition. Because the first dialysis is so critical, the physician usually prescribes a slow blood flow and only 2 hours of dialysis. If the patient is very fluid overloaded, has a high BUN, or is a child, the physician may order mannitol to prevent hypotension and avoid a complicated first dialysis. This helps prevent the occurrence of the dialysis disequilibrium syndrome.

PREDIALYSIS ASSESSMENT
What is predialysis assessment?

Before initiation of hemodialysis, the patient and machine are both evaluated. The patient's physiologic status is assessed to ascertain the need to adjust dialysis orders or prescribed medications. The machine parameters are assessed to ensure that the prescribed procedure is implemented correctly.

What is included in the patient's preassessment?

Preassessment includes the following:
- Fluid status (respiratory rate/effort, JVD, heart sounds, breath sounds, presence of edema)
- Weight
- Blood pressure, sitting and standing
- TPR, including apical/peripheral pulse evaluation
- Skin color, temperature, turgor, and integrity
- Vascular access patency and freedom from bleeding and infection
- Interpretation of physical assessment and laboratory data for appropriate intervention and medication administration

What other checks should be done on the dialysis machine before patient use?

It is necessary to ensure that machine functions have been checked and that they work correctly: All extracorporeal alarms should be tested to ensure that they respond appropriately. Arterial pressure, venous pressure, and air detector alarms should all cause the blood pump to stop and the venous line clamp to close. In addition, conductivity and temperature of the dialysate should be tested to ensure that they are within the proper range. These alarms must be working at all times so that if any problems arise, the dialysate will be diverted from the dialyzer and a major complication avoided. Finally, there should be an adequate amount of dialysate concentrate to complete the patient's treatment.

What is included in machine preassessment?

Preassessment includes the following:
- Dialyzer membrane check for patency and integrity
- Blood tubing intact without leaks
- Appropriate prescribed dialyzer
- Dialysate fluid composition as ordered and within safe limits (12.8 to 14.8 mho) as read by a Myron-L meter
- Appropriate prescribed dialysate potassium and calcium

- Temperature within limits (35° to 37° C)
- Correlation of machine conductivity with an external meter reading of dialysate (Myron-L or Western)
- Dialysate delivery system free of sterilant or disinfectant agents
- Extracorporeal blood circuit free of air
- Blood pump properly occluded
- Dialyzer bloodline tubing free of kinks or crimps
- Blood pump segment of tubing properly seated in the pump segment
- Physician's orders reviewed to ensure adherence to dialysis prescription
- All alarms programmed and set within limits
- Dialysis quality water evaluated for chloramines

What is sodium modeling/variation and when is it applicable?

During dialysis small solutes, primarily urea, are removed from the extracellular fluid (ECF) resulting in a fall in ECF osmolality. This fall in ECF osmolality causes a shift of water into cells, aggravating hypotension. One way of preventing this phenomenon is by replacing the lost osmoles (urea) with sodium. This can be done automatically by the dialysis machine and may prevent or minimize hypotension.

Sodium variations allow the dialysis treatment to be modified by increasing the concentrate-to-water ratio slightly, resulting in a rise in dialysate sodium. This feature allows the dialysis staff to initiate hemodialysis with a high-dialysate sodium concentration and use progressively lower sodium-containing dialysate, decreasing to the original baseline level in a programmed time and profile. These maneuvers are intended to reduce the incidence of hypotension and cramping. By varying the level of sodium in the dialysate, the drop in osmolality of the patient's serum is more gradual. The fluid that is in the interstitial spaces in the tissues does not transfer into the vascular spaces as fast as the dialysis machine is able to remove it. The result of this is fluid depletion of the vascular space and the resultant side effects of hypotension. The sodium variation system keeps the vascular space filled enough to prevent this fluid depletion from occurring. There are several machines available to perform this treatment function. The Fresenius 2008H has three sodium variation system profiles. They are step decrease, linear decrease, or exponential decrease. Fig. 11-1 illustrates these system profiles. The baseline is determined by the basic setting of the mechanical acid/acetate and bicarbonate concentrate pumps. With this method of sodium modeling, there is a significant variation in the dialysate potassium level. If the dialysate sodium is increased from 140 to 160 mEq/L (about 14%), the dialysate potassium concentration will also increase by 14%. If the baseline concentrate has 3 mEq/L of potassium and is increased by 14%, the new potassium concentrate would be 3.4 mEq/L. If there is a decrease in the dialysate sodium to 120 mEq/L (decrease of 14%), the new potassium concentrate will be 2.6 mEq/L. Increasing sodium in the dialysate has assisted many patients in the prevention of hypotension, cramping, and disequilibrium syndrome during dialysis. The physician writes the orders for the sodium modeling for each patient.

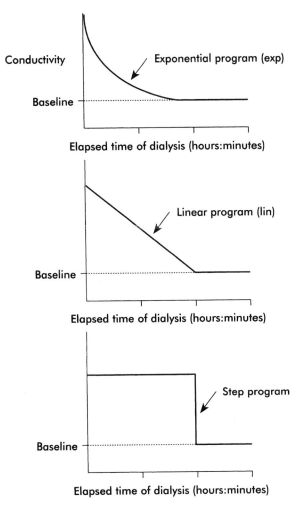

Fig. 11-1 Sodium variation system profiles. The exponential program causes the conductivity to decrease toward the baseline over the programmed time in a smooth curve. The linear program is a straight-line reduction from the program maximum to the baseline level. The step program allows for a single large step to be performed. *(From Gotch FA, et al: Measurement of whole body UF on urea mass transfer coefficients: implications for Na⁺ urea modeling in dialysis, Presentation at the American Society of Nurses, 1984.)*

Are there complications of sodium modeling?

Some patients experience increased interdialytic thirst, weight gain, and BP when sodium modeling is used. Adjustment of the dialysate sodium concentration may be required.

Why is it necessary to do such a thorough assessment of the patient and the machine before initiation of the dialysis treatment?

The accuracy of assessment and the appropriateness of the interventions directly affect the patient's outcome and will ensure that the goal of adequacy of dialysis is achieved.

What is ultrafiltration (UF)?

UF is the removal of fluid during dialysis. It is the result of hydrostatic force across the dialysis membrane. The difference in hydrostatic pressure, blood to fluid, is the transmembrane pressure, or TMP. The rate of UF is the sum total of positive and negative pressures plus the filtration factor, known as the UF coefficient (k_{UF}), of each individual dialyzer. The k_{UF} ranges from 0.5 to 80.0 mL/hr/mm Hg, depending on specific dialyzer characteristics (see Chapter 7).

What information does one need to calculate UF?

All of the following questions must be answered:
- What is the patient's dry weight?
- What weight loss is needed (in kilograms)?
- What is the target postdialysis weight?
- How much fluid will the patient receive orally and/or intravenously during the treatment?
- What is the k_{UF} of the dialyzer?
- How much saline will be infused to rinse the blood circuit?
- What is the length of time the patient is to be dialyzed?

How is fluid removal calculated?

The following steps are taken in calculating fluid removal:

1. *Add*   Amount of weight to be removed in milliliters
   Amount of fluid intake in milliliters during treatment
   + Amount of IV fluid to be removed in milliliters
   ———————————————————————————
   Total amount of fluid to be removed in milliliters

2. *Divide* $\dfrac{\text{Total amount of fluid to be removed in milliliters}}{\text{Number of hours of dialysis}} = \text{mL/hr}$

3. *Divide* $\dfrac{\text{Total from step 2}}{k_{UF} \text{ of dialyzer}} = \text{TMP}$

An example of how to calculate fluid removal is as follows:
Dialyze for 3 hours; remove 2.3 kg, conventional dialyzer k_{UF} equals 4.

1. *Add*

	Weight to be removed in millimeters	2300 mL
	Oral intake	600 mL
+	Saline rinsed back	100 mL
	Total amount of fluid to be removed	3000 mL

2. *Divide*

$$\frac{\text{Fluid to be removed (3000 mL)}}{\text{Number of hours of dialysis (3 hr)}} = 1000 \text{ mL/hr}$$

3. *Divide*

$$\frac{\text{Total from step 2 (1000 mL)}}{k_{UF} = 4} = 250 \text{ TMP}$$

In a conventional dialysis delivery machine, the TMP must be set manually. Most systems now provide a programmable function for controlled UF. This controlled UF allows the machine to adjust and control the fluid removal.

What is sequential UF and dialysis?

The application of UF as a means of fluid removal during dialysis was instituted by Alwall in 1947. The concept of convective transport rather than diffusion (see Chapter 6) is currently put to use in the hemofiltration approach. Several dialyzers have membranes or fibers of sufficient permeability and strength to give UF of several liters per hour at safe transmembrane pressures.

Application of UF alone before conventional dialysis with minimal UF is known as sequential or isolated UF and dialysis. During the UF phase blood circulates normally through the dialyzer, but the dialysis fluid does not. The UF resulting from the negative pressure gradient across the membrane is collected at the outflow side and measured. Patients tolerate fluid removal by this method at a rate and quantity greater than with conventional dialysis without hypotension or symptoms. Severely hypertensive patients are able to achieve better BP control than would otherwise be obtainable. This therapy is particularly useful for maintenance dialysis patients with chronic large fluid gains (see Chapter 15 for more information).

What is UF profile and how is it used in the dialysis treatment?

UF profiling is an option on some dialysis machines, which varies the rate of fluid removal during the patient's dialysis treatment. The Fresenius 2008H has four preset profiles and four blank screens for customizing profiles. With UF profiling, the entire UF goal is removed, but at a variable rate. An example of this would be removing the greater proportion of fluid during the first half of the treatment. The greatest amount of available fluid volume is available at this time in the treatment. As the treatment progresses and the patient is ultrafiltrated, the rate of fluid removal is decreased, allowing time for the intravascular space to refill. This can help to prevent complications such as hypotension and cramping. The UF profile is helpful for patients with either high or low predialysis blood pressure, patients with large interdialytic weight gain, and patients such as those with diabetes mellitus who have difficulty with plasma refilling. The UF profile system works well in conjunction with the sodium variation system.

What is high-efficiency dialysis?

High-efficiency dialysis is performed with a special dialyzer with a large surface area. This dialyzer has a permeable membrane that allows solutes in the low to middle molecular weight and up to 5000 Da to be removed. The k_{UF} ranges from 5 to 15 mL/hr/mm Hg. With this higher k_{UF}, an UF control system is essential to control fluid loss. In addition, cardiovascular instability becomes more of a problem because of the rapid fluid removal and accompanying hypotension. Therefore a bicarbonate delivery system is imperative to allow for fluid removal while maintaining cardiovascular stability. Blood flow rates are from 300 to 500 mL/hr and dialysate flow is from 500 to 1000 mL/hr.

What is a high-flux dialysis?

High-flux dialysis is performed with a special dialyzer with a synthetic, highly permeable membrane that allows small- and large-molecular-weight solutes to be convected across the membrane. The major difference in high-efficiency and high-flux dialysis is the membrane. High-flux membranes have solute clearance in the molecular weight range of 5000 Da (insulin) to 12,000 Da (β_2-microglobulins, β_2M). The membrane surface area ranges from 0.6 to 2.0 m^2. Water permeability is much higher in high-flux than in high-efficiency membranes and much higher than with conventional membranes, thus resulting in possible backflow of dialysate. The k_{UF} for high-flux membranes ranges from 20 to 80 mL/hr/mm Hg. A fluid delivery system with UF control is required. High-flux dialysis requires a blood flow rate of 300 to 500 mL/min. Bicarbonate dialysate is required for cardiovascular stability. Usually dialysate flow is at 500 or 800 mL/min. Because the membrane is so permeable, very stringent water quality is imperative (see Chapter 7 on dialyzers, Chapter 8 on water treatment, and Chapter 9 on dialyzer preparation and reprocessing). The equipment and bicarbonate dialysate containers must be disinfected regularly.

INTRADIALYTIC ASSESSMENT AND MONITORING
What is intradialytic monitoring?

Intradialytic monitoring is the ongoing assessment of the patient and equipment during the hemodialysis treatment. The patient and the machine are monitored every hour by the caregivers. Monitoring is done more frequently in unstable patients. The vital signs and machine monitors are assessed. Machine parameters are listed in Box 11-1.

The patient must also be monitored for consciousness and the caregiver must always do a visual check to make sure that the patient's access is visible and the needles and lines are secure.

These parameters are adjusted as needed in accordance with the treatment goals. All assessments are logged on the dialysis flow records. In computerized fluid delivery

Box 11-1
MACHINE PARAMETERS

Arterial pressure
Venous pressure
Fluid removal
Dialysate flow
Blood flow
Visual check of the dialyzer, blood tubing, and connections
Visual checks of the machine monitor setting
Heparin pump
Visual check of the air/foam alarm status
Visual check of the patient's access that needles are visible and secure

---

systems, the machine parameters are automatically monitored and recorded on the dialysis flow sheets.

Are any other patient assessments done during dialysis?

An important one, not subject to numerical recording, is the general condition and response of the patient during the procedure. Nausea, apprehension, shortness of breath, restlessness or agitation, irritability, itching, flushing, twitching, irrational behavior, sensation of faintness, and complaints of pain are some of the many signs or symptoms that can occur. A person on regular dialysis has an individual pattern of response, and any change in the pattern is significant. Acute dialysis patients must be evaluated more often because of their less stable condition and unknown response to therapy. All observed clinical conditions are documented on the chart and reported to the physician. Sometimes reactions or complications are reported to the continuous quality improvement (CQI) committee for the purpose of ongoing monitoring or corrective action.

Is there any way of knowing how well you are cleaning a patient's blood during a treatment?

There is a noninvasive assessment tool that can monitor the amount of clearance the patient is receiving during the actual dialysis treatment. One such tool is the OnLine Clearance Adequacy Monitoring Program, which is available on several types of machines in the market today. For example, the Fresenius 2008H and 2008K machines use a monitoring system called OnLine Clearance. This monitoring tool uses sodium chloride, which has a molecular weight of 58, as a surrogate marker for urea, which has a molecular weight of 60. Sodium can move across the dialyzer membrane similarly to urea. The online clearance test occurs in two phases. The first phase or half of the test involves raising the dialysate sodium above the normal sodium concentration in the blood. The dialysate sodium is raised as high as 15.5 ms/cm. Because of the concentration gradient now created, sodium will cross the dialyzer membrane into the blood. The second half of the OnLine Clearance test involves lowering the dialysate sodium to 13.5 ms/cm, allowing diffusion to again take place with the sodium moving from the blood compartment into the dialysate compartment. Conductivity monitors are at both the dialyzer inlet and outlet flow paths. The difference between the two conductivity readings generates a clearance value. Because of the similarities in urea and sodium chloride, a prediction of the degree of urea removal can be made. The machine performs up to six OnLine Clearance tests during a 4-hour treatment. This allows the dialysis nurse or technician to actually see how well the treatment prescription is working for that patient. The patient's volume of urea distribution is entered into the OnLine Clearance program before treatment is initiated because this is used to determine effective clearance. Certain variables contribute to the patient not being dialyzed optimally and these include: poor needle positioning, clotting of the dialyzer, access recirculation, or blood/dialysate flow rates incorrectly set. The OnLine Clearance program is a tool that can greatly improve the adequacy of patients' treatment, which will in turn help to improve the quality of their lives. One advantage to using these types of tools is the dialysis caregiver will know whether during that treatment if you are providing optimal adequacy and also be able to troubleshoot early in the treatment to correct problems.

What are potential hemodialysis complications?

During the hemodialysis procedure many potential complications can occur to both the patient and the equipment. These complications may result from the process itself or from complex interactions between the patient and the dialysis procedure.

What is the most common complication during the hemodialysis treatment?

The most common complication is hypotension related to rapid decrease of circulating blood volume caused by UF. Lack of vasoconstriction caused by antihypertensive medications or other cardiac factors are other causes of hypotension.

The ingestion of food during the dialysis treatment may contribute to hypotension due to splanchnic vasodilation. This is commonly referred to as postprandial hypotension and usually occurs about 2 hours after eating. It is prudent for the patient not to eat during his treatment for this reason, and also loss of consciousness may occur with untreated hypotension, placing the patient at risk for obstructing his airway if he is eating.

What causes hypotension as dialysis is begun?

Hypotension at the beginning of dialysis occurs in some patients with a relatively small blood volume (children, small women). This is the result of volume shifts as the dialyzer is filled with the patient's blood. It is much less frequent with small-volume dialyzers than with larger ones. This type of reaction is rarely serious and usually does not last long. It will respond to the infusion of small amounts of saline or albumin. Careful technique in starting the dialysis will minimize the occurrence of these episodes.

What about hypotension occurring later during dialysis?

Later hypotension is usually attributable to removal of fluid from the vascular space (UF) in excess of the patient's ability to compensate for this. The hypotension may be asymptomatic until there has been a fall of 40 to 55 mm Hg in systolic pressure. It usually responds to fluid replacement. Most modern dialysis machines remove fluid at a steady rate set by the practitioner. Removing more than 1% of a patient's dry body weight as fluid per hour often results in hypotension.

Some patients with gross edema become hypotensive early during a dialysis. Why does this occur?

Patients with gross fluid overload may have heart failure or a low serum albumin. The dialysis removes fluid from the vascular compartment, but the low serum protein does not exert sufficient oncotic pressure to mobilize fluid from the interstitial space. There is another group of patients in whom cardiac failure or hypoproteinemia are not obvious causes, who have problems with overhydration, and who have vascular instability during dialysis. These people, during conventional dialysis with UF, become symptomatically hypotensive with tachycardia, nausea, and vomiting. The causes are likely to be multifactorial. Changes in serum osmolality, effects of acetate if this is used as the buffer, and norepinephrine depletion have been suggested or demonstrated. Infusion of hypertonic saline, mannitol, or use of a higher than usual sodium in the dialysis fluid may be beneficial. Sequential UF followed by dialysis may also give good results.

How is hypotension prevented and treated intradialytically?

Sodium modeling and UF profile discussed earlier, are excellent methods of preventing severe hypotension. Blood pressure monitoring, with careful observation and/or the use of an inline hematocrit monitor is also helpful in reducing hypotensive episodes. If hypotension is treated early by placing the patient in the Trendelenburg position, by decreasing the UF pressures, or by giving replacement fluid, more serious complications may be avoided. It is helpful to be aware of the signs of hypotension such as the patient complaining of feeling hot or lightheaded. Some patients will complain of blurred vision or nausea. It is prudent to check a patient's blood pressure whenever he or she complains of these symptoms. The treatment for hypotension is administering a normal saline bolus, placing the patient in Trendelenburg, decreasing the UF rate, and using a volume expander if ordered.

What is the Crit-Line instrument?

The Crit-Line monitor is an arterial inline medical instrument that provides continuous measurement of absolute hematocrit, percent blood volume change, and oxygen saturation in real time. It measures blood volume change based on the hematocrit because these two values have an inverse relationship. As fluid is removed from the intravascular space, the blood density increases. This is displayed in percent of blood volume change on a gridlike graph on the Crit-Line screen (Fig. 11-2). With this device,

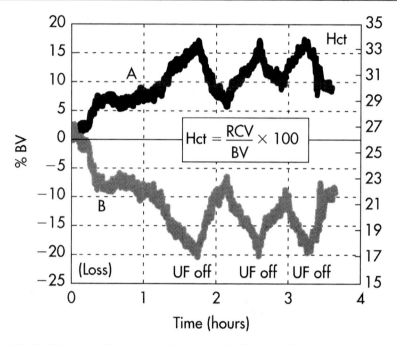

Fig. 11-2 A, (black line) Absolute hematocrit. **B,** (gray line) Percent of blood volume change. *(Courtesy In-Line Diagnostics, Farmington, Utah.)*

it is possible to maximize UF safely and prevent hypotension, cramping, and other intradialytic complications associated with volume depletion. A disposable blood chamber is attached to the arterial side of the dialyzer and a photometric technology is utilized. This device will also measure access recirculation. The Crit-Line is Clinical Laboratory Improvement Act (CLIA) exempt.

Does hypertension occur during dialysis?

A small minority of patients develop a rise in BP during dialysis. Some have a gradual rise throughout the run, whereas others experience an elevation soon after starting. In some patients the rise in pressure is the result of increased cardiac output as fluid overload is relieved. In other instances there may be an increase in peripheral vascular resistance on a reflex or hormonal basis. Angiotensin-converting enzyme (ACE) inhibitor therapy or bilateral nephrectomy may be indicated in cases in which high renin levels are present, whereas the hypertension in very young and elderly patients may respond to a lower blood flow rate and the use of a smaller surface area dialyzer.

Are arrhythmias common during dialysis?

As more older patients and persons with complicating diseases enter ESRD programs, arrhythmias become frequent. They are most often caused by underlying heart disease.

The physician should make the presence of such problems and their significance known to the dialysis personnel. Evaluation of a new, or different, rhythm developing during dialysis requires an electrocardiogram. The patient should be queried as to medications, and a review of recent serum potassium, calcium, and magnesium values should be made. Patients with myocardial damage may develop arrhythmias of various types in response to volume change or a shift in electrolytes, particularly potassium. Patients receiving digitalis may pose particular problems.

What if a patient develops chest pains during dialysis?

Some patients have chest pain that comes on during dialysis. Often these persons have a history of underlying heart disease, and the pain must be presumed to be angina. It may go away if blood flow is slowed or saline is infused. Often a tablet of nitroglycerin or other medication for angina taken just before hookup will prevent the symptoms. Some patients on occasion have a vague chest distress or low back pain. The mechanism is obscure but often seems related to blood volume change or decreased hematocrit. When new or unexpected chest pain occurs in a patient with no known history of cardiac disease, it is always advisable to obtain an electrocardiogram.

What causes muscle cramping during dialysis?

The cause is probably fluid shift or osmolar change, although pH change may play a role. Use of sodium modeling may be preventive, and infusion of hypertonic saline or a 50% dextrose solution usually brings relief once cramps occur. Heat and pressure over the painful area are temporary measures. In patients in whom there may be preexisting small-vessel disease (usually older men), oral administration of quinine before dialysis may reduce or prevent cramping. Many patients respond to 400 units of vitamin E taken 30 minutes before dialysis.

What are other serious complications during hemodialysis?

Other complications that can occur are hemolysis and air embolism.

What is hemolysis?

Hemolysis is the lysis (break up) of the red blood cells resulting in the release of intracellular potassium. Hemolysis may be caused by chemical, thermal, or mechanical events. Chemical causes of hemolysis include exposure of the blood to chemicals such as sodium hypochlorite, formaldehyde, copper, or nitrates. Thermal hemolysis is from the exposure of blood to overheated dialysate. Dialysate temperatures greater than $42°$ C are considered dangerous. Mechanical causes of hemolysis include kinking of the bloodlines, overoccluded blood pumps, excessive negative pressure from a small-gauge needle with a high blood flow rate, or a poorly positioned needle. Other causes of hemolysis include dialyzing the patient against a hypotonic bath and blood transfusions. Hemolysis may be either acute or chronic. It may be slight and require no immediate treatment, or it may be a life-threatening emergency. Acute hemolysis during the dialysis treatment is a medical emergency. The patient may also experience symptoms after going home from dialysis treatment and present in the emergency department. For unknown reasons, pancreatitis will sometime occur following an episode of acute hemolysis.

What are the symptoms of hemolysis?

With hemolysis, the blood in the extracorporeal circuit may appear transparent and "cherry soda pop" in color; however, the blood may appear very dark and opaque. Other symptoms of hemolysis are burning sensation in the access extremity, usually the venous needle, from the release of large amounts of potassium from the ruptured red blood cells (RBCs). The patient will often complain of abdominal pain or cramping, low back pain, chest pain, nausea and vomiting, shortness of breath, or indigestion. Cardiac changes may be seen as the potassium is released from the cells, causing arrhythmias and bradycardia with hypo- or hypertension. An acute drop in hematocrit will be seen as the RBCs rupture.

What steps should be taken if you suspect hemolysis in your patient?

Monitors should detect a hypotonic dialysate solution or high dialysate temperature; however, machines are not infallible. Careful monitoring by dialysis personnel is essential to avoid this potentially life-threatening complication. If hemolysis is suspected, the bloodlines should be clamped immediately, the blood pump stopped, and the patient's symptoms treated. The dialysate should be sampled for pH and conductivity. A blood sample from the patient should be obtained and checked for hematocrit, electrolytes, free hemoglobin, and haptoglobin. If hemolysis is suspected, a blood sample in a serum separator tube when centrifuged will have red serum. It is important to remember to never reinfuse hemolyzed blood cells. Returning hemolyzed blood could cause hyperkalemia. The patient's symptoms should be treated and the physician notified.

Describe an air embolism.

Air embolism occurs when air or a large amount of foam (microbubbles) is introduced into a patient's vascular system. Air embolism can occur when arterial or venous lines become disconnected or when blood or saline infusion bags run dry. The resultant vacuum causes microbubbles, or foam. Dialysis personnel are responsible for setting and monitoring the air detector throughout the entire dialysis procedure.

What symptoms are associated with an air embolism?

The patient may complain of chest pain or tightness or shortness of breath, and may cough. If the patient is sitting upright, air may be introduced into the cerebral venous system and cause neurologic symptoms such as visual problems, loss of consciousness, and convulsions.

What action is taken if a patient receives an infusion of air?

When a patient receives air, treatment must be immediate. The bloodlines are clamped and dialysis is stopped. The patient is placed on the left side in the Trendelenburg (head down) position. This position decreases the movement of air to the brain and traps air in the right atrium above the tricuspid valve. This minimizes foaming, which occurs primarily in the right ventricle of the heart. It is important to maintain the patient's airway and to administer oxygen if needed. The patient must be moved as little as possible and must be maintained in the Trendelenburg position. It takes several hours for all of the air, particularly the nitrogen, to be totally reabsorbed. A chest x-ray examination should be done to evaluate the amount of air present in the heart.

What is Disequilibrium syndrome?

This is a situation that produces neurologic and other symptoms soon after a patient begins dialysis treatments. Urea has the ability to move freely between the cells and the serum. Theories suggest that when a patient who is very uremic is dialyzed for the first time, as the urea is removed, the plasma becomes more hypotonic, causing water to shift from the plasma into the brain tissue, which is less hypotonic and contains higher amounts of urea. This usually occurs in patients with very high blood urea nitrogen levels or those with acute renal failure. As the water flows to the higher urea concentration, the brain cells begin to swell, causing the neurologic symptoms that include headache, nausea, vomiting, restlessness, and twitching to the more severe tremors, disorientation, and convulsions. Treatment includes the administration of a hypertonic solution such as hypertonic saline, 50% dextrose, or mannitol. The patient's symptoms should be treated. Delivering a less effective treatment by using lower blood and dialysate flow rates, decreasing treatment time, or running the patient with a concurrent flow will help to minimize these symptoms until the blood urea nitrogen levels stabilize.

What happens during a dialyzer reaction?

Dialyzer reactions are sometimes referred to as "first-use syndrome" because some patients, when exposed to the dialyzer membrane for the first time, develop allergic-type symptoms. Dialyzer reactions are now more commonly referred to as type A and type B reactions.

Type A reactions are the more severe of the two and often present with anaphylactic type symptoms. These reactions usually occur within the first 5 minutes of treatment with the patient experiencing the following symptoms: dyspnea, chest and back pain, feeling of warmth, sense of impending doom, and cardiac arrest. Less threatening symptoms include itching, urticaria, coughing, sneezing, watery eyes, and abdominal cramping. Type A reactions are usually caused by the factory sterilant ethylene oxide (Eto). This type of reaction is less common today because some dialyzer manufacturers are using alternative sterilization methods such as gamma irradiation as a sterilant, E-Beam, or steam sterilization. For those using dialyzers sterilized with Eto, proper priming of the dialyzer may help to prevent pockets of Eto remaining in the fibers to be released during the patient's dialysis treatment.

Type B reactions are less threatening but more commonly seen. The symptoms usually occur as soon as the patient's blood is exposed to the dialyzer and returned to the patient. Symptoms include chest pain, hypotension, and occasionally back pain. The treatment for both types is based on symptoms. The treatment should be discontinued until a determination is made as to the cause of the symptoms and the physician is notified. Oxygen is generally administered for difficulty breathing. Intravenous antihistamines may be ordered or epinephrine for anaphylaxis. Blood pressure support may also be necessary for hypotension.

What is a formaldehyde reaction?

A formaldehyde reaction occurs when the patient's blood is exposed to the sterilant. This may occur when a formaldehyde-filled dialyzer is incorrectly rinsed of the sterilant or from improper testing for the presence of residual formaldehyde. Symptoms include a bitter peppery taste in the mouth, anxiety, burning in the venous needle, numbness around the mouth or lips, chest/back pain, and shortness of breath. It is important to recognize and treat formaldehyde reactions immediately because hemolysis of red blood cells may also occur. The treatment should be stopped and the patient's symptoms should be taken care of. Approximately 10 mL of blood should be removed from each needle so that the patient receives no further formaldehyde. Proper rinsing of the system and attention to safety testing for residual will help alleviate this complication.

What causes a pyrogen reaction to occur?

A pyrogen reaction may occur from an improperly sterilized dialyzer, bacteria in the water system or dialysate, break in aseptic technique, or improper access preparation. A pyrogen is a fever-producing substance, usually an endotoxin, which is a by-product of dead bacterial cell walls. Bacteria are too large to cross the dialyzer membrane, but an endotoxin is small enough to cross, causing the symptoms. A patient will experience chills after the commencement of the dialysis treatment along with a decrease in the systolic blood pressure. Headache, fever, myalgia (muscle pain), nausea, and vomiting may also be experienced. The symptoms will usually subside after the patient's treatment is discontinued. The hypotension and fever may need to be treated. Blood cultures may be ordered. It is imperative to practice scrupulous infection control technique when accessing your patient's catheter or internal access. Dialyzers should never be used if they have been recirculating for longer than the manufacturer's directions and facility's policy allow. Care must be used to disinfect dialysate jugs, mixing tanks, and machines per facility policy. It is important to rule out septicemia, as the symptoms are very similar to those of a pyrogen reaction.

What are potential hemodialysis equipment problems?

Hemodialysis equipment is designed to protect the patient from complications that may occur during the treatment. However, machines are not infallible and will periodically malfunction. A malfunction of the temperature control device can cause hyperthermia, resulting in hemolysis. If not detected, this condition could cause death. Its opposite, hypothermia, can also occur; this condition can cause extreme chills and violent shaking.

Are there other equipment complications?

Yes. Other complications may occur when dialyzers and bloodlines become disconnected, leak, or clot. Most machine complications can be prevented by careful monitoring. Machine maintenance also plays an important role in the prevention of machine-related accidents. Chapter 7 discusses the equipment and its preventive maintenance.

What is arterial pressure?

Arterial pressure is a measurement of the extracorporeal blood circuit pressure between the patient's needle site and a site proximal to the blood pump. It is not the equivalent of the patient's systemic arterial pressure but the negative pressure created by the blood pump. Arterial monitoring guards against excessive suction on the vascular access. For example, if the patient's arterial pressure has been reading (–) 100 mm Hg and it suddenly increases to (–) 200 mm Hg, this could indicate a clotted or dislodged needle, a drop in the patient's systemic BP, or a kink in the arterial line. If the arterial negative pressure increases or decreases, as long as the monitor is properly set, the alarm will be activated and the blood pump will shut off. This audible and visual alarm alerts the caregiver of a dialysis complication and always requires immediate attention. The alarm will remain activated, and the blood pump will not work until the abnormality is corrected. A high negative arterial pressure must always be assessed and steps taken to correct the problem. High negative arterial pressure may be damaging to the vascular access and may cause hemolysis in the patient.

What is venous pressure?

Venous pressure is a measurement of the extracorporeal blood circuit pressure at some point after the dialyzer and before the blood reenters the patient's body. The monitoring line is usually attached to the top of the venous bubble trap. Venous extracorporeal pressure measures the resistance of the blood returning to the patient via the venous needle. For example, if the patient's venous pressure reading suddenly increases from 50 to 150 mm Hg, this increase would indicate that the venous line may be kinked, the bubble trap may be clotted, the venous needle may be clotted or misaligned, or the vascular access may be in danger of failing. If, however, there is a sudden and dramatic decrease in venous pressure, the venous needle may have been pulled out, the transducer may be wet, or the arterial chamber may be clotted. The venous pressure alarm is similar to the arterial pressure alarm in that once activated, the abnormal condition must be corrected before the machine will allow the blood to continue through the blood circuit.

Note: All alarms must be set properly at the initiation of dialysis. This ensures that if any complication occurs, an audible and visual alarm will be activated and alert caregivers to a potential problem.

What effect does the dialysis solution (dialysate) flow rate have on the dialyzer clearance?

Dialysis solution flow rate affects clearance of small solutes such as urea. The usual dialysis solution flow rate is 500 mL/min, although some types of dialysis equipment (e.g., Sorb System's Redy 2000) use 250 mL/min. The slower flow rate leads to slightly lower dialyzer urea clearance. Dialysis solution flow rates of greater than 500 mL/min are used to increase clearance for high-efficiency dialysis. Higher dialysate flow rate can be used to enhance urea clearance when the blood flow rate is reduced for any reason. According to Nissenson, "little clinical benefit is achievable using presently available equipment at blood flow rates greater than 500 mL/min. There is a point where the relationship between dialysis solution flow rate and dialyzer clearance levels off with the higher dialysis solution flow rates."

Why should ESRD patients control their food and oral fluid intake during dialysis treatment?

There are several reasons for controlling intake. First, the amount of fluid removed by UF is the net change in weight from the predialysis to the postdialysis weight. If the patient consumes large amounts of food and drink, this net weight change does not reflect a realistic fluid loss. The quantity of food or fluid ingested during dialysis should always be taken into consideration when calculating how much fluid to ultrafiltrate during the dialysis procedure. If it is permissible for patients to eat during dialysis, it is best to limit this to very small snacks. Food in the digestive tract causes pooling of blood and may cause hypotension and vomiting and increased risk of aspiration. Still, with more efficient dialysis and removal of fluid, ESRD patients have fewer restrictions with respect to oral intake than formerly. See Chapter 14 for more on nutrition.

What about the consumption of ice chips as a water substitute?

Ice has two advantages: (1) its coldness and (2) the time required for it to melt in the mouth. These factors make it more effective in alleviating the sensation of thirst. A 200-mL glass filled with ice chips yields about 150 mL of water. Therefore the patient will consume less fluid by eating ice chips than by drinking water.

POSTDIALYTIC THERAPY ASSESSMENT
What is postdialytic assessment?

Postdialytic assessment is the total evaluation of the patient, the treatment, and an interpretation of the predialytic goals. Factors to be included are listed in Box 11-2.

<table>
<tr><td>Box 11-2</td></tr>
</table>

PATIENT PARAMETERS EVALUATED AFTER DIALYSIS

Patient's weight and weight loss

Vital signs, e.g., temperature, pulse, respiration (TPR) and blood pressure (BP)

Resolution/improvement of problematic predialysis parameters (improvement of fluid status)

Total of infusions given; both saline and blood

Patient's subjective physical assessment, e.g., any pain or complaints

Access assessment

Bleeding status

<table>
<tr><td>Box 11-3</td></tr>
</table>

ITEMS FOR MONTHLY EVALUATION OF END-STAGE RENAL DISEASE (ESRD) PATIENTS

Nutritional status, dry weight control, diet and fluid control

Kt/V and/or urea reduction ratio (URR)—dialyzer, blood flow, hours of treatment

Chemistries: dialysate K and Ca

Vital signs and blood pressure: sodium modeling

Access: complications, aneurysm

Any bleeding in relation to heparin dose

Physical assessment

Bowel habit changes

Sleep habits

Sexuality

Medication review

Psychosocial review for general problems (social or financial)

Are there other postdialytic assessments?

The dialysis prescription plan is assessed for any changes that will be implemented in the next dialysis. Finally, the date for the next dialysis is scheduled.

MONTHLY ASSESSMENTS
What is the purpose of monthly assessments for ESRD patients?

Each patient's prescription should be evaluated monthly to review his or her status and determine the adequacy of dialysis treatment (Box 11-3).

Summary

There are multiple types of assessment in the treatment of the ESRD patient. Each assessment is used to improve patient outcomes and decrease the mortality and morbidity. The NKF-K/DOQI has established guidelines to enhance and promote the assessment of the ESRD patient for improved outcome.

12 Anticoagulation and Heparin Administration

Blood tends to clot when it encounters any surface that is not the lining of a normal blood vessel. This mechanism is vital to preserving the life of the individual. Thus blood will clot soon after entering the extracorporeal circuit of the hemodialysis system, rendering treatment impossible, unless the ability to clot is interrupted. There are several methods to prevent coagulation of the extracorporeal circuit—each with advantages and drawbacks for patient and/or practitioner. It is essential that the dialysis practitioner be familiar with more than one method to safely and effectively meet the needs of each individual hemodialysis patient.

What is anticoagulation?

Anticoagulation is the blocking, suppression, or delaying clotting of the blood. Clot formation occurs when blood contacts "foreign" surfaces, such as it does when it enters the bloodlines and dialyzer. Normally blood does not clot within the vascular system. However, clots can form under certain conditions, most commonly after an injury, when the clot serves to seal the damaged vessel and prevent further blood loss.

What causes blood to clot?

Clotting is a part of a complex body process called hemostasis. This process involves (1) retraction and contraction of the injured vessel, (2) the ability of blood platelets to stick to the injured area, and (3) a complex interaction of coagulation factors, resulting in a formed clot. These coagulation factors are present in normal blood and are identified by roman numerals I to V and VII through XIII. Platelets are damaged by contact with a foreign surface. Platelet factor III is released, causing platelets to stick and start the clotting process. Plasma factors XI and XII are also activated by contact with a foreign surface and contribute to clotting.

Why doesn't blood clot within the normal vascular system?

The lining of the blood vessels, the endothelium, is smooth, allowing the blood to flow freely through the vessels. The other surfaces of cells—vascular endothelial cells, platelets, and red cells—are gelatinous and hydrophilic, with a high water content. They have low interfacial tensions and have little tendency to adhere when intact.

Why is anticoagulation needed during dialysis?

Blood coagulates when it comes into contact with foreign surfaces such as dialyzers and bloodlines. To avoid this, anticoagulants are used. The first anticoagulant was hirudin, obtained from the heads of medicinal leeches. In 1916, McLean found an anticoagulant in the liver of animals. This extract he called heparin, but it was not purified for human use until 1936. Its potency was finally standardized in the United States in 1966.

What is the nature of heparin?

Heparin is an acid mucopolysaccharide and is neutralized by strong basic compounds such as protamine sulfate, toluidine blue, and quinidine, causing it to lose its anticoagulant properties. Heparin for clinical use includes a number of fractions, with molecular weights (MWs) ranging from 8000 to 14,000 Da. Heparin composed only of low MW (4000 to 6000 Da) is available in the United States and, although more expensive, has the benefit of single-dose administration, less bleeding risk, and less effect on circulating lipases, potentially resulting in lower triglyceride and cholesterol levels in long-term hemodialysis patients. This latter factor may be significant, because high triglyceride and cholesterol levels are associated with cardiovascular disease.

How does heparin prevent coagulation?

Heparin combines with a blood protein fraction called heparin cofactor (antithrombin III). The complex of heparin-antithrombin III combines with and inactivates thrombin, activated factor X, and activated factor XI, thus preventing clotting at all three stages of coagulation (Fig. 12-1). The conversion of prothrombin to thrombin is inhibited as well

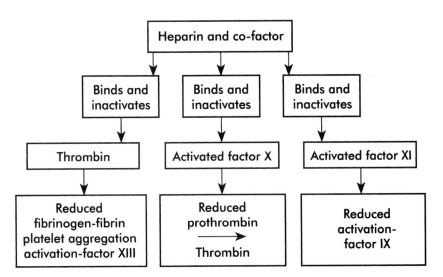

Fig. 12-1 Schematic diagram of heparin effect.

as the conversion of fibrinogen to fibrin. Peak anticoagulant activity is reached 5 to 10 minutes after injection. The half-life is about 90 minutes for doses usually used in dialysis. The mechanism of heparin inactivation is not completely clear; it is metabolized by the liver and is also taken up by the reticuloendothelial system.

Are there different kinds of heparin?

Most heparin is derived from pork intestinal mucosa or from beef lung. Pork mucosal heparin is more abundant, less expensive, and most commonly used. The U.S. Pharmacopoeia (USP) unitage—i.e., units of activity per mL—for both forms is the same, but there is a difference in their anticoagulant actions on a weight basis—that is, 1 mg of porcine heparin has more anticoagulant activity than 1 mg of beef lung heparin. The rare patient who develops a sensitivity to pork mucosal heparin may need to be switched to heparin derived from beef lung.

What drugs interact with heparin?

Some medications such as aspirin, nonsteroidal antiinflammatory agents, and dextran may enhance the effectiveness of heparin and cause bleeding. Cardiac glycosides, nicotine, quinine, and tetracycline interfere with or decrease heparin's effectiveness.

What is the unit measurement of heparin?

The official USP unit is that quantity of heparin that prevents clotting of 1 mL of sheep plasma for 1 hour under specified conditions.

The heparin concentration commonly used in dialysis is 1000 units/mL. The same number of units of either lung or mucosal heparin produces an equivalent degree of anticoagulation. It should be noted that the international unit values used in Britain and Europe differ slightly from the USP unit in anticoagulant activity.

How is the heparin dosage determined?

The patient's heparin dosage is prescribed by the physician and is generally based on the patient's dry weight. Dosage adjustments need to be made if the patient has a change in weight, changes in the length of treatment, or dialyzer membrane changes. Erythropoietin may increase heparin requirements, necessitating an increase in the prescribed amount. The heparin dosage must be low enough to reduce the risk of bleeding yet high enough to prevent clotting of the extracorporeal circuit. With adequate heparinization, the patient will have better clearance of solutes through the dialyzer membrane. Adequate heparinization will also help the dialyzer to clear more thoroughly, allowing the patient to receive as many red blood cells as possible when the patient's blood is returned to him or her at the end of the treatment. Because chronic outpatient dialysis units are not able to monitor clotting times due to Clinical Laboratory Improvement Act (CLIA) mandates, dialysis personnel have to be attentive to indications that the patient may require more or less heparin requirements. Clotting of the dialysis system, poor clearance of the dialyzer posttreatment, and inadequate urea clearance may all indicate a need of additional heparin dosing. Excessive bleeding or bruising posttreatment may indicate a need to decrease heparin dosing.

What techniques are used in heparin administration?

Systemic heparinization is when an initial loading dose of heparin is given predialysis treatment. It is typically a dose ordered by the physician and based on body weight. An initial bolus of heparin is administered intravenously after the needles are placed and no further heparin is administered. Dialysis personnel may administer additional heparin based on the patient's orders if the system appears to be clotting during the dialysis treatment.

Describe the intermittent intravenous heparin technique.

An activated clotting time (ACT) test is first performed. Normal is about 60 to 90 seconds. An intravenous priming dose of heparin is given at the beginning of dialysis, and smaller doses are repeated intermittently throughout the procedure. The usual objective is to maintain the ACT at about three times the baseline. In acute dialysis, when the patient could have a problem with bleeding, heparin dosage is set to give a clotting time between 150 and 180 seconds. Alternatively, given the CLIA limit on performing clotting times, the circuit can be rinsed at 30- to 60-minute intervals with about 100 mL of saline, the fibers and air-blood interface of both drip chambers inspected for signs of early clotting, and the heparin dose adjusted as needed. Naturally, the ultrafiltration (UF) goal must be increased to remove this extra fluid infusion.

The priming dose, most often around 25 to 50 units/kg of body weight, is given either through the venous side of the vascular catheter or via the last needle placed, if the patient has a graft or fistula. The latter method is intended to prevent any oozing of blood or hematoma formation if there is any difficulty with the initial needle insertion. In the few minutes before the patient is attached to the dialyzer, the entire blood volume will become anticoagulated. This is called *systemic heparinization.*

Describe the continuous infusion technique of intravenous heparin.

A priming, or "loading," dose of heparin is given as previously described. Heparin is then slowly injected into the extracorporeal system at a constant rate by an infusion pump. This is continued throughout the dialysis, usually at a rate of 1000 to 2000 units/hr. Clotting is evaluated at intervals, usually by saline flushes and visual inspection of drip chambers and/or dialyzer fibers, and the heparin infusion rate is adjusted accordingly. The infusion is normally stopped 30 minutes to 1 hour before the end of the treatment to allow the clotting time to begin its return to normal, especially for those patients from whom needles must be removed postdialysis.

What is the danger of bleeding when heparin is used for hemodialysis?

There is always a danger of bleeding when heparin is used. Uremic patients tend to bleed easily. One must be particularly concerned about any patient who has had surgery within the preceding 24 to 48 hours or is scheduled for surgery immediately postdialysis, who has recently been injured, has pericarditis, or may have a hemorrhagic lesion of the gastrointestinal tract or uterus.

Are there special techniques for using heparin in hemodialysis when there is danger of bleeding?

Three approaches have been used for this situation: regional heparinization; low-dose, or "tight," systemic heparinization; or no-heparin/saline flush techniques.

What is regional heparinization?

In regional heparinization, an anticoagulant is infused continuously into the inlet (arterial) line of the dialyzer while simultaneously neutralizing it by infusing an antidote into the outlet (venous) line before the blood returns to the patient.

In the past, heparin was used as the anticoagulant and protamine sulfate, a low–molecular-weight protein derived from salmon sperm, was infused into the venous line. Protamine, a strongly basic protein, bound the acidic heparin and thus neutralized its effect on the coagulation system. However, because of a number of difficulties—precise balancing of dosage of each infusion, a tendency toward rebound anticoagulation several hours postdialysis, and protamine-induced anaphylaxis—this method is rarely used today.

An alternative method of regional anticoagulation involves the use of sodium citrate. Regional citrate anticoagulation works by binding the ionized calcium present in the extracorporeal circuit; calcium ions are essential for clot formation. This technique involves infusing trisodium citrate into the arterial line. A calcium-free dialysate must be used. Since returning blood with a decreased ionized calcium to the patient would be dangerous, the process is reversed by the infusion of calcium chloride into the venous line as close as possible to the vascular access connection.

The major disadvantages of this technique are that frequent laboratory tests must be done to check the patient's total calcium level as well as clotting times. Metabolism of the citrate produces bicarbonate. Plasma level of bicarbonate will increase, occasionally to significantly alkalotic levels. (An alternative version uses a large volume of dilute sodium citrate, normal dialysate, and no calcium infusion. The disadvantages are minimized, but UF goals must be adjusted to remove the extra fluid.)

Both types of regional anticoagulation require a high level of experience, skill, and attention to detail. With the low-dose/"tight" systemic and heparin-free techniques available today, regional methods are generally reserved for the most critically ill acute dialysis patients.

What is low-dose, or "tight," heparinization?

Low-dose, or "tight," heparinization consists of monitoring the patient with frequent clotting times and administering only enough heparin to keep the clotting time at 90 to 120 seconds by ACT. Low-dose, or "tight," heparinization is usually the most practical technique for managing the patient who is at risk for bleeding. These would include patients who have recently had surgery, those who are menstruating, or if the patient is having the central venous catheter removed posttreatment. A baseline clotting time is drawn through the first dialysis needle inserted, and this acts as a guide to the size of the priming dose and maintenance heparin requirements. After the administration of the minimal priming dose, usually 10 units/kg, heparin dosage is adjusted to provide an ACT of 110 ± 10 seconds.

In some centers, low-dose, or "tight," heparin is used for the patient's first dialysis treatment. After several treatments a consistent dose of heparin can be established. However, due to CLIA restrictions, anticoagulation methods that require the use of clotting time determinations present a problem.

Can patients be hemodialyzed without heparin?

Heparin-free dialysis has become the method of choice when treating actively bleeding patients and in those with an increased risk of bleeding, pericarditis, coagulopathy, or thrombocytopenia.

Several techniques can be utilized, but most commonly the following are used:
- The bloodlines and dialyzer are rinsed with saline containing 3000 units of heparin/L. The saline priming dose with the heparin is then discarded. No heparin is used for the saline prime of dialyzers for patients who are at very high risk of bleeding (e.g., patients with liver disease).
- The blood flow rate is set as high as possible, 350 to 450 mL/min if it can be tolerated.
- The dialyzer is rinsed with 100 to 200 mL of saline as often as every 15 minutes but at least every hour. This is done by occluding the "arterial" line and infusing the saline rapidly. The dialyzer is visually inspected if possible for clotting during the rinse. The extra saline should be added to the UF goal unless the patient needs the extra fluid volume.

Some facilities do not prime the system with heparin when the patient is running heparin free and will only utilize half hourly or hourly saline rinses to monitor for clotting in the dialyzer or venous drip chamber.

Can blood be transfused into at-risk patients during heparin-free dialysis?

Blood transfusions can complicate heparin-free dialysis, especially because they commonly involve packed red blood cells (RBCs). The transfused blood increases the viscosity of the blood in the dialyzer and may infuse clinically significant amounts of normal (i.e., nonuremic) clotting factors. A modification of the standard method for blood transfusion involves the use of a large-bore three-way stopcock inserted between the patient's access and the tip of the venous bloodline (Fig. 12-2). The stopcock is positioned to run three ways simultaneously so that the transfused blood enters the flow of dialyzed blood returning to the patient; the blood bag is either elevated 1 m

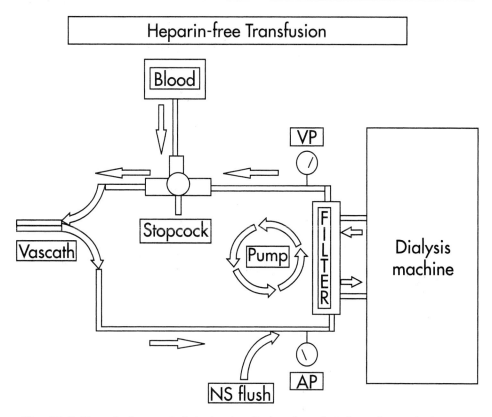

Fig. 12-2 Transfusion and dialysis circuit showing direction of transfusion and blood flow. *(From Sepulveda S, Davis L, Schwab S: Blood transfusion during heparin-free hemodialysis,* Kid Int *51:2018-2021, 1997.)*

above the patient or fitted with a pressure bag inflated to 300 mm Hg. The other parameters—saline flushes, blood flow rate, etc.—remain the same as used in heparin-free dialysis.

How can vascular catheter patency be protected between treatments?

Although the anticoagulation methods need not be altered for use with vascular catheters, the method used for the "heparin lock" to preserve catheter patency between treatments has significant clinical implications. It is essential to keep sufficient heparin within the catheter lumen to prevent clotting, yet prevent any of the heparin from entering the circulation of an at-risk patient. The following method should be used. After dialysis, flush each lumen (side) of the catheter with 10 mL normal saline to clear it of blood cells, then rapidly instill a volume of 5000 units/mL heparin sufficient to exactly displace the saline in the catheter lumen and clamp the lumen immediately. The key is to inject precisely the volume of 5000 units/mL heparin that the catheter can hold so that there is no excess to go into the patient and to inject it fast enough so that it does not mix with the saline and become diluted. This volume can be determined by noting the individual volume printed on each vascular catheter and injecting exactly that amount. Some facilities prefer not to use 5000 units/mL heparin to close the patient's catheters and will instill 1000 units/mL heparin.

What are contributing factors that prevent hemorrhage during hemodialysis?

Success in preventing hemorrhage during the dialysis procedure rests on the general management of the patient and the care with which the dialysis is done. The bleeding tendency of uremic patients is correctable with adequate dialysis. The technique used for anticoagulation during dialysis is an important part of the process because any coagulation in the extracorporeal circuit will impair treatment outcome. Thus the timely institution of an adequate dialysis program is an important initial factor in the prevention of hemorrhage, but subsequent success depends on careful and continuous attention to all of the factors related to optimal treatment adequacy.

How is the effect of heparin measured clinically?

Heparin effect is estimated by the increase in the length of time necessary for a clot to form. There are several laboratory methods for this, including Lee-White clotting time, activated partial thromboplastin time (APTT or PTT), and ACT, discussed later. The clinician should be aware of the impact of CLIA (1992). Although CLIA was intended to apply to noncertified employees doing lab tests in doctors' offices, its broad wording encompasses all lab tests done by nonlaboratory-certified personnel in any setting. Thus CLIA effectively prohibits dialysis staff from performing clotting time determinations on acute and chronic hemodialysis patients unless provision is made for appropriate staff and equipment certification.

Which tests are best for clinical hemodialysis?

Normally one of three tests is used for monitoring clotting times during dialysis. The first of these is the Lee-White clotting time, which is performed by putting 0.4 mL of blood into a tube and inverting the tube every 30 seconds until the blood clots. Because of the long clotting times involved, poor standardization, and poor reproducibility, it is the least desirable method to use during dialysis. Normal clotting times with this test are 6 to 17 minutes.

The second test is the PTT. This test must be performed in the laboratory and is reliable only at lower levels of anticoagulation.

The third test is the ACT. It is similar to the PTT but uses siliceous earth in the tube to hasten the clotting process. The test is done by an automated method that has

Box 12-1	
PROTOCOL FOR ACTIVATED CLOTTING TIMES	
Regular control	150 to 180 sec
Moderate control	105 to 150 sec
Tight control	90 to 120 sec

excellent reproducibility. Evaluation of heparin effect can be done in 180 to 275 seconds. Because of this, the ACT test is easily used in dialysis units. Blood samples are drawn from the "arterial" line before the infusion of heparin, reflecting the status of the patient's circulation rather than the extracorporeal circuit. Box 12-1 gives a protocol for clotting time using the ACT method.

13 Medication Problems and Dialysis

Dialysis patients routinely take an average of 10 different medications and experience adverse drug reactions at least three times more frequently than the general population (Jick, 1977; St Peter et al, 1997). To optimize drug outcomes, health professionals must be prepared to recognize and manage problems associated with medication use. Table 13-1 lists several problematic reactions to medications that clinicians encounter in providing care to patients on dialysis and other patients with renal impairment.

All these problem areas are complex and require consideration of multiple factors unique to each situation, including patient characteristics (e.g., severity of renal impairment, acuity or chronicity of renal failure, comorbidities, age, nutritional status), drug properties (e.g., pharmacokinetics, pharmacodynamics, dose, route), and the dialysis procedures (e.g., type, equipment, duration). The purpose of this chapter is to emphasize the pharmacologic principles common to managing these problem areas and overview each problem area briefly.

How do drugs cause renal impairment?

The rate of drug-induced nephrotoxicity ranges from a fraction of 1% in the general population to as high as 90% in at-risk patients (Bailie, 1995). There are several reasons the kidneys are particularly vulnerable to damage by drugs. The kidneys only constitute 0.4% of body weight, but receive 20% to 25% of total blood flow. This disproportionate blood flow exposes kidneys excessively to drugs in the blood. In addition, drugs are concentrated as the tubular filtrate passes through the nephron and water is reabsorbed. Tubular transport systems further concentrate drugs in the filtrate. Enzymes in the kidney may metabolize drugs to metabolites that are nephrotoxic. In renal insufficiency, the remaining functional nephrons are even more susceptible to nephrotoxins.

Drugs contribute to nearly 30% of acute renal failure in hospitalized patients (Davidman et al, 1991). The most commonly implicated pharmacologic nephrotoxins are antibiotics (aminoglycosides, cephalosporins, pentamidine, amphotercin B), radiocontrast agents used for radiologic studies, cyclosporine, cisplastin, angiotensin-converting enzyme (ACE) inhibitors, and nonsteroidal antiinflammatory drugs (NSAIDs). Because of the development of new agents (e.g., lower osmolar radiocontrast agents), changing drug use patterns (e.g., decreased use of aminoglycosides), and the shift of care from inpatient to outpatient settings, NSAIDs and ACE inhibitors are increasingly

Table 13-1	Problem Areas Involving Drugs
Problem area	**Corresponding responsibility of dialysis personnel**
Drugs can damage kidneys, initiating or worsening renal failure.	Monitor renal function of patients on drugs or drug combinations that can damage kidneys. Identify patients at high risk for renal damage from drugs. Avoid or use extreme caution with drugs that damage renal function in high-risk patients and those with existing renal disease. Initiate hydration and other documented measures to minimize nephrotoxicity.
Pharmacologic activity of drugs is altered by renal failure.	Adjust dosages to compensate for altered pharmacokinetic and pharmacodynamic activity. Monitor for therapeutic failure, adverse effects, or toxicity of all drugs used. Anticipate more adverse effects in patients with renal impairment.
The amount of medication removed from the body during dialysis varies, depending on the characteristics of the drug and dialysis conditions.	Using references and formulas, estimate how much drug is removed by dialysis. Calculate dosage adjustments and/or postdialysis replacement dosage. Monitor clinical response to calculated doses and alter the dosage as indicated.
Some poisons or drugs taken in overdose can be removed wholly or in part by dialysis.	Know which poisons and overdosed drugs can be removed by various dialysis procedures. Implement dialysis to treat poisoning and overdose, providing appropriate supportive care and observation during the procedure.
Medications may increase risks associated with the dialysis procedure.	Know what medications the patient is taking. Monitor for excess effects of the medication.

predominant causes of transient acute renal failure. In chronic outpatient settings, end-stage renal failure can occur due to combination analgesics—which consist of either aspirin or an NSAID combined with acetaminophen, caffeine, and/or codeine. Although the agents specifically cited here are the most frequent causes of renal damage, numerous other medications from diverse drug categories cause renal damage. Whenever a patient evidences renal impairment, a careful analysis of the drug profile for potential drug nephrotoxicity should be conducted. Nephrotoxins should be avoided in patients with renal insufficiency or used with appropriate dosage adjustments and meticulous monitoring.

Describe the mechanisms by which these drugs usually cause renal damage.

Several mechanisms of renal damage by drug nephrotoxins have been identified (Zarama and Abraham, 1997), but most nephrotoxins damage the kidneys through more than one. Hemodynamic mechanisms involve inhibition of regulatory and compensatory processes, nonspecific renal vasoconstriction, or altered colloid oncotic pressure. A primary example of hemodynamic mechanisms for nephrotoxicity includes transient acute renal failure from inhibition of the renin-angiotensin-aldosterone system by ACE inhibitors in patients with renal artery stenosis. A second example is the inhibition of prostaglandin-dependent renal blood flow by NSAIDs in patients with conditions associated with decreased renal blood flow (e.g., volume depletion and congestive heart failure). Renal vasoconstriction is a hypothesized mechanism of renal damage from propranolol, mannitol, combination of triamterene and indomethacin, and the initial months of cyclosporine therapy. Dextran-40 can elevate oncotic pressure and impair glomerular filtration.

Another mechanism of damage is renal vascular alterations, such as thrombotic microangiopathy, that may result from oral contraceptives, cyclosporine, mitomycin C, cisplatin, and quinine. Glomerular alterations that result in nephrotic syndrome and glomerulonephritis are more often immune than toxic effects. The most common drug-induced glomerular alteration is membranous nephropathy that occurs with oral and parenteral gold therapy and penicillamine. Less common glomerular toxicities include the following: minimal change nephrotic syndrome associated with NSAIDs, ampicillin, rifampin, phenytoin, and lithium; focal segmental glomerulosclerosis secondary to heroin abuse; and membranoproliferative glomerulonephritis from hydralazine, interferon-alpha, and interleukin-2. Toxic drug effects resulting in acute tubular necrosis are most often caused by aminoglycosides, radiographic contrast media, cisplatin, amphotericin B, pentamidine, and foscarnet. Tubulointerstitial disease takes several forms and is commonly manifested as one of the following conditions: an acute allergic interstitial nephritis from antibiotics (e.g., penicillins, cephalosporins, tetracyclines, sulfonamides, fluoroquinolones), NSAIDs, diuretics, and anticonvulsants; chronic interstitial nephritis from lithium and cyclosporine; and papillary necrosis from analgesics (e.g., NSAIDs, aspirin, and acetaminophen used alone or in combination) or high-dose dapsone therapy.

Obstructive nephropathies from drugs include uric acid nephropathy during chemotherapy; rhabdomyolysis from phencyclidine, adrenergic drugs including terbutaline, cocaine, vasopressin infusion, erythromycin, and systemic cholesterol-lowering drugs, especially HMG CoA reductase inhibitors (e.g., lovastatin, atorvastatin, simvastatin); and urinary tract outflow obstruction from anticholinergic drugs (e.g., tricyclic antidepressants, disopyramide), cyclophosphamide, and methysergide.

How can renal damage from such drugs be minimized or avoided?

Naturally, drugs with potential to cause renal damage should be avoided or used cautiously in patients with high risk for renal impairment. Conditions that predispose to renal damage by drugs include use of multiple nephrotoxins, sodium or fluid depletion, preexisting renal disease, and low renal blood flow in patients with diseases like congestive heart failure and cirrhosis (Davidman et al, 1991; Zarama and Abraham, 1997). Often drug-induced renal damage is reversible if the drug is discontinued and supportive care initiated before permanent effects occur. Giving saline intravenously may decrease damage by some nephrotoxins such as cyclosporine and cisplatin by diluting the concentration of the drug in the renal tubule. Misoprostol, a prostaglandin analog, may prevent NSAID nephropathy. Drugs with the least nephrotoxic potential should be selected. For example, acetaminophen, aspirin, nonacetylated salicylates, sulindac, or nabumetone may have less nephrotoxicity than other NSAIDs. Finally, drugs should be given in the lowest effective doses for the shortest possible duration.

How does renal failure itself alter response to medications?

The changes that accompany renal failure can alter drug response by two major mechanisms: pharmacodynamics and pharmacokinetics. Medications chemically interact with receptors on cell membranes or on enzymes to cause their effects. This interaction is known as pharmacodynamics and can be thought of as what the drug does to the body. Adverse effects (also called side effects or toxic effects) occur when a drug or metabolite acts at receptors other than the target receptors or when excess drug is present at the target receptor. Uremic substances in the blood or altered electrolyte concentrations resulting from renal failure can modify the drug-receptor interaction, resulting in altered drug effect. Altered receptor sensitivity is thought to be responsible for increased central nervous system effects of narcotics, sedatives, and hypnotics, as well as for the resistance to effects of epinephrine and other catecholamines that occurs in uremic patients. Altered electrolyte and acid-base balance also affect the response to such medications as antiarrhythmics, digoxin, phenothiazines, and antidepressants.

The magnitude and persistence of drug action depend on the duration and concentration of the drug in proximity to the receptor. This relationship of time and drug concentration is known as pharmacokinetics and can be thought of as how the body acts on the drug through the processes of absorption, distribution, metabolism, and excretion. How renal failure affects pharmacodynamics is not well understood. On the other hand, many of the effects of altered pharmacokinetics in patients on dialysis have been sufficiently studied to develop mathematical formulas for calculating drug dosage. Decreased renal excretion is the most obvious alteration in pharmacokinetics resulting from renal dysfunction, but each of the other pharmacokinetic processes may also be altered.

What are the pharmacokinetic parameters that reflect alterations caused by renal failure?

Several measurement parameters can be computed for each drug to represent its pharmacokinetic profile. These include bioavailability, volume of distribution, clearance, and elimination half-life. Bioavailability, which is abbreviated F for fraction, is the measure of drug absorption. Bioavailability is the percentage of the administered dose that gets absorbed into the systemic circulation.

Each drug has a unique pattern of distribution throughout the body, represented as its apparent volume of distribution (V_d). Volume of distribution is the hypothetical volume that would be required to contain the dosage of drug at its concentration in the plasma. For example, if 500 mg of a drug were administered to a patient and an hour later the concentration of the drug in a sample of his plasma was 0.001 mg/mL, the V_d would be 500 L. Stated another way, if each milliliter of plasma had 0.001 mg in it, 500 L would be required to contain 500 mg. Although V_d is an abstraction, it can be interpreted to reflect the distribution characteristics of a drug. If the V_d is 5 L (0.06 L/kg), it is likely most of the drug stays in the intravascular space. If the V_d is more than 46 L (0.7 L/kg), the drug is sequestered in the peripheral tissues, usually dissolved in fatty tissues or bound to tissues. Drugs with large volumes of distribution are poorly dialyzable because most of the drug is outside the bloodstream and therefore not exposed to the dialysis membrane. V_d is used in the calculation of loading doses.

The two modes of elimination, metabolism and excretion, are measured as drug clearance (CL). Clearance is defined as the rate of removal of a drug in proportion to its concentration in the plasma. Clearance is reported as the volume of plasma cleared of the drug per unit of time. Therefore, if the plasma concentration of a drug is 0.002 mg/mL and the body eliminates 2 mg/hr, the clearance is 1 L/hr or about 17 mL/min. (This is because, in such cases, 1000 mL or 1 L of plasma is needed to contain 2 mg at a concentration of 0.002 mg/mL.) Like volume of distribution, clearance is a useful abstraction, rather than a concrete reality. CL is useful for calculating the maintenance dose of a drug. In the patient with renal impairment and lower clearance, lower maintenance doses are needed.

Elimination half-life ($t_{1/2}$) is an indicator of how long a drug stays in the body. It is the time required for half of the drug to be eliminated and is manifested clinically as the time required for the concentration in the blood to decline 50%. Half-life is prolonged by large V_d or by slow CL, which are both pharmacokinetic changes common in renal failure. The relationship among half-life, volume of distribution, and clearance is:

$$t_{1/2} = 0.7 \times V_d/CL$$

What factors affect absorption of medications in patients with renal failure?

In uremia the breakdown of urea in the gastrointestinal tract may raise pH and slow absorption of acid drugs, such as aspirin, iron preparations, and diuretics. Gastroparesis and gastrointestinal responses to uremia (nausea, vomiting, and diarrhea) may significantly alter the absorption of oral medication. Antacids, commonly used to bind dietary phosphate in ESRD, diminish absorption of drugs by forming unabsorbable compounds with drugs like digoxin, iron preparations, and some antibiotics (e.g., tetracyclines and fluoroquinolones). Drugs used to suppress gastric acid secretions such as H_2 blockers (e.g., cimetidine, ranitidine, famotidine), antacids, and proton pump inhibitors (omeprazole, lansoprazole) affect the absorption of some drugs. For example, ketoconazole, which requires an acid environment for absorption, decrease bioavailability in patients taking drugs that suppress gastric acidity, whereas oral penicillins, which are inactivated by gastric acid, improve absorption when patients take these agents.

Orally administered drugs pass through the liver before reaching the main circulation, and large portions of a dose of drugs like morphine, propranolol, and codeine are metabolized during this "first pass" through the liver. Because the first-past effect reduces the bioavailability (F) of orally administered morphine, the oral dose of morphine must be much larger than the injected dose to achieve the same amount of pain relief. In uremia, the fraction of drug metabolized by this first-pass effect may be decreased, unchanged, or increased because some metabolic by-products of uremia change the activity of liver enzymes. Thus bioavailability of drugs is highly variable in renal failure.

Drugs are absorbed across the peritoneum when administered into the dialysate. Antibiotics are frequently given via this route, which results in high concentrations at the site of a peritoneal infection. Some patients have experienced improved diabetic control with intraperitoneal administration of insulin. Administration of drugs by the peritoneal route will result in a different plasma profile than oral or parenteral administration, usually with delayed onset, decreased peak plasma concentration, and prolonged duration of action. Presence of peritonitis will alter the bioavailability of drugs administered peritoneally.

What factors affect distribution of medications in patients with renal failure?

Once a drug is absorbed into the blood, some molecules bind to proteins in the plasma. Drugs that are highly bound to plasma proteins in the blood usually have small V_d because most of the drug molecules are attached to plasma protein, which normally cannot exit the blood vessels. Drugs that predominantly exit from the blood and bind to muscles or dissolve in fatty tissue in the periphery have large V_d. In general, drugs with small V_d have short half-lives because they are mostly in the plasma, which frequently passes through the liver and kidney (and dialysis machine), where they are eliminated. Conversely, drugs with a large V_d have longer half-lives and less susceptibility to removal by dialysis. Edema and ascites often increase V_d and will increase the half-life of drugs that normally have small distribution volumes.

Plasma protein binding of acidic drugs to albumin may be decreased in renal failure as a result of either decreased concentration of albumin or decreased capacity of the albumin to bind to drugs. Changes in protein binding can alter V_d and the drug effect because only the free drug is pharmacologically active. Decreased albumin binding is thought to contribute to the central nervous system toxicity of acid drugs like theophylline, phenytoin, penicillin, phenobarbital, and salicylates in uremia. Some alkaline drugs (e.g., lidocaine, phenothiazines, propranolol, quinidine, and tricyclic antidepressants) that bind to glycoprotein also undergo increased or decreased binding in renal disease, but the clinical relevance of these changes is not as well studied as albumin binding. Although changes in V_d and plasma protein binding theoretically could have substantial effect on drug response, current research suggests the effects of altered V_d in renal disease are usually minimal. There are a few exceptions, in which these changes require modification in the approach to patient care. An example is decreased protein binding of phenytoin during renal failure, which must be considered in clinical management. Measured serum concentrations of phenytoin that reflect total (bound + free) drug concentration in the plasma often are reported in the subtherapeutic range in patients with renal failure. This is because the amount of phenytoin bound to albumin is decreased, but the fraction of unbound drug is increased. Because the unbound drug is the active portion, lower drug concentrations of phenytoin are desirable for patients in renal failure to achieve the desired effect (Aweeka, 1995). In some centers both free and total phenytoin drug concentrations are measured to avoid toxicity. In patients without renal disease, protein binding is about 90% of the total drug, whereas in ESRD binding of phenytoin ranges from 65% to 80%. Another approach to interpretation of phenytoin levels in ESRD patients is to use a correction formula that adjusts the reported phenytoin plasma concentration for albumin level, renal function, and decreased affinity of phenytoin for albumin in ESRD (Liponi et al, 1984).

What factors affect elimination of medications in patients with renal failure?

Some drugs are cleared almost exclusively in their original chemical form by renal excretion; these drugs are said to be excreted unchanged. Other drugs undergo alteration of chemical structure by enzymes, a process called biotransformation or metabolism. Most drugs are cleared by a combination of hepatic metabolism and renal excretion. Metabolites (form drugs take after chemical alteration by metabolism) are usually more water soluble than the original drug and are usually eliminated by the kidneys. Active metabolites retain the ability to bind to a receptor and elicit the same effect as the original drug. Inactive metabolites are usually insignificant because they do not stimulate the target receptor. Toxic metabolites are those that cause an adverse effect at a site different from the target receptor.

When a drug that is normally cleared unchanged by the kidneys is repeatedly administered to a patient with renal insufficiency, it begins to accumulate in the blood and may cause adverse effects. Increased portions of the drug may be eliminated by alternate routes such as hepatic metabolism or through the lungs, bile, or sweat glands. Metabolites of drugs accumulate in renal insufficiency, and active or toxic metabolites contribute to adverse effects. An example is normeperidine, a metabolite of meperidine, which causes stupor or seizures when it accumulates. Box 13-1 includes examples of

Box 13-1

EXAMPLES OF DRUGS WITH ACTIVE OR TOXIC METABOLITES

Acetaminophen	Diazepam	Methyldopa
Allopurinol	Enalapril	Nitroprusside
Amiodarone	Fluoxetine	Procainamide
Azathioprine	Glyburide	Propoxyphene
Buspirone	Levodopa	Quinidine
Cefotaxime	Meperidine	Triamterene
Cimetidine	Metronidazole	Verapamil

drugs with active or toxic metabolites that may accumulate in renal failure. If viable alternatives exist, drugs with active or toxic metabolites are avoided in patients with renal failure. When drugs with active or toxic metabolites are used in renal failure, decreased dosages may be required and clinical monitoring must be vigilant. For example, patients with renal impairment taking allopurinol for gout or cancer require lower dosages than those with normal renal function because an active metabolite of allopurinol can cause exfoliative dermatitis when it accumulates in the body. Although far less important than active metabolites, inactive metabolites may also have consequences. For example, the accumulation of inactive metabolites may cause interference with laboratory tests.

Impaired renal function may also affect liver metabolism, decreasing elimination of some drugs (e.g., morphine, clonidine) and increasing metabolism for a few others (e.g., phenobarbital and phenytoin). Renal impairment alters metabolism through accumulation of uremic substances that can induce (speed up) or inhibit (slow down) drug-metabolizing enzymes in the liver. Insulin is metabolized by enzymes in the kidney, so it is more slowly cleared in severe renal disease. Liver metabolism is dependent upon genetic inheritance, diet, environmental pollution, and concurrent administration of other medications; thus the effects of renal dysfunction are likely to be highly variable from drug to drug and person to person. Effects on renal elimination are more predictable: the greater the proportion of drug or its active metabolites eliminated by the kidneys, the more likely that altered dosing will be required for patients with renal impairment and those on dialysis.

How does dialysis affect pharmacokinetics of drugs and poisons?

The kidneys eliminate drugs through several processes. Although dialysis is not a substitute for all these renal processes, some drugs are removed by dialysis. Dialysis may also affect other pharmacokinetic parameters. For example, changes in total body water from pre- to postdialysis will affect the V_d of some drugs. Characteristics of drugs that promote removal by dialysis are as follows: (1) small molecular size, (2) small V_d, (3) water solubility, and (4) low protein binding. If protein binding exceeds 90%, the drug will be negligibly eliminated by dialysis. Drugs are more likely to be removed when the dialyzer membrane is highly permeable and its surface area is large and the blood flow rate and dialysate flow rate are high. Peritoneal dialysis generally provides little drug removal because dialysate flow rate is slower than with other methods, although a greater amount of protein-bound drug can be removed due to large protein losses seen with this mode. Continuous therapy with hemofiltration or continuous hemodialysis for critically ill patients can remove substantial fractions of drugs. Removal of drugs by hemofiltration procedures is determined by the ultrafiltration rate and degree of protein binding. Treatment of drug overdose and poisoning involves application of these principles to decrease serum concentration of the toxic drugs or substance (Winchester and Kriger, 1995). Similarly, poisons with high protein binding or large V_d are not dialyzable. Although many standard references classify a drug as dialyzable or not dialyzable, dialyzability is not an all-or-nothing characteristic. Some drugs are virtually entirely removed by dialysis; others have negligible removal. Many drugs fall somewhere in the middle. The type of dialysis equipment and length of dialysis greatly influence whether a drug is removed. Classification of dialyzability as yes or no is based on an expert's opinion of whether removal is clinically significant—that is, sufficient to remove an overdose—or whether the patient will require dosage replacement.

How should drugs and dosages be selected for the patient with renal impairment or ESRD?

Drug selection for the patient with renal impairment requires consideration of the effect of the drug on kidney function, electrolyte balance, and uremia. Agents that will worsen the disease state or increase metabolic load (Box 13-2) are avoided or used with caution. A drug that increases metabolic load burdens the failing kidney with chemicals that accumulate in renal disease, such as urea, sodium, potassium, or acids. For the patient with ESRD these substances must be removed by dialysis and may affect well-being or cause serious adverse effects, such as cardiac arrhythmia from hyperkalemia. Drugs with nephrotoxic properties are also used with caution in patients with renal impairment. Meticulous monitoring should be incorporated into the patient care plan for patients with renal impairment taking medications that are nephrotoxic or increase metabolic load. Medications should be avoided for self-limiting conditions and those that can be managed by nonpharmacologic methods. Whenever possible, a single agent that can manage several conditions should be selected. For example, in the absence of contraindications such as renal stenosis, an angiotensin-converting enzyme (ACE) inhibitor would be a prudent choice for the patient with both hypertension and congestive heart failure. Well-studied established agents are usually preferred over newly marketed drugs. All other therapeutic considerations being equal, drugs with reliable laboratory assays for drug level are advantageous because the drug level data can enhance clinical monitoring.

The need for and extent of dosage modification in renal impairment depend on the pathophysiology of the disease process and its severity, as well as the pharmacology of the drug. Guidelines for dosage reduction of many drugs can be found in standard drug

---

Box 13-2

EXAMPLES OF DRUGS PRODUCING METABOLIC LOADS

Sodium load

Ampicillin (IV)

Azlocillin (IV)

Antacids

Carbenicillin (IV)

Cephalothin (IV)

Moxalactam (IV)

Polystyrene sulfonate
  (Kayexalate)

Ticarcillin (IV)

Potassium Load

Blood transfusion

Neuromuscular-blocking drugs

Potassium penicillin G (IV)

Salt substitutes

Spironolactone

Triamterene

Magnesium

Laxatives

Antacids

Urea

Dexamethasone

Prednisone

Tetracycline

Acid

Acetazolamide

Aspirin

Methenamine mandelate

Alkali

Antacids

Carbenicillin

---

references such as the *Physicians' Desk Reference,* drug handbooks, and package inserts. Many nephrology textbooks and other sources provide summary tables that include pharmacokinetic parameters in ESRD (e.g., V_d, CL, $t_{1/2}$), recommended dosage adjustments for various levels of renal function, and guidelines for postdialysis replacement doses. An example of a reference table format is shown in Table 13-2. Most of these data and guidelines are based on studies in patients with stable chronic renal failure on maintenance dialysis and may not apply to the unstable acute renal failure patient. Each of the following five steps of dosage selection is defined and discussed in subsequent sections:

1.   Assessment of relevant patient variables
2.   Determination of loading dose
3.   Determination of maintenance dose
4.   Determination of postdialysis replacement dose
5.   Monitoring of drug levels and clinical response

What are the unique assessment requirements related to drug dosing in renal failure?

In addition to the standard assessment of drug allergies, previous drug history, comorbidities, concurrent medications, and baseline laboratory and clinical findings that precede initiation of a new drug in any patient, patients in renal failure require estimation

Table 13-2   Sample Reference Chart for Pharmacokinetic Parameters, Dosage Adjustment, and Dialyzability

Drug name	V_d L/kg	Half-life (hr) Normal	Half-life (hr) ESRD	Cl (mL/min) Normal	Cl (mL/min) ESRD	% Excreted unchanged	Protein bound %	Dialyzable	Method	GFR mL/min >50	GFR mL/min 10-50	GFR mL/min <10
Antimicrobials												
Amphotericin B	0.46	24	40	15	9	5	95	No	I	24	24	24-36
Cephalozin	0.14	1.8	27	60	5	85	80	Yes	I	8	12	24-48
Erythromycin	0.57	2	5	310	90	15	80	No	I	Unch	Unch	Unch
Fluconazole	0.71	32	98	—	—	80	10	Yes	I	24	24-48	48-72
Gentamicin	0.24	2	60	95	2	85	<10	Yes	I	8-12	23	12-24
Penicillin G	0.18	0.7	13	205	10	80	65	Yes	D	Unch	75	25-50
Tetracycline	1.5	9	80	131	14	55	50	—	I	3-12	12-24	24-48
Cardiac Drugs												
Captopril	3	1.9	3.5	1277	69	50	30	Yes	D	Unch	75	50
Clonidine	3.2	8	40	315	65	50	25	No	D	Unch	Unch	50-75
Digoxin	7.1	36	100	160	35	>90	25	Yes	I	24	36	48-96
Hydralazine	1.6	3	>16	430	<80	10	87	No	I	8	8	8-16
Propranolol	3	3.5	3.5	695	695	0	93	No		Unch	Unch	Unch

CNS Drugs: Antiseizure, Analgesics, Hypnotics												
Acetaminophen	1	2	2	400	400	2	15	Yes	I	4	6	8
Pentazocine	—	2	2	—	—	10	65	No	D	Unch	75	50
Phenytoin	0.57	18	9	25	125	5	90	Yes		Unch	Unch	Unch
Phenobarbital	0.75	70	100	9	6	50	55	No	I	Unch	Unch	12-16
Secobarbital	1.42	25	—	4.6	—	Variable	70			Unch	Unch	Unch
Valproate sodium	0.3	12	—	10	—	Variable	95	No		Unch	Unch	Unch
Anticoagulants, Miscellaneous												
Glipizide	0.16	3-7	—	52	—	7	95	No		Unch	Unch	Unch
Heparin	0.06	1	1.5	50	30	50	>90	No		Unch	Unch	Unch
Warfarin	0.11	33	30	3	3	<1	97			Unch	Unch	Unch

D, Dosage adjustment indicated as percent of usual dose; *I*, interval extension as hours between doses; (—), data not available; Unch, unchanged from usual dose and interval.

Sources: Aronoff and Erbeck, 1994; Aweeka, 1995; Bennett et al, 1994; Brater, 1995; Cutler, Forland and Hammer, 1995; Golper and Bennett, 1995; Swan and Bennett, 1997.

of residual renal function and determination of ideal body weight. Because weight may fluctuate between dialysis procedures and because daily dosage requirements usually correspond to lean body weight rather than actual weight in obese or edematous patients, ideal weight is calculated for men as 50 kg plus 2.3 kg for each inch in height over 5 feet. For women, ideal body weight is 45.5 kg plus 2.3 kg for each inch over 5 feet (Aronoff and Erbeck, 1994). Renal function can be determined in the stable patient by laboratory determination of creatinine clearance or estimation of creatinine clearance (CL_{cr}) using the Cockroft-Gault formula:

$$CL_{cr} = \frac{(140 - \text{Age in years}) \, (\text{Lean body weight in kg})}{72 \, (\text{Serum creatinine in mg/dL})}$$

For women the estimate of CL_{cr} is 85% of the calculated value, so the results of the equation above are multiplied by 0.85 to estimate creatinine clearance in women. The Cockroft-Gault formula yields artifactual results for patients on dialysis, so it is not a reliable estimate in these patients.

In addition to assessing residual renal function, the efficiency of extrarenal mechanisms for drug elimination, especially liver function, should be evaluated because concurrent hepatic impairment may necessitate more stringent dose reduction.

What is a loading dose and when is it indicated?

Loading doses are indicated when it is necessary to attain therapeutic plasma concentrations rapidly. Even in patients with normal renal function, loading doses can be dangerous, so this approach should be reserved for serious or life-threatening situations. This technique is most commonly employed in critical care settings. Loading doses are listed in references for some drugs or can be calculated as the product of the desired plasma concentration or "blood level" (Cp) and the volume of distribution of the drug (Swan and Bennett, 1997).

$$\text{Loading dose (mg/kg)} = V_d \, (\text{mL/kg}) \times Cp \, (\text{mg/mL})$$

The computed dose in mg/kg is then multiplied by the patient's ideal weight.

What is a maintenance dose and how is it determined?

Maintenance doses are given regularly, usually once or more daily, but possibly less often in renal failure. Maintenance doses replace the drug eliminated since the previous dose and sustain therapeutic plasma concentrations. If no loading dose is given, plasma concentrations take four half-lives of repeated maintenance dosing to reach steady state. Steady state occurs when the amount of a drug absorbed and the amount eliminated per unit of time are equal. Before steady state, peak plasma concentrations increase with each subsequent dose. At steady state, the mean plasma concentration levels off after four half-lives and peak and trough concentrations are effectively equal from dose to dose at steady state. Generally, dosages should not be adjusted upward until steady state. Because of prolonged half-life for many drugs in renal failure, it may take days to weeks for drugs to reach steady state in these patients. Because the purpose of a maintenance dose is to replace the eliminated drug, the decreased drug clearance in renal impairment requires reduced maintenance doses for agents eliminated unchanged by the kidneys and for agents with active metabolites eliminated by the kidneys. There are three main approaches to dosage reduction: (1) decreased amount of drug given at usual intervals, (2) usual dose of drug with extended time between doses, and (3) a combination of decreased amount and interval extension (Swan and Bennett, 1997). Extension of the time interval between doses causes wide fluctuations between peak and trough levels and is not indicated for drugs with a narrow therapeutic range or where a low serum concentration at the end of the dosing interval may be dangerous. The dosage reduction or combined approach is indicated when more constant serum concentrations are desirable. On dialysis days the recommended dose, as well as replacement doses, should be administered after the procedure is completed. For drugs removed by peritoneal dialysis, the additional dose is added to the usual daily maintenance dose.

Recommended maintenance doses are included in standard references, usually by level of creatinine clearance (or glomerular filtration rate), as illustrated in Table 13-2. These tables offer little individualization of dosage for the patient in renal failure because wide ranges of creatinine clearance are grouped together and the dosage recommendations may be the same for patients with tenfold differences in creatinine clearance. The wide variety of formulas used to calculate individualized maintenance doses include the following:

- *Ratio method.* Ratio methods involve the derivation of a dosage adjustment factor based on the ratio of some parameter in the patient with renal impairment compared with that of a person with normal renal function. One approach uses the ratio between the half-life in normal renal function and the half-life in renal impairment. For a drug with a half-life of 3 hours with normal renal function and 6 hours with renal failure, the ratio would be 3:6, or 1:2. Multiplying the usual dose by this ratio or dividing the usual interval by this ratio derives the therapy for renal failure: A drug usually given 300 mg every 12 hours would be given 150 mg every 12 hours or 300 mg once per day in renal failure. The ratio of creatinine clearance of the patient to normal creatinine clearance can also be used to determine dosage (Brater, 1995). The dosage adjustment factor Q can be computed as follows (Matzke and Frye, 1997):

$$Q = 1 - [f_e(1 - KF)]$$

  where f_e is the fraction of the drug eliminated unchanged by the kidneys, and KF is the ratio of the patient's creatinine clearance to normal creatinine clearance. The usual dose is multiplied by Q to derive an individualized dose for a particular patient with renal impairment. It is also possible to derive the dosage adjustment factors from nomograms. Nomograms are graphs showing relationships among variables. Standardized nomograms have been developed and published for determining dosage in renal failure.
- *Pharmacokinetic method.* The pharmacokinetic method involves measurement of pharmacokinetic parameters for a particular patient. After the patient receives

one or more doses, blood samples are taken from which the V_d, $t_{1/2}$, and CL are derived. These parameters are individualized to the patient and provide the most accurate indications of that patient's drug disposition. From these parameters, the maintenance dose can be computed using the following formula (Brater, 1995):

$$\text{Maintenance dose} = CL \ (\text{L/hr}) \times C_p \ (\text{mcg/mL}) \times t(\text{hrs})$$

where CL is the patient's drug clearance, C_p is the desired plasma concentration, and t is the dosing interval. The pharmacokinetic method is often paired with therapeutic drug monitoring, which involves determination of the plasma concentration of the drug at steady state to validate the dosage selected, and at regular intervals thereafter. Therapeutic drug monitoring can also be used with the other dose calculation methods. Although the pharmacokinetic method yields the most accurate and individualized results, it is useful only when a reliable assay is available for the drug. It is commonly used with drugs with narrow therapeutic margins such as gentamicin, digoxin, and antiarrhythmic drugs.

- *Drug-specific method.* Another method to determine maintenance dose is based on studies on individual drugs published in the literature. The studies establish the relationship between pharmacokinetic parameters (e.g., V_d, total body clearance) and some continuous index of renal function, such as creatinine clearance. For example, the relationship for total clearance and clearance for ganciclovir has been reported as (Sommadossi et al., 1988):

$$CL \ (\text{mL/min/1.8 m}^2) = 1.25 \ (CL_{cr}) + 8.57$$

- Using the creatinine clearance (CL_{cr}) for the patient, the total clearance of ganciclovir can be estimated with this formula. The result of this calculation is then used to calculate the maintenance dose of ganciclovir, using the formula listed above in the pharmacokinetic method.

How is postdialysis replacement dosage determined?

Standard references and texts include recommendations for average postdialysis replacement for drugs that are substantially removed during dialysis. These recommendations vary by procedure because peritoneal dialysis and hemodialysis removes different amounts of drug. For example, for the β-blocker nadolol, which is renally excreted, a 40-mg dose is recommended following hemodialysis, but no supplementation is needed for peritoneal dialysis. Much of the data on which these reference tables were based was collected before recent advances in dialysis equipment affecting membrane function and blood flow rates, so it is likely that standard references underestimate the amount of drug removal during dialysis. Hemofiltration also removes different amounts of drug compared with other dialysis procedures, but research on dosage replacement after this procedure is limited. For drugs with long half-lives, regular maintenance doses may not be needed if the postdialysis replacement dose includes the drug eliminated between dialysis treatments, as well as that removed during the procedure.

For some drugs, the dialysis clearance values have been studied and published in the literature. These drug-specific values can be used to compute the replacement dose. Differences in dialysis equipment (type of membrane, surface area, blood flow rate, length of procedure) must be considered in determining replacement doses from these published values. For patients who have authorized reuse of dialysis filters, dialysis drug clearance may be lower when the filter has had multiple uses (Matzke and Frye, 1997). For increased accuracy, dialysis clearance rates can also be individually calculated based on laboratory measurement of dialysate and serial plasma concentrations. Other procedures base calculations of dialysis clearance on measures of drug concentration in the blood going into the filter and blood leaving the filter.

What are considerations for monitoring drug levels?

All of the methods for determining dosages include physiologic and mathematic assumptions that may not reflect an individual patient's unique and changing physiologic status, so the formulas and guidelines should be considered beginning estimates of dosage requirements to be followed by dosage titration based on patient response. For drugs with valid and reliable laboratory assays, determination of plasma concentration (i.e., therapeutic drug monitoring) can be a useful tool for dosage adjustment. This is often called blood levels, which is an inaccurate term because the test is not run on whole blood but rather on plasma or serum, and the concentration of the drug is not level but fluctuates throughout each dosing cycle. Therefore it is very important that blood samples for drug levels be collected at the correct time. For peak concentrations, blood is usually drawn 1 to 2 hours after an oral dose or 30 to 60 minutes after a parenteral dose, although timing may vary depending upon the characteristics of the drug and route of administration. Trough concentrations are based on blood drawn immediately before the next dose. For some drugs, such as aminoglycosides, both peak and trough values may be collected because the peak value corresponds to therapeutic effect and the trough value may reflect risk of adverse effects with these agents.

Plasma concentrations are interpreted by comparing the patient's measured value to the published therapeutic range for a drug. However, there are several pitfalls in interpreting plasma concentrations. Not all patients get therapeutic or toxic response at the same concentration. It has been estimated that up to 50% of elderly with digoxin concentrations in the therapeutic range are actually experiencing toxic effects and that many older adults are adequately treated with concentrations in the subtherapeutic range. In addition, decreased serum protein binding common in renal disease may also complicate the interpretation of laboratory reports of drug concentration. Laboratories generally report concentrations of total drug, including both bound and free fractions. A change in the ratio of bound to free drug can result in a reported normal serum concentration, when the concentration of free (active) drug is actually at toxic levels. Conversely, a patient may be adequately treated even though the reported serum concentration is subtherapeutic, because the portion of unbound active drug is increased. Some physicians order both total and free drug concentrations and compare the published reports of the normal percentage of drug binding to that reported for an individual patient.

Therefore, even when data on serum concentration are available, clinical data such as the patient's subjective information, physical examination findings, and laboratory results should be used to regulate dosage. Interference with laboratory results by drugs and drug metabolites can be enhanced when drugs accumulate in renal insufficiency. Drug interaction with the laboratory test should be considered when reported laboratory values are inconsistent with the clinical presentation. Box 13-3 lists examples of drug test interactions relevant to dialysis patients. The mechanism of these interactions is interference by the drug or its metabolites with one of the reagents used in the laboratory test. When an abnormal value for one of these common tests is reported, intervention based on the laboratory result should not be initiated until the patient's drug therapy is reviewed for interacting drugs. The laboratory director should be consulted about the resolution of the drug test interaction because an alternate assay methodology could circumvent the interaction.

The importance of clinical monitoring and observation cannot be overstated. Knowledge of the usual pattern of responses of the patient enables the clinician to recognize at an early stage deviations that suggest the need to evaluate the drug regimen.

Can drugs affect the dialysis procedure?

Several drug groups can affect the dialysis procedure. Many patients on dialysis take antihypertensive medications, which can contribute to hypotension during the dialysis procedure. Epoetin therapy is associated with a decrease in the prolonged bleeding time seen in some patients with ESRD and may increase heparin requirement during dialysis

---

Box 13-3
EXAMPLE OF DRUGS THAT INTERFERE WITH LABORATORY TESTS

Serum Creatinine
Ascorbic acid
Aspirin
Cefoxitin
Cimetidine
Levodopa
Methyldopa
Trimethoprim

Serum Uric Acid
Ascorbic acid
Acetaminophen
Aminophylline

Levodopa
Methyldopa
Salicylates

Urinary Protein (dipstick method)
Acetazolamide
Aspirin
Cephalosporins
Contrast media
Penicillins
Sulfonamide antibiotics
Tolbutamide

in some patients. Vascular access thrombosis may be more frequent in those on epoetin, but there is no evidence of increased thrombosis with native arteriovenous fistula (St Peter et al, 1997).

MEDICATION CONSIDERATIONS
Antianemics

People with uremia or on maintenance dialysis are anemic and have considerably lower hematocrit values. Causes include (1) failure of production, or inhibition of action, of erythropoietin, a hormone produced by the kidney that stimulates the bone marrow to produce red blood cells; (2) a shortened life span of the red blood cells; (3) impaired intake of iron; (4) blood loss, including a tendency to bleed from the nose, gums, gastrointestinal tract, uterus, or skin, caused by platelet abnormalities; and (5) blood loss related to the dialysis procedure itself.

How does dialysis influence the anemia?

Incomplete blood recovery after dialysis, dialyzer leaks, and frequent blood sampling contribute to anemia. The patient who is receiving adequate dialysis, is in a good nutritional state, and has adequate iron stores and intake will usually stabilize with a hematocrit between 20% and 30%. It is unusual for the hematocrit to go much higher except in persons with polycystic kidney disease, in whom there may be greater than normal production of erythropoietin.

As the hematocrit improves on dialysis, the patient begins to feel better. These people still have considerably fewer red blood cells than normal and become dyspneic and tire easily. Other symptoms attributable to anemia include poor exercise tolerance, weakness, sexual dysfunction, anorexia, and inability to think clearly.

What is EPO?

Epoetin alfa (EPO) (Epogen, Procrit) is a recombinant form of the hormone erythropoietin, which is produced by the normal, healthy kidney. It was introduced in 1989 and had a profound effect on the ESRD patient.

In appropriate doses it will raise the hematocrit to normal levels. Any ESRD patient with a hematocrit less than 30% should receive EPO. The target hematocrit should be 33% to 36%, depending on patient symptoms.

How is EPO given?

EPO is given either intravenously or subcutaneously, usually three times per week at the end of a regular dialysis treatment.

What are some causes of suboptimal response to EPO therapy?

The National Kidney Foundation (NKF) K/DOQI clinical practice guidelines for anemia of chronic kidney disease identifies the most common cause of inadequate response to EPO therapy as iron deficiency. Nine conditions are cited as potential reasons for a patient's nonresponse. The four most common conditions are infection and inflammation, chronic blood loss, osteitis fibrosa, and aluminum toxicity. The remaining five causes are less common and should only be considered after the first four have been ruled out as causes. These include: hemoglobinopathies (such as sickle cell anemia), folate/vitamin B_{12} deficiency, multiple myeloma, malnutrition, and hemolysis.

Hemoglobin (Hgb) levels in the K/DOQI target range of 11 to 12 g/dL are associated with improved outcomes, including increased energy/activity levels and quality of life, along with decreased risk of hospitalization and mortality.

What are the complications of EPO?

The major complication of EPO is an elevation in blood pressure due to the increased blood viscosity secondary to the increased red blood cell mass. This usually occurs during the initial 12 weeks of therapy, while the hematocrit is rising, and is treated with antihypertensive medications and fluid removal with dialysis.

As the hematocrit rises, the efficiency of dialysis falls somewhat because the red blood cells do not release their toxins (e.g., creatinine, potassium) very readily as they pass through the dialyzer. Close attention to blood chemistries is essential in patients receiving EPO, and some adjustment of the dialysis prescription may be necessary.

When should transfusions be given?

The routine administration of blood at a certain hematocrit value is not done. If the patient suffers a large blood loss from a dialyzer leak or from hemorrhage, the blood should be replaced. If the patient becomes short of breath or excessively fatigued or has angina, a transfusion will often relieve the symptoms. In general, increasing the dose of EPO to improve the anemia is more desirable than transfusion.

What are some of the complications of transfusions?

The most common complications include the following:
- Incompatibility reactions caused by major or minor blood group incompatibility may occur. Chest or back pain, chills, and fever occur soon after blood is started. If this occurs, the transfusion should be stopped immediately. A blood specimen should be drawn from the patient for evidence of hemolysis and for recheck of type and crossmatch. Chills or fever should be treated symptomatically. Intravenous steroids may be used if symptoms are severe.
- Allergic reactions to leukocytes, platelets, or protein of the donor blood may occur. Manifestations include chilling, fever, or skin eruption developing about 30 to 60 minutes after the start of the transfusion. These are treated by slowing the rate of infusion. An antihistamine, such as diphenhydramine (Benadryl), 20 to 50 mg, or steroids should be given intravenously if symptoms are severe.
- Infections—whether caused by hepatitis A, B, or C; cytomegalovirus; Epstein-Barr virus; or human immunodeficiency virus (HIV)—may

be transmitted by blood. The onset is from 1 to 4 months after the
transfusion.
- Preformed antibodies may result from minor incompatibility or allergic reactions. These are particularly important to the patient awaiting a renal transplant. Some dialysis units with transplantation affiliation give a limited number of transfusions on a regular basis. This has an enhancing effect on graft survival.

What can be done to minimize the anemia?

A good dietary intake of protein is important. Adequate iron intake is essential if the patient's iron stores are depleted before starting EPO. Maintenance iron therapy is needed in most patients to ensure adequate iron stores and an optimal response to EPO. Oral iron supplements are rarely adequate. They often cause gastrointestinal upset, nausea, gas, vomiting, or anorexia. Intravenous iron, such as iron dextran, can be given in 100-mg doses, usually for a total course of 1 g, depending on the adequacy of iron stores. In patients on EPO, iron deficiency is almost inevitable because iron is used rapidly under EPO stimulation of red blood cell (RBC) production and is continually lost from the patient. Patients on EPO may benefit from regular administration of small doses of parenteral iron. Folic acid and vitamin B_{12}, both of which are important in RBC formation, are water soluble and theoretically could be depleted by dialysis. Although there is little evidence that these vitamins are seriously deficient, it is the usual practice to give a supplement, particularly of the former.

When is EPO administered?

EPO is administered intravenously (IV) during hemodialysis to stimulate red blood cell production. A predialysis hematocrit is used to monitor anemia and determine EPO administration. Each dialysis unit should follow its own protocol. The amount of EPO required is determined by hematocrit, hemoglobin, and individual patient response. Adequate iron stores and folic acid are required for erythropoietin to be effective. (A serum ferritin of 300 to 500 ng/mL is considered optimal per K/DOQI guidelines.) Although EPO is given mostly IV during hemodialysis, K/DOQI suggests that the subcutaneous route of administration is as effective or more effective than the IV route. The Anemia Work Group recommends that subcutaneous EPO be the preferred route of administration. When given subcutaneously, the site of injection should be rotated. Most hemodialysis patients prefer the IV route because of the discomfort generated by subcutaneous administration.

When is iron therapy required?

The need for iron therapy is determined by two things: First, the serum iron value is divided by the total iron binding capacity, times 100. This is called the transferrin saturation, or TSAT, and correlates with the amount of iron available for erythropoiesis. (Optimal TSAT is 25% to 35%. Less than 20% indicates absolute iron deficiency; more than 50% indicates risk of iron overload, according to K/DOQI guidelines published by the National Kidney Foundation.) Second, if the serum ferritin level is less than 100 ng/mL, iron therapy is prescribed, usually by the IV route.

How is iron administered?

Iron is administered orally and/or IV. Oral iron should not be taken with phosphate binders, which diminish its effect. When oral iron is prescribed, the patient should be instructed to always take the medication with food to avoid gastrointestinal distress. Patients will usually need to supplement oral iron with the IV form at intervals to maintain adequate stores for erythropoiesis. IV iron is given during hemodialysis. The dosage is determined by the patient's starting hematocrit and TSAT. If TSAT is less than 20% and serum ferritin is less than 100 ng/mL, K/DOQI guidelines recommend 50 to 100 mg of iron IV once per week for 10 hemodialysis treatments. However, each facility should follow its own policy. IV iron should be held if the TSAT is greater than 50% or serum ferritin is greater than 800 ng/mL in accordance with K/DOQI guidelines. Iron dextran (Infed) was used most commonly before the newer iron products (Ferrlecit [sodium ferric gluconate] and Venofer [iron sucrose injection]) became available. Today, the newer forms of IV iron have been shown to cause a lower incidence of anaphylaxis than previous generations of IV iron. A test dose is recommended before administering iron dextran products, whereas the other irons do not require a test dose. Various side effects may occur from the administration of IV iron from hypotension (which is usually related to the rate of administration) to cramping, nausea, headaches, and hypersensitivity reactions. IV iron should always be administered according to the manufacturer's instructions.

Can a patient receive too much iron?

Iron overload or hematochromatosis may occur from multiple transfusions, excessive iron intake via diet or medications, receiving iron therapy for anemia not related to iron deficiency, or in those patients with certain genetic markers predisposing them to iron overload. Nausea and vomiting, diarrhea, and elevated liver enzymes may be present.

ANTIHYPERTENSIVES
What is hypertension?

A blood pressure (BP) greater than 140/90 mm Hg is classified as hypertension. Hypertension is commonly seen in the chronic kidney disease (CKD) patient and can be a cause or result of the disease. Hypertension can be attributed to volume overload, increased rennin secretion, uremic toxins, dietary sodium, and secondary hyperparathyroidism. Hypertension can cause left ventricular hypertrophy and other cardiac complications. Both nonpharmacologic and pharmacologic treatment options must be employed to manage the hypertension associated with CKD. A variety of antihypertensive medications are available to treat the patient. It is not unusual for the patient to be prescribed more than one antihypertensive for treatment.

The National Heart, Lung, and Blood Institute classifies two levels of high blood pressure: stage 1 and stage 2 (Table 13-3).

Table 13-3	Categories for Blood Pressure Levels in Adults* (in mm Hg)	
Category	**Systolic (top number)**	**Diastolic (bottom number)**
Normal	Less than 120	Less than 80
Prehypertension	120-139	80-89
High Blood Pressure		
Stage 1	140-159	90-99
Stage 2	160 or higher	100 or higher

*For adults 18 and older who:
Are not on medicine for high blood pressure
Are not having a short-term serious illness
Do not have other conditions such as diabetes and kidney disease
Note: When systolic and diastolic blood pressures fall into different categories, the higher category should be used to classify blood pressure level. For example, 160/80 mm Hg would be stage 2 high blood pressure. There is an exception to the above definition of high blood pressure. A blood pressure of 130/80 mm Hg or higher is considered high blood pressure in persons with diabetes and chronic kidney disease. National Heart Lung and Blood Institute. Diseases and Conditions Index. High Blood Pressure.

Antihypertensive medications are divided into different categories because their mechanisms of action vary by drug. Most of these medications are used for the control of high blood pressure; however, some of the medications are used in the treatment of heart failure, angina, and cardiac dysrhythmias.

WHAT ARE THE DIFFERENT TYPES OF ANTIHYPERTENSIVE MEDICATIONS?
ACE inhibitors

ACE inhibitors work by blocking an enzyme in the body that is responsible for causing the blood vessels to narrow. When the blood vessels are relaxed, blood pressure is lowered. ACE inhibitors also lower the amount of salt in the body, which assists in decreasing the blood pressure. ACE inhibitors have renoprotective effects and are thought to prevent the progression of renal disease in the compromised patient.

ACE inhibitors do cause a number of side effects including dry persistent cough, increased serum creatinine, rash, increased serum potassium, and angioedema. Examples of ACE inhibitors are quinapril (Accupril), ramipril (Altace), captopril (Capoten), benazepril (Lotensin), trandolapril (Mavik), fosinopril (Monopril), lisinopril (Prinivil and Zestril), and enalapril (Vasotec).

Angiotensin-receptor blockers (ARBs)

ARBs are an alternative medication to ACE inhibitors. ARBs block the enzyme angiotensin II, which causes vasoconstriction. ARBs are as effective as, but do not cause the cough sometimes associated with, the ACE inhibitors. Some potential side effects of this medication are headaches, angioedema, and hyperkalemia. Examples of ARBs are losartan (Cozaar), valsartan (Diovan), irbesartan (Avapro), and candesartan (Atacand).

β-Blockers

β-Blockers work by slowing the nerve impulses that travel through the heart. When this happens, the heart has less of a demand for blood and oxygen, which makes it work less hard, thereby decreasing blood pressure. Bradycardia, fatigue, cold hands and feet, weakness, dizziness, dry mouth, wheezing, and swelling of the hands and feet are side effects that might occur from taking a β-blocker.

β-Blockers include timolol (Blocadren), esmolol, (Brevibloc) carteolol (Cartrol), nadolol (Corgard), propranolol (Inderal) metoprolol (Lopressor and Roprol-XL), labetalol (Normodyne and Trandate), acebutolol (Sectral), atenolol (Tenormin), and pindolol (Visken).

Calcium Channel Blockers

Calcium channel blockers slow the rate at which calcium passes into the heart muscle and into the vessel walls. This relaxes the vessels, which allow blood to flow more easily through them, thereby lowering blood pressure. Side effects of calcium channel blockers are headaches, lower leg and ankle edema, fatigue, and stomach discomfort. Examples of calcium channel blockers are amlodipine (Norvasc), bepridil, diltiazem (Cardizem, Cardizem CD, cardizem SR, Dilacor XR, Tiamate, and Tiazac), felodipine (Plendil), isradipine (DynaCirc, DynaCirc CR), nicardipine hydrochloride (Cardene, Cardene SR), nifedipine (Procardia, Procardia XL, Adalat, Adalat CC), nisoldipine (Sular), and verapamil (Calan SR, Covera-HS, Isoptin, Isoptin SR).

Diuretics

Diuretics are recommended as the first line of treatment for high blood pressure. They are usually recommended as one of at least two medications to control hypertension. Diuretics work by restricting the reabsorption of water, promoting diuresis, and removing excess sodium and water from the body. This reduction in total body water reduces blood pressure. Several different types of diuretics work on different areas of the kidneys.

Side effects include frequent urination, weakness, increased thirst, and reduced levels of some electrolytes in the blood (potassium, sodium, and magnesium). Examples of diuretics include chlorthalidone (Hygroton), chlorothiazide (Aldoclor, Diupres, Diuril), hydrochlorothiazide and hydrochlorothiazide combinations (Aldoril, Capozide, Dyazide), bumetanide (Bumex), furosemide (Lasix), and torsemide (Demadex).

CATION EXCHANGE RESIN
What medication is used to treat hyperkalemia?

Sodium polystyrene sulfonate, or Kayexalate, is used in the treatment of hyperkalemia. Kayexalate is a cation exchange resin that replaces potassium ions for sodium ions, mostly in the large intestine. This exchange or lowering of the serum potassium may take hours to days, so this is not an effective method of treating severe hyperkalemia. Kayexalate is administered either orally or by retention enema. Some ESRD patients take Kayexalate regularly to control hyperkalemia. Side effects of this medication may include constipation, diarrhea, nausea, vomiting, hypokalemia, hypomagnesemia, or hypocalcemia, because it is not selective to just potassium.

INTRADIALYTIC PARENTERAL NUTRITION

Intradialytic parenteral nutrition is a form of nutritional support for the patient who has hypoalbuminemia and consists of an emulsion of amino acids, lipids, and dextrose. See Chapter 14 for more information.

LEVOCARNITINE
What is the role of levocarnitine?

Levocarnitine, an amino acid derivative, is sometimes deficient in the patient with ESRD undergoing dialysis therapy. Levocarnitine is similar in shape and size to creatinine, so it can be dialyzed out during the dialysis treatment. Another reason for the deficiency is that the dialysis patient's diet is lacking in red meat and dairy products, which provides a good source for this amino acid. The patient who has been on dialysis for several years will experience a decrease in plasma and skeletal muscle carnitine. Levocarnitine is essential for fatty acid and energy metabolism. Many organs, including the heart, muscle, liver, and kidney rely on levocarnitine as an energy source. Levocarnitine (Carnitor) is a medication used for carnitine deficiency. The benefits of levocarnitine supplementation in dialysis patients are decreased muscle cramps and weakness, decreased intradialytic hypotension, and increased cardiac output and exercise capacity. See Chapter 14 for additional information on carnitine.

PHOSPHATE BINDERS

Disturbances of calcium and phosphorus metabolism are common in patients who develop renal insufficiency gradually and are often apparent even before dialysis is required. During the progression of renal failure there is loss of ability to excrete phosphate. Phosphate ions accumulate in the body fluids and lead to a reciprocal decrease of serum calcium. The parathyroid glands seek to maintain a normal concentration of calcium in body fluid and respond by increasing production of parathyroid hormone (PTH). This causes calcium to be reabsorbed from the bones, resulting in loss of bone density and strength. In addition, the active form of vitamin D, needed for normal bone metabolism, is manufactured in the kidney and is deficient in ESRD patients. Dialysis does not fully correct the disordered calcium-phosphorus metabolism, and progressive osteodystrophy (the term for several bony manifestations) is a serious problem for many ESRD patients.

What is the function of oral calcium as a phosphate binder?

Oral calcium (usually as calcium carbonate), when taken immediately after a meal, binds phosphorus in the stomach so that it passes out with the stool, thereby not contributing to raising the serum phosphorus. This helps control the calcium-phosphorus product. If the calcium is taken too long after eating or on an empty stomach, it may contribute to making the patient hypercalcemic. If a high serum phosphorus with a low serum calcium is left untreated, the parathyroid glands become stimulated and result in loss of calcium from the patient's bones.

How are phosphate binders taken?

Phosphate binders need to be taken with every meal and with snacks containing protein. It is best not to take phosphate binders when oral iron or antibiotics are taken because the efficacy of these medications becomes reduced. Patient compliance with the regular use of phosphate binders is problematic. A major factor contributing to noncompliance with phosphate binder therapy is the number of medications the ESRD patient takes on a regular basis. The addition of phosphate binders, which need to be taken with every meal, is cumbersome, and add to the already sizable number of pills the patient must take. Some of the binders leave a chalky taste in the mouth and may cause constipation, which becomes a deterrent to some patients taking the medication.

Are there different types of phosphate binders?

Several different types of phosphate binders are available to control excess phosphorus in the bloodstream. Aluminum-based phosphate binders (aluminum hydroxide [Alucaps]) were the first type of binders to be used in the ESRD patient. Aluminum-based binders are extremely effective in keeping serum phosphorus levels low because of their high phosphorus-binding ability. These binders, however, have the ability to cause high serum aluminum levels or aluminum toxicity. Aluminum-based binders are therefore seldom used in the ESRD patient today. Calcium-based binders (calcium acetate [Calcichew, Titralac, PhosLo], calcium carbonate) are more commonly used and serve a dual role of decreasing serum phosphorus as well as supplementing calcium in the patient with hypocalcemia. Attention must be given to the patient's monthly laboratory studies to ensure he or she is not becoming hypercalcemic.

A new phosphate binder is available that is both calcium and aluminum free (sevelamer hydrochloride [Renagel]). Sevelamer works in the gastrointestinal tract, where positively charged hydrogel binds with negatively charged phosphate from the diet. The complex formed does not cross the gastrointestinal tract but is instead excreted in the feces. Because sevelamer contains no calcium, the patient will be able to have phosphorus control while keeping the calcium phosphorus product at an acceptable level. Sevelamer must be taken with every meal and when eating between meals.

VITAMINS AND VITAMIN ANALOGS
What are the indications for administering vitamin D analog 1,25-dihydroxyvitamin D_3 (Calcitriol)?

Calcitriol is used to treat hypocalcemia in patients receiving chronic dialysis. It is the active form of vitamin D_3. It increases calcium levels and has been shown to reduce elevated PTH levels, preventing secondary hyperparathyroidism and improving renal osteodystrophy.

How and when is calcitriol administered?

Calcitriol in the intravenous form (Calcijex) is administered during a hemodialysis treatment as an intravenous bolus. An oral form of calcitriol (Rocaltrol) is available.

Are there any adverse effects of treatment with calcitriol?

Hypercalcemia can result from calcitriol treatment. Serum calcium and phosphorus must be evaluated on a regular basis to avoid hypercalcemia that could lead to generalized vascular calcification and soft tissue calcification (eyes, skin, and heart).

When is calcitriol withheld?

Hold the calcitriol (Calcijex) when the serum calcium is between 10.5 and 12.5 mg/dL and the product (calcium mg/dL times the phosphorus mg/dL) is greater than 70. Conversely, hold the calcitriol if the serum calcium is greater than 12.5 mg/dL, even if the product is less than 70.

What is Paricalcitol (Zemplar) injection?

Paricalcitol (Zemplar) is a recent synthetic analog of vitamin D for treatment of secondary hyperparathyroidism. Paricalcitol is given IV to ESRD patients to decrease PTH levels with minimal effect on calcium and phosphorus; however, the calcium phosphorus product should continue to be monitored for elevations. Hypercalcemia will promote digitalis toxicity, so laboratory studies should be monitored closely in the patient taking digitalis. Paricalcitol should never be used in patients with vitamin D toxicity, or hypercalcemia. It is an aggressive treatment of secondary hyperparathyroidism.

What is doxercalciferol (Hectorol)?

Doxercalciferol (Hectorol) is a synthetic vitamin D analog used to suppress PTH and manage secondary hyperparathyroidism. Doxercalciferol is available in either an intravenous or oral form. Hypercalcemia, hyperphosphatemia, and oversuppression of the parathyroid gland are possible adverse effects associated with the use of this medication. The dosing is based on PTH levels along with the monitoring of the serum calcium and phosphorus.

When is deferoxamine mesylate (Desferal) used?

Deferoxamine mesylate (Desferal) is a chelating agent used to remove excessive metals from the bloodstream. It was originally formulated to treat iron overload. Deferoxamine has been found to be useful as an aluminum chelating agent in dialysis patients, and acts to remove aluminum from the tissues so it can be dialyzed out or adsorbed by a special cartridge. The dosage of deferoxamine varies for different patients. The dosage is usually based on body weight and is ordered by the physician. Deferoxamine is usually mixed with 200 mL of normal saline infused during the last 2 hours of the dialysis treatment three times a week. Deferoxamine should be held for 2 weeks after infusion of intravenous iron. Deferoxamine administration may cause visual and auditory disturbances when administered over prolonged periods at high doses. Flushing, urticaria, hypotension, tachycardia, and shock may occur during IV administration, so the patient must be carefully observed during administration.

14 Nutrition Management

Nutrition plays a critical role in the management of renal disease. The diet will vary considerably depending on the type and stage of renal disease as well as on patient and treatment modality-specific factors. A "renal diet" that can be applied to all patients does not exist. Each situation must be evaluated individually. Certain commonalities may apply to patients with chronic and acute renal disease.

Why is diet important for people with renal disease?

Diet therapy offers the following potential benefits:
- It may be helpful in delaying the need for dialysis.
- Diet can help attenuate many of the complications of renal disease (e.g., phosphorus restriction to aid in prevention of bone disease).
- Adequate protein and calorie nutrition can influence morbidity and mortality in patients with renal disease.
- Quality of life for people with end-stage renal disease (ESRD) may be improved by individualization of diet to suit lifestyle, ethnic, and socioeconomic variables.

What is the role of the registered dietitian?

The registered dietitian assesses each patient's needs and makes recommendations to the nephrologist as to the diet prescription. Patient and family are taught specifics of the diet by the dietitian, who monitors nutrition-related parameters and reevaluates needs. The dietitian is responsible for the primary diet education, and functions as a member of the interdisciplinary team. Communication between the dietitian, nurses, technicians, physician, and social worker as to changes in a patient's medical condition, dialysis treatment, medications, psychosocial situation, and nutritional status is critical to providing optimal patient care.

What diet concerns are there before initiation of dialysis?

Before dialysis, the diet is constructed to achieve several goals. One goal is to delay the need for dialysis by slowing the decline of renal function. At present, studies are inconclusive as to whether protein or phosphorus restriction can help slow the progression of renal disease. Kidney Disease Outcomes Quality Initiative (K/DOQI) clinical practice guidelines for chronic kidney disease (CKD) suggest that patients with a glomerular filtration rate (GFR) less than 60 mL/min/1.73 m^2 should undergo assessment of dietary protein and energy intake and nutritional status.

In addition to possible delay in the progression of renal disease, protein restriction, when employed with an adequate caloric intake, can be helpful in minimizing nitrogenous wastes and can aid in the control of uremic symptoms. Diet management can often be effective in delaying the need for dialysis until the GFR falls below about 15 mL/min, at which time some type of renal replacement therapy is necessary. Preservation of nutritional status by the provision of adequate calories to maintain or achieve a desirable body weight and avoid endogenous protein catabolism is of prime importance during this period.

Phosphorus control, by limiting high-phosphorus foods and/or the use of phosphate-binding medications, is often necessary when the GFR falls below 20 mL/min. (Phosphorus control is discussed later in this chapter.)

Another diet concern before the initiation of dialysis is sodium control for the patient who is edematous or hypertensive. But potassium restriction is generally not necessary until urine output falls below 1000 mL/day; therefore, restriction may not be necessary until after dialysis is initiated.

What are the diet modifications for hemodialysis?

The need for dietary modification once hemodialysis begins is highly individualized depending on such factors as height, weight, nutritional status, the level of residual renal function, laboratory data, intercurrent illnesses, and prescribed medications. Maintenance of good nutritional status, as evidenced by adequate anthropometric measurements and biochemical indices, is critically important during this period. Achieving and maintaining a normal serum albumin level is the number one goal of nutrition therapy for the hemodialysis patient. Various studies have demonstrated that the primary biochemical predictor of mortality in hemodialysis patients is a low serum albumin. In the absence of proteinuria or significant liver disease, albumin levels can be maintained with provision of adequate protein and calories. Although the diet is highly individualized, certain diet commonalities do apply to most patients on hemodialysis.

What amount of protein is appropriate for hemodialysis patients?

Protein requirements, as suggested by current research, are thought to be 1.2 ± 0.2 g/kg/day, with the upper end of the range for protein-malnourished patients. In general, at least 50% of this protein should be derived from high biologic–value protein sources such as meat, fish, or poultry. Such protein sources contain a full complement of essential amino acids. Examples of low biologic–value protein are fruits, vegetables, and grains; however, a carefully planned vegetarian diet can be used without compromise of nutritional status (Fig. 14-1). The protein needs of hemodialysis patients are higher than those of the general population, in part because of the loss of 5 to 10 g of amino acid during each hemodialysis treatment.

CLIENT EDUCATION TIPS ON PROTEIN INTAKE

THERE ARE TWO DIFFERENT TYPES OF PROTEIN

One is called animal or high biological protein, which contains ALL essential amino acids.

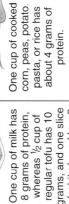

The other type is vegetable or low biological protein, which contains SOME amino acids.

THE HEMODIALYSIS AND THE PERITONEAL MEMBRANE ARE NOT SELECTIVE, WHICH MEANS THAT VITAL AMINO ACIDS AND VITAMINS AS WELL AS UNWANTED WASTES ARE REMOVED

If you are on HEMODIALYSIS, you should aim for **1.2 grams of protein per kg of body weight;** e.g., if you weigh 65 kg (143 lb), your protein intake should be about 78 grams per day.

If you are on PERITONEAL DIALYSIS, you should aim for **1.3 grams of protein per kg of body weight;** e.g., if you weigh 70 kg (154 lb), your protein intake should be about 91 grams per day.

EXAMPLES OF PROTEIN SOURCES

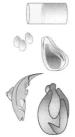

3.5 oz. of extra lean ground beef has 24 grams of protein, whereas rib eye has 28 grams of protein.

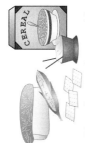

Half of a chicken breast (3.5 oz.) has 29 grams of protein. Turkey white meat (3.5 oz) has 30 grams of protein.

One can of Ensure has 13 grams of protein, whereas 1 scoop of Promod has 5 grams, and one egg has 6 grams of protein.

15 large cooked shrimp have 17 grams of protein. A 3 oz. can of white tuna in water has 22 grams of protein.

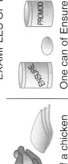

One cup of milk has 8 grams of protein, whereas ½ cup of regular tofu has 10 grams, and one slice of white bread has 2 grams of protein.

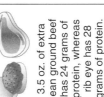

One cup of cooked corn, peas, potato pasta, or rice has about 4 grams of protein.

Fig. 14-1 Renal teaching aids: tips on protein intake. *(From Black JM, Hawks JH, Keene AM: Medical-Surgical Nursing: Clinical Management for Positive Outcomes, ed. 7, Philadelphia, 2005, Saunders. Modified from Darlene Michl, Sidney, British Columbia.)*

What calorie level is advisable?

Energy requirements for hemodialysis patients are not well defined, although they are generally accepted to be 35 kcal/kg/day for maintenance. With stress or malnutrition, calorie needs may be as high as 40 to 45 kcal/kg. For the obese patient, 25 to 30 kcal/kg may be appropriate.

What about potassium control?

Almost all foods contain potassium, and certain fruits and vegetables are particularly rich sources. Once urine output falls below 1 L/day, and in some cases before this happens, potassium should be controlled in the diet. An intake of approximately 70 mEq or 2730 mg of potassium is safe for most hemodialysis patients. The specific dietary potassium intake depends on the size of the patient, the level of potassium in the dialysate, and other factors that may affect the serum potassium level. Factors other than dietary indiscretion may contribute to hyperkalemia, including severe acidosis, constipation, catabolism, insulin deficiency, and the use of certain medications such as β-adrenergic–blocking agents and angiotensin-converting enzyme (ACE) inhibitors. The potassium content of selected foods may be found in Appendix C.

How much sodium is acceptable?

An intake of approximately 87 mEq or 2000 mg/day of sodium is appropriate for most hemodialysis patients. Adjustments can be made depending on blood pressure, urine output, and the presence or absence of edema. Hypertension in ESRD patients is largely volume related, and dry weight should be constantly reassessed in the hypertensive patient. Renin-mediated hypertension is present in a small percentage of dialysis patients. Appropriate antihypertensive medications, rather than further sodium and fluid restriction, are necessary for this subgroup. The sodium content of specific foods may be found in Appendix C.

What level of fluid intake is acceptable?

Generally, the recommended fluid intake is an amount equal to urine output plus approximately 500 to 700 mL/day. Fluids contained in foods such as fruits and vegetables are not usually counted in this total. Foods that are liquid at room temperature, such as Popsicles and ice, are counted in the daily fluid allotment. The volume of fluid in solid foods, approximately 500 to 800 mL, is roughly equivalent to insensible fluid losses; therefore remaining "visible" fluid intake will correlate with interdialytic weight gain. An acceptable interdialytic weight gain is 1.5 kg, or less than 3% of body weight. Excessive fluid contributes to high blood pressure and results in left ventricular hypertrophy.

What about phosphorus and calcium intake?

Phosphorus intake should be limited to 600 to 1200 mg/day. Because phosphorus content of the diet correlates with protein intake, it may be necessary to include some high-phosphorus food to achieve an adequate protein intake. Phosphorus is also controlled by the intake of phosphate-binding antacids such as calcium carbonate or calcium acetate. Aluminum-containing antacids should be avoided to minimize risk of aluminum bone disease. The calcium-containing antacids are given with meals and snacks, and ideally are titrated to the phosphorus content of the diet. Calcium content in the diet is typically low because foods high in phosphorus also tend to be rich sources of calcium. Calcium supplements, aside from that in the phosphate-binding antacids, may not be necessary to maintain calcium balance when either oral or intravenous 1,25-dihydroxycholecalciferol is used. Calcium requirements vary considerably depending on the phosphate intake, use of vitamin D, the calcium content of the dialysate, and the presence of hyperparathyroidism. This is discussed in greater detail in Chapter 13.

Are vitamin supplements necessary?

Patients on dialysis may be at risk for deficiencies of certain water-soluble vitamins because of poor nutrient intake, drug-nutrient interactions, altered vitamin metabolism, and dialysis losses. Although evaluation of specific requirements and recommendations is ongoing, supplementation with US Recommended Daily Allowance (US RDA) amounts of vitamins B_1, B_2, B_{12}, biotin, pantothenic acid, and niacin, as well as 800 to 1000 mcg of folic acid and 10 mg of pyridoxine (B_6) daily, is reasonable. The recommendations for folic acid, B_{12}, and B_6 continue to be reevaluated in light of information concerning the amino acid intermediate, homocysteine. Elevated levels of homocysteine have been demonstrated to be a risk factor in cardiovascular disease and can be present in patients with ESRD. High doses of folic acid, and in some studies B_6 and B_{12}, have been shown to normalize homocysteine levels and therefore may have a cardioprotective effect. The efficacy of high-dose supplementation of these B vitamins and the appropriate dosages are yet to be determined in the dialysis population. Vitamin C supplementation is limited to 60 mg/day. Higher doses of vitamin C should be avoided to prevent accumulation of oxalate, an ascorbic acid metabolite. Supplemental vitamin A should be avoided because of potential toxicity related to decreased renal degradation of retinol-binding protein in renal failure.

What about the need for trace minerals?

Trace mineral requirements are not well defined for the dialysis patient, and at present routine supplementation is not appropriate. Zinc deficiency may be present in some patients on dialysis, although the best method of measuring stores is yet to be determined in this population. In a patient who exhibits signs of zinc deficiency—such as hypogeusia (loss of sense of taste), delayed wound healing or alopecia—a time-limited trial of zinc supplementation may be reasonable. Selenium is another trace metal undergoing investigation into the possible role of selenium deficiency in promoting comorbid conditions such as cardiovascular disease and cancer in the dialysis population. The optimal method of assessing selenium status and appropriate dosing remain to be defined.

How is iron deficiency assessed?

Iron deficiency is a common finding in dialysis patients receiving human recombinant erythropoietin and concomitant utilization of iron for erythropoiesis. Before the use of erythropoietin, iron overload was common in this population as a result of multiple blood transfusions (each unit of transfused blood contains approximately 200 to 250 mg iron). Routine assessment of iron stores by serum ferritin and percent transferrin saturation (iron divided by total iron-binding capacity) should be included in any erythropoietin therapy protocol.

A low mean corpuscular volume may be a late indicator of iron deficiency. If a deficiency is present, intravenous iron administration or oral iron supplementation is warranted. Increasing the iron content of the diet generally does not provide adequate replacement once iron deficiency is identified. Various oral forms of iron are available but may cause gastrointestinal upset. Guidelines for administering intravenous iron and erythropoietin therapy are described in Chapter 13.

Do people on dialysis have to control fat intake?

Dyslipidemia, typically seen as hypertriglyceridemia, combined with low high-density lipoprotein (HDL) cholesterol and normal total serum cholesterol, is the most common lipid abnormality found in dialysis patients. Some patients may present with elevated serum cholesterol, defined as serum cholesterol greater than 200 mg/dL. For these people, it may be appropriate to prescribe a low-cholesterol, low-fat diet.

Obesity may exacerbate hypertriglyceridemia. Therefore, in the obese dialysis patient, weight control may be of benefit in helping to control triglyceride levels. A regular aerobic exercise program may also be of benefit in helping control both cholesterol and triglyceride levels. Carnitine, discussed later in this chapter, and fish oil supplements also have been shown to help lower triglyceride levels.

What about sugar and carbohydrates?

Restriction of sugar and carbohydrates is not appropriate or necessary for most people on dialysis. Exceptions are diabetics or those who are overweight, or who have hypertriglyceridemia that may respond to total calorie restriction. Often sugars and other carbohydrates need to be increased to provide adequate calories in the diet.

How is nutritional status monitored?

One category of assessment tools is anthropometric measurements, which include height, weight, ideal or desirable body weight, weight changes, and other measurements such as triceps skinfold (to assess fat stores) and midarm muscle circumference (to measure somatic protein stores). A second category is biochemical data. Serum albumin correlates with protein nutriture in stable hemodialysis patients in the absence of a nephrotic syndrome or liver disease, although levels are influenced by volume status. Data from the US Renal Data System indicate that low serum albumin, as indicative of overall nutritional status, is associated with increased mortality in patients on hemodialysis. Serum albumin appears to be a less reliable indicator of nutritional status in patients on peritoneal dialysis and does not correlate well with mortality risk in these patients. Other biochemical parameters such as serum transferrin, serum IGF-1 concentration, prealbumin levels and low serum creatinine with low creatinine kinetics have been used to assess nutritional status, although each parameter has limitations.

Subjective data such as food diaries or diet recall obtained by a skilled interviewer can provide valuable information. A method called subjective global assessment (SGA) has been used to quantify nutritional status and includes physical assessment, functional impairment, gastrointestinal symptoms, as well as anthropometric indices.

What is urea kinetic modeling (UKM)?

UKM is used to prescribe and monitor dialysis therapy and to assess protein intake. Although optimal methods for performing UKM and determining results are not agreed on in the dialysis community, formal UKM has become a standard of practice for both hemodialysis and peritoneal dialysis programs. UKM is usually performed using a computer because the mathematical computations are elaborate. Data entered into the computer are blood urea nitrogen (BUN) levels from before and after a given dialysis treatment (some methods also include predialysis BUN from the subsequent dialysis treatment), and for patients who urinate, residual urea clearance is included. Information about the dialysis treatment (blood flow, dialysate flow, dialyzer clearance data, length of treatment, and interdialytic interval) and patient-specific data (pre- and postdialysis weights, height, sex, and hematocrit) are also incorporated in the calculations.

What do the results mean?

One result derived from UKM is the Kt/V, which refers to the following:

K = Clearance of dialyzer for a given dialysis treatment and, if applicable, a measurement of any residual urine urea clearance

t = Length of time for a given dialysis treatment

V = Volume of distribution of urea for a given patient that equates with total body water

The goal for delivered Kt/V is thought to be at minimum 1.2 for thrice-weekly dialysis for both adults and children. Goal Kt/V for twice-weekly dialysis is undefined. Levels less than 1.2 may indicate inadequate dialysis and are associated with increased morbidity and poor prognosis on dialysis. Whether or not Kt/V can be too high and whether higher levels of Kt/V improve morbidity and/or mortality remains to be evaluated.

What other methods are available for estimating adequacy of dialysis?

Percent urea reduction or urea reduction ratio (URR) is another method used to assess dialysis adequacy. A reduction of BUN of 65% during a given dialysis treatment roughly correlates with a Kt/V of 1.2 for patients on dialysis three times a week. URR is not a substitute for formal UKM because it does not reflect the contribution of residual renal function, does not reflect protein catabolic rate (PCR), and does not provide a means of evaluating the validity of results.

How is URR calculated?

$$\% \text{ URR } = 100 \times (1 - Ct/Co)$$

where   Ct   =   Postdialysis BUN

Co   =   Predialysis BUN

What is the PCR?

PCR refers to a given patient's protein intake expressed in grams of protein per kilogram normalized body weight, assuming the patient is stable—that is, neither anabolic nor catabolic. The goal PCR is between 0.8 and 1.4 g protein per kilogram and is probably optimal at the upper end of the range.

What is the basis for interpreting the results of UKM?

Interpretation was based originally on the National Cooperative Dialysis Study (NCDS) published in 1983, in which an attempt was made to correlate patient outcome with amount of dialysis delivered. Both hospitalization and morbidity increased with high BUN levels in the presence of inadequate protein intake. The NCDS data later underwent a mechanistic analysis by Gotch and Sargent, from which the concept of Kt/V was derived. Since that time the generally accepted goals for Kt/V have continued to be reevaluated and revised upward.

What about UKM for peritoneal dialysis?

Studies comparable to the NCDS are not available in the peritoneal dialysis population. Guidelines are available for determining urea clearance and weekly creatinine clearance as well as PCR for this treatment modality. For continuous ambulatory peritoneal dialysis (CAPD), the delivered dose of peritoneal dialysis (PD) should be a Kt/V of at least 2.0 per week and a total creatinine clearance (Ccr) of at least 60 L/week/1.73 m². For nocturnal intermittent peritoneal dialysis (NIPD), the weekly delivered dose should be a total Kt/V of at least 2.2 and a weekly total Ccr of at least 66 L/1.73 m². For continuous cyclic peritoneal dialysis (CCPD), Kt/V of at least 2.1 and Ccr of at least 63 L/1.73 m² should be used.

Peritoneal equilibration testing (PET) is performed to assess the clearance capabilities of a given patient's peritoneal membrane and determine the optimal peritoneal dialysis regimen. See Chapter 17 for further information about PET.

What can be done for the patient who is unable to eat?

The first step in helping a patient who is unable to eat is to determine why he or she cannot eat and how to correct it. This often can be best addressed by a team approach including nurse, dietitian, technician, physician, and social worker. Among the possible causes are underdialysis/uremia, gastroparesis, depression, intercurrent illness, poor dentition, constipation, side effects of medications, depression or socioeconomic factors that influence the ability to obtain, prepare, or store foods. These are but a few causes of poor nutritional intake. Inadequate intake and poor nutritional status should not be accepted as "normal" for dialysis patients. Each problem should be assessed and investigated because there's often an etiology that can be remedied.

Once the identifiable causes of poor intake have been alleviated, certain strategies can be employed to augment nutrient intake. Commercially available supplements or homemade equivalents may be appropriate for some patients. The dietitian can evaluate the need for such supplements and recommend an appropriate type. Eating five or six small meals per day instead of two or three large ones may improve intake for some patients. The social worker can be helpful in enrolling a patient in a program such as Meals on Wheels or in involving the family in promoting food intake. Specific cultural habits and preferences are also incorporated in formulating a nutrition care plan. Medications to augment appetite have been used safely and effectively in patients with cancer and acquired immunodeficiency syndrome (AIDS). These medications have not been well studied in the dialysis population but may be used when other strategies to augment oral intake have failed. Enteral nutrition via nasogastric, percutaneous endoscopic gastrostomy or jejunostomy tubes should also be considered as an alternative method of providing support in the patient who is unable to eat but has a viable gastrointestinal tract. If, despite these efforts, a patient continues to deteriorate nutritionally, intradialytic parenteral nutrition may be appropriate.

What is intradialytic parenteral nutrition (IDPN)?

IDPN is a form of nutrition support by which protein, fat, and carbohydrate can be given during the dialysis treatment. Typically, a 1-liter solution of amino acids, lipid solution, and dextrose is infused during a dialysis run through the venous drip chamber. This provides 800 to 1000 calories and 60 to 90 g of amino acids. The advantage is that nutrients can be provided with a concomitant removal of volume, and a central line is not necessary because the dialysis access serves as the line of administration. Although this method cannot meet a patient's entire nutritional needs, it can provide supplemental nutrition for patients who are unable to take adequate intake by mouth, for whom enteral feeding is not an option, and for whom a central line is contraindicated. Approximately 90% of the amino acids infused are retained during this process. Potential side effects include hyperglycemia and reactive hypoglycemia.

Is there a comparable method of administering nutritional support for patients on peritoneal dialysis?

Amino acid dialysate (AAD) has been used in patients on peritoneal dialysis, in which amino acids are substituted for a portion of dextrose in peritoneal dialysis solutions. It is typically given during one exchange in a 24-hour period and serves as both an osmotic agent as well as a protein source. It has been shown to improve protein nutritional status in patients on this modality; however, increased BUN concentrations and metabolic acidosis have been described as potential side effects. Cost factors may prohibit its widespread use.

What can be done for constipation?

Constipation is a common problem for people on dialysis and is often related to medication taken for phosphate binding. The usual recommendations for this problem given to people not on dialysis, such as increasing fluid intake, consuming relatively large amounts of bran products, and eating foods such as prunes and other fruits and vegetables, may not be appropriate for dialysis patients. Medications such as stool softeners or substances such as sorbitol, which draws fluid into the intestinal tract, may be necessary to alleviate constipation. In chronic renal failure, stool output is a major route of potassium excretion, allowing for 30 to 40 mEq of potassium excretion each day. In a patient with hyperkalemia that cannot be easily accounted for by increased potassium intake, constipation should be considered as a possible etiologic factor.

How does the diet differ for patients on peritoneal dialysis (PD)?

The diet for patients on continuous ambulatory peritoneal dialysis (CAPD), continuous cycling peritoneal dialysis (CCPD), and other peritoneal dialysis modalities differs from that of patients on hemodialysis in several ways.

Protein. Protein needs are higher for patients on PD as a result of dialysate protein losses that average about 9 g/24 hr. Levels of 1.2 to 1.5 g of protein per kilogram of body weight are prescribed and are often difficult to achieve, although there is evidence that some patients maintain positive nitrogen balance on lower protein intakes. As with hemodialysis, the general recommendation is that at least 50% of the protein should be derived from high biological value sources; however, it is possible to maintain good protein nutriture with a carefully planned vegetarian diet. Protein supplements may be used when needs cannot be met by high-protein foods alone.

Calories. Although calorie needs are the same for both hemodialysis and peritoneal dialysis patients, those on peritoneal dialysis absorb 150 to 1000 calories per day from the dextrose in the dialysate. This may provide a particular advantage in the patient who has energy malnutrition or may be problematic in the obese or hypertriglyceridemic patient.

Sodium/fluid. Typically, dietary sodium and fluid can be liberalized for the PD patient as compared with the same patient on hemodialysis because the dextrose content of the dialysis solution can be adjusted with each exchange to remove varying volumes of fluid. A sodium intake of 4 g, and a fluid intake as guided by thirst, can often provide acceptable fluid management, provided that dialysis can be adjusted to maintain euvolemia.

Potassium. Potassium control tends to be less of a problem in patients on peritoneal dialysis in part because the constant glucose infusion combined with endogenous insulin production drives potassium intracellularly. Supplemental potassium may be indicated in approximately 10% of peritoneal dialysis patients. Hyperkalemia may be present in others.

Phosphorus. Control of serum phosphorus presents a challenge for patients on PD. An obligatory higher phosphorus intake is often necessary to achieve an adequate dietary protein intake, as foods that are high in protein tend to be high in phosphorus. Requirements for phosphate binding medications may therefore be higher.

Vitamins and other minerals. Needs for these other nutrients are generally thought to be the same as for patients on hemodialysis.

What is the diet for acute renal failure?

There is no set diet for acute renal failure because nutritional requirements vary considerably depending on comorbid conditions, degree of renal compromise, and presence of anuria or oliguria.

High mortality rates continue to be associated with acute renal failure, and protein-calorie malnutrition is thought to be one predictor of outcome. Although aggressive nutritional support has yet to be demonstrated to improve outcome, protein and calorie intake should be provided to meet increased needs associated with hypercatabolism. Protein requirements may be 1.5 g protein per kilogram per day or higher and can be determined using nitrogen balance studies. Both essential and nonessential amino acids should be used in most situations requiring parenteral nutrition. Calorie requirements vary considerably and can best be determined in the intensive care unit setting using indirect calorimetry.

Do the various treatment modalities influence the provision of parenteral nutrition?

Yes. The use of continuous arteriovenous or venovenous hemofiltration with or without dialysis allows for provision of large volumes of fluid necessary to give adequate amounts of parenteral nutrition in the hypercatabolic acute renal failure patient. Renal replacement therapy, however, also contributes to the catabolic state because loss of nutrients (amino acids) and high-flux membranes increase these losses, in comparison with low-flux membranes. In addition, membrane characteristics, in particular bioincompatability, may further enhance catabolism.

What is carnitine and should it be routinely supplemented in patients on dialysis?

Carnitine is synthesized in the body from the essential amino acids lysine and methionine and plays a role in transporting long-chain fatty acids into the mitrochondria. Although methods of measuring carnitine in various metabolic pools in the body are imprecise, free plasma carnitine and muscle carnitine concentrations may be low in patients on dialysis. Carnitine has been used to lower triglyceride levels, help with muscle cramps and muscle weakness, and decrease red blood cell fragility in patients on dialysis. The question of optimal dose and whether supplementation should be routine remains to be addressed.

Can the chronic kidney disease (CKD) patient use herbal remedies?

In recent years, people have become increasingly aware of alternative therapies in medicine and diet. Supplementing diets with herbals, vitamins and minerals, and other supplements may provide some health benefits; however, these products must be used with caution in the CKD patient. Declining renal function causes changes in the pharmacokinetics of many medications, which leads to altered absorption, distribution, metabolism, and excretion. These changes necessitate dosage adjustments to prevent the patient from being exposed to toxic levels of certain medications. Without reliable information about the pharmacokinetic behavior of herbal remedies, supplements, and their potentially active or toxic metabolites in renal failure, their safe use remains almost impossible in this population (Dahl, 2001). Some believe these remedies are safe because they are labeled as "natural" and not viewed as drugs. Unfortunately, some of these remedies and natural products can have a deleterious effect on the kidneys and other organs of the body. Acute renal failure secondary to interstitial nephritis is associated with the use of certain Chinese herbal drugs, *Aristolochia*, in particular. Juice from the noni plant *(Morinda citrifolia)*, which is promoted to increase mental clarity and improve physical performance, contains excessive potassium and should not be used by the CKD patient. The ingestion of star fruit, has been associated with harmful outcomes in the CKD patient, causing neurologic symptoms, seizures, and intractable hiccups.

In the United States, herbal remedies are not regulated by the US Food and Drug Administration (FDA). The consumer then must trust that the manufacturer has prepared and advertised his product in good faith. Some herbal remedies have a direct toxic effect on the kidneys and some may affect electrolyte balance, blood pressure control, and anticoagulation. Some products may interfere with efficacy of antirejection medications used in transplant patients. It is critical to question patients regarding their use of herbal supplements and alternative therapies because they are sometimes reluctant to reveal this information. Assessing for herbal remedy use should become part of the nursing assessment done on the CKD patient. Healthcare workers should become familiar with herbal remedies and their effects on the kidneys and the CKD patient. CKD patients should be encouraged to discuss the use of any herbal remedy with their nephrologist before use. Table 14-1 provides information on herbal remedies, their uses, and adverse effects.

What about the needs of pediatric patients?

The basic concepts of diet management apply to pediatric patients with chronic renal failure with one key exception: meeting the needs of protein, calories, and other nutrients to facilitate growth and development.

In summary, dialysis therapy, for the patient with either acute or chronic renal failure, can provide optimal patient outcomes when combined with effective and appropriate nutrition management. Although diet management is ultimately the responsibility of the patient or caretaker, members of the interdisciplinary team play a vital role in educating and reinforcing diet information that is tailored to the individual and monitored for effectiveness.

Table 14-1	Herbal Remedies: Benefits and Adverse Effects	
Herb	**Health benefit**	**Adverse effects**
Aloe	Used as laxative	May cause cramps and diarrhea. Electrolyte imbalances, particularly hypokalemia, may occur over time. May interfere with absorption of some medications
Aristolochic acid	Weight loss	May cause permanent kidney damage or urinary tract malignancies
Echinacea	Treats upper respiratory infections and flu, antiseptic, aids in digestion, used for migraines, antipyretic	Should not be used by patients with a transplant or those with acquired immunodeficiency syndrome Allergic reactions are possible
Ephedra	Used as a decongestant Central nervous system stimulant	Not recommended for dialysis or transplant patients. Should not be used by patients with heart disease, hypertension, thyroid disease, or diabetes. May increase blood pressure and heart rate. Other effects include heart palpitations and increased risk of stroke Should not be used when taking antihypertensives or antidepressants
Garlic	Improves blood lipid levels Reduces hypertension Increases bleeding/ clotting time Diuretic	Should not be taken if using antihypertensives or anticoagulants May increase bleeding tendencies May decrease clotting times and cause heartburn

Data from Bickform A: *Therapies for kidney patients,* Tampa, FL, 2000, American Association of Kidney Patients; Allen D, Bell J: Herbal medicine and the transplant patient, *Nephrol Nurs J* 29(3): 269–274, 2002; Myhre M: Herbal remedies, nephropathies, and renal disease, *Nephrol Nurs J* 2000.

Continued

Table 14-1	Herbal Remedies: Benefits and Adverse Effects—cont'd	
Herb	**Health benefit**	**Adverse effects**
Ginkgo biloba	Antioxidant Improves concentration, memory, vertigo, depression, and headache	Should not be used if taking anticoagulants Headache, gastrointestinal problems, dizziness
Ginseng	Used as a stimulant or relaxant. Regulates glucose in type 2 diabetes. May improve anemia, depression, and appetite. Enhances immunity	Should not be taken by those who have a transplant. May cause headaches, insomnia, anxiety, skin rash, and morning diarrhea
Hawthorn	Used for heart disease Decreases angina episodes	May interfere with blood pressure and heart medications
Licorice root	Used for the treatment of peptic ulcers and respiratory infections, cough suppressant, expectorant Antiinflammatory	Should not be taken by those with kidney disease, glaucoma, or by those on antihypertensives, digitalis, corticoids, or diuretics. May cause sodium and water retention, and significant potassium losses
St. John's wort	Used to treat moderate depression Antibacterial/antiviral Enhances wound healing; diuretic	Not recommended for patients with renal failure May cause headache, flulike symptoms, cough, fatigue, dry mouth, confusion, increased sensitivity to light, and gastrointestinal irritation. Should not be taken with antidepressants. May lower cyclosporine levels

15 Acute Renal Failure and Dialysis

Dialysis is often necessary for the treatment of acute renal failure. The most common indications include uremia, hyperkalemia, acidosis, fluid overload, and drug overdose.

What is acute renal failure (ARF)?

ARF is the rapid deterioration of renal function. It is usually reversible if diagnosed and treated early. Signs and symptoms of ARF are a urine output of less than 400 mL/day (oliguria), or less than 20 mL/hr for an adult, as well as an increase in blood urea nitrogen (BUN) and creatinine, hyperkalemia, and acidosis.

What are the types of ARF?

ARF is divided into three categories: prerenal, intrarenal, and postrenal (Box 15-1) (see Chapter 3).

Prerenal. Prerenal renal failure accounts for approximately 70% of ARF cases. Prerenal events result in a decrease in blood flow to the kidney. Examples include congestive heart failure, hypovolemia, sepsis, myocardial infarction, prolonged hypotension, and vascular disorders of the renal artery or vein.

Intrarenal. Approximately 25% of ARF cases are caused by intrarenal factors. Any event that damages the kidney tissue, structure, and function is categorized as intrarenal ARF. The damage, which may involve the glomeruli, the tubules, or both, interferes with the ability of the kidneys to carry out their normal functions. The most common cause of intrarenal failure is damage to the tubules. This is called acute tubular necrosis (ATN). ATN is caused by severely reduced blood flow leading to prolonged ischemia, or by direct toxic insult to tubular cells. In oliguric ATN, urine flow falls to about 20 mL/hr, and BUN and serum creatinine, phosphate, and potassium levels rise. With nonoliguric ARF, the patient may remain in better fluid balance, but elimination of waste products is impaired. Ischemic injury to the kidneys can occur when the mean arterial blood pressure drops below 60 mm Hg for more than 30 minutes. Massive hemorrhage, transfusion reaction, sepsis, cardiovascular collapse, or major trauma can cause ischemic renal injury.

Substances that injure the kidneys are called nephrotoxins. The most common are medications such as antibiotics and nonsteroidal antiinflammatory agents

Box 15-1
ETIOLOGIES OF ACUTE RENAL FAILURE

Prerenal (Decreased Renal Perfusion)
Hypovolemia
- Hemorrhage
- Shock
- Third-spacing (edema, ascites)
- Burns
- Dehydration (GI losses, overuse of diuretics)

Decreased cardiac output
- Cardiogenic shock
- Dysrhythmias
- Cardiac tamponade
- Congestive heart failure
- Myocardial infarction

Thromboembolic obstruction of the renal vasculature

Intrarenal (Damage to the Nephron)
Acute tubular necrosis
- Ischemic
  Prolonged prerenal acute renal failure
  Transfusion reaction
  Rhabdomyolysis
- Nephrotoxic
  Prolonged postrenal acute renal failure
  Antibotics (aminoglycosides, carbenicillin, amphotericin B)
  Contrast media
  Heavy metals (lead, mercury)
  Carbon tetrachloride
  Insecticides, fungicides
  Cytotoxic drugs (certain chemotherapeutic agents)
  Hemolytic-uremic syndrome
- Inflammatory
  Acute glomerulonephritis
  Acute pyelonephritis

From Copstead LC, Banasik JL: *Pathophysiology,* ed 3, St Louis, 2005, Mosby.

Box 15-1
ETIOLOGIES OF ACUTE RENAL FAILURE—Cont'd

Postrenal (Obstruction)
Benign prostatic hypertrophy
Calculi (stones)
Urinary tract infection
Tumors
Strictures
Altered bladder contraction (neurogenic bladder from medication or injury/disease)

(NSAIDs). Other medications, including anesthetics and cancer chemotherapy agents, as well as street drugs, are toxic to the kidney in varying degrees. Radiologic contrast dye used for intravenous pyelography, cardiac catheterization, and computed tomography (CT) is potentially nephrotoxic. Other nephrotoxins include hemoglobin (from hemolysis of red cells) and myoglobin from muscle breakdown (rhabdomyolysis), because of crush injury, heatstroke, or seizure.

Postrenal. Postrenal causes account for approximately 5% of ARF cases. Postrenal failure is usually the result of obstruction in the flow of urine anywhere from the kidney to the urinary meatus. The obstruction can be functional or mechanical. Functional causes include diabetic nephropathy, medications such as ganglionic blocking agents that block the autonomic nerve supply to the urinary system, and neurogenic bladder subsequent to spinal cord injury or cerebrovascular accident (CVA). Tumors, stones, prostatic hypertrophy, and urethral strictures are some mechanical causes of postrenal failure.

Does a patient with ARF have urine output?

Some patients with ARF have significant urine output, referred to as nonoliguric renal failure. Most patients progress through several stages from oliguria to anuria to polyuria, depending on the phase of ARF (Table 15-1).

Oliguric-anuric phase. Oliguria is defined as urine volume less than 400 mL/24 hours. Anuria is a urine output of less than 50 mL/24 hours. This phase can last from 2 days to 30 days or longer. The longer the oliguria/anuria continues, the more the prospect of returning to normal urine output worsens. Proper management of fluid volume is essential.

Diuretic phase. This phase begins when the urine output reaches 1 L/24 hours. The renal indices may stabilize, and then start to approach normal with gradual return of renal function. A 24-hour urine volume can increase to as much as 4 to 5 L. Accurate evaluation of the patient's status to avoid dehydration leading to hypoperfusion of the kidneys is mandatory. Laboratory values are monitored

Table 15-1	Phases of Acute Renal Failure				
Phase	Definition	Approximate time span	Renal blood flow (%)	Urine (% of normal)	Filtration (%)
Oliguric	< 400 mL/day	1 to 2 wk	25	5	10
Diuretic	>400 mL/day to stable laboratory values	2 to 10 days	30-50	150-200	10-50
Convalescent	Stable laboratory values to normal function	3-12 mo	100	100	100

From Copstead LC, Banasik JL: *Pathophysiology*, ed 3, St Louis, 2005, Mosby.

closely with the expectation that they will return to normal in the late phase of ARF.

Convalescent phase. This period begins with the stabilization of serum chemistries and gradual return of normal kidney function. This phase may last from 3 to 6 months. Return to normal glomerular filtration rate (GFR), if it occurs, may take up to a year.

What are the clinical presentations of ARF?

These include all the symptoms, signs, and findings of rapidly developing uremia (see Chapter 4).

What biochemical changes are present in ARF?

The damaged kidneys are unable to excrete the products of normal body metabolism. There is elevation of the serum urea and creatinine, and altered electrolyte levels. Increased hydrogen ion concentration causes acidosis and a low serum pH. Hyperkalemia or hypokalemia, hypocalcemia, hyperphosphatemia, hypermagnesemia, and a low bicarbonate may be observed.

How is ARF treated?

Many treatment options are available depending on the cause of the renal failure, the severity of symptoms, and the overall condition of the patient. Options include hemodialysis, isolated ultrafiltration, peritoneal dialysis, continuous renal replacement therapy (CRRT), and charcoal hemoperfusion.

What are the indications for treatment?

The most common indications for acute dialysis include the following:

Uremia. Acute dialysis is initiated when a patient becomes symptomatically uremic (see Chapter 4), regardless of BUN or creatinine level. Dialysis may be started prophylactically when the BUN reaches 100 mg/dL, even if the patient has few or no symptoms.

Pulmonary edema. Acute pulmonary edema is a life-threatening complication of ARF that necessitates immediate dialysis. Acute pulmonary edema can result from fluid overload directly attributable to ARF or as the result of an acute myocardial infarction or from overzealous administration of fluid.

Hyperkalemia. Hyperkalemia is a result of the damaged kidney's inability to secrete potassium and the release of intracellular potassium (because of acidosis and tissue breakdown). Hemodialysis is effective in lowering potassium and is initiated when rapid reduction of plasma potassium is indicated. Peritoneal dialysis is an acceptable treatment option, although its effects are slower than that of hemodialysis. Hyperkalemia can be managed in an emergency, while waiting for hemodialysis, by intravenous administration of glucose and insulin in combination with intravenous sodium bicarbonate. These shift extracellular potassium into the cell, where it cannot cause cardiac arrhythmia. Calcium gluconate may be given intravenously to reduce myocardial irritability. Sodium polystyrene sulfonate cation exchange resin (Kayexalate) by mouth or by enema can be administered when slower correction of potassium is acceptable or in the initial management of hyperkalemia.

Acidosis. Metabolic acidosis is caused by inability of the kidneys to excrete hydrogen ion and to reabsorb bicarbonate. Acidosis can be treated temporarily by intravenous sodium bicarbonate. Hemodialysis may be required because of the added sodium, which increases the danger of volume overload.

Neurologic changes. Toxic effects of uremia can result in central nervous system changes. Headache, insomnia, and drowsiness are early symptoms; confusion, convulsions, and coma may occur later. Dialysis is indicated when any of these serious symptoms are seen, and preferably before they occur.

Drug overdoses and poisonings. Dialysis is indicated for the treatment of some drug intoxications. Drugs normally excreted by the kidneys, or water-soluble drugs of low molecular weight, will diffuse rapidly across cellulosic dialysis membranes. Such drugs are readily removed with hemodialysis. Examples include ethanol, lithium, methanol, and salicylates. Water-soluble drugs with high molecular weight such as vancomycin and amphotericin B diffuse across cellulosic membranes much more slowly and are less well removed. If the intoxicant is protein bound (e.g., digoxin and acetylsalicylic acid) or lipid soluble (e.g., glutethimide), hemodialysis is not useful. However, both of these intoxicants are removed by hemoperfusion with a charcoal cartridge or with a plasma membrane filter.

What type of vascular access is used for acute dialysis?

The most common access to the circulation for acute dialysis is a double-lumen venous catheter. The catheter may be placed in the subclavian, internal jugular, or femoral vein. Insertion of a catheter into the subclavian or internal jugular vein must be followed by an x-ray examination to determine correct placement, and to rule out pneumothorax or hemothorax before the catheter is used (see Chapter 10).

Can an arteriovenous (AV) fistula or graft be used for acute dialysis?

Patients with an AV fistula or graft may require acute dialysis, and the fistula or graft may be used after its patency is determined (see Chapter 10 for additional information).

How often are patients dialyzed?

Frequency of dialysis is determined by the patient's response to treatment. Patients may be hemodialyzed daily for a few days until the BUN, serum creatinine, potassium level, and acidosis are considered acceptable. Daily dialysis may be necessary for volume overload, or if parenteral nutrition is to be given.

What complications may occur with ARF?

Congestive heart failure (CHF) is a common occurrence. It is most often caused by hypertension, volume excess, and/or anemia.

Hypertension. Fluid removal by dialysis may correct the hypertension. Antihypertensive medication may be necessary.

Hypotension. Hypotension may result from blood loss, a strict fluid restriction, sepsis, myocardial infarction or pericarditis. To prevent additional kidney damage, the underlying cause of the hypotension must be corrected to maintain adequate renal perfusion. The use of a vasopressor such as dopamine may be necessary.

Anemia. In acute renal failure the release of erythropoietin is decreased. The usual response to therapy with recombinant erythropoietin or epoetin (EPO) requires 3 to 4 weeks, so it is not of immediate help. Uremic red cells also have a shortened life span. Blood loss from bleeding is often present (see Chapter 4 for additional information about complications).

What is the most serious complication of ARF?

Infection is the leading cause of death in ARF. Uremia causes immune suppression, which predisposes the patient to sepsis. Strict aseptic technique must be used for all invasive procedures, including initiating and discontinuing dialysis, starting an intravenous line, and caring for the bladder catheter.

Are there special considerations when dialyzing a patient for the first time?

An infrequent syndrome known as the "first-use" syndrome results from an allergic-type reaction to new dialyzers and is characterized by itching, hypotension, chest and back pain, and breathing difficulties. In severe cases, cardiopulmonary arrest may occur. Symptoms are usually manifested during the first 15 to 30 minutes of dialysis. Cuprophan dialyzers are most often implicated. Cellulose acetate, modified cellulosic and synthetic membranes (polysulfone, polyamide, and polyacrylonitrile) are less likely to cause first-use syndrome.

What is the treatment for first-use syndrome?

When the symptoms are severe, the blood must not be returned to the patient, and the dialyzer is discarded. The physician should be notified and an assessment of symptoms, particularly cardiopulmonary status, performed. The use of a more biocompatible membrane may be necessary. When the symptoms are less severe, symptomatic treatment (e.g., nasal O_2 or oral diphenhydramine [Benadryl]) is adequate. In this situation, dialysis can continue because the symptoms usually subside after the first hour.

Are there special precautions when dialyzing someone with ARF?

Patients requiring acute dialysis are generally critically ill with multisystem failure. A thorough and accurate total assessment of the patient is essential before initiating dialysis (see Chapter 11). The nephrology nurse must be highly cognizant of changes, be prudent in assessing and monitoring the patient's vital signs, and respond appropriately.

Controlled anticoagulation with heparin may be necessary to minimize clotting of the dialyzer; however, dialysis can be performed with little or no heparin. Careful monitoring of clotting times may be necessary to prevent complications related to heparinization during hemodialysis. A baseline clotting time must be obtained before the start of dialysis; a normal activated clotting time (ACT is 60 to 90 seconds). The Clinical Laboratory Improvement Act (CLIA) now requires quality control checks for ACT machines to meet CLIA requirements. These requirements are resource intensive and may not permit bedside monitoring of ACT levels during dialysis (see Chapter 12).

The physician determines the technique of anticoagulation. "Tight" or no heparin may be used for patients at high risk for bleeding. In tight heparinization, clotting times are performed every 30 minutes. The ACT is kept at 1.25 times the baseline with additional heparin, as indicated when the ACT falls below the 1.25 baseline value. With systemic heparinization, generally the ACT values are allowed to range from 2.5 to 3 times the baseline.

"No heparin" dialysis requires a blood flow between 250 and 300 mL/min, or significant dialyzer clotting will occur. The dialyzer is flushed every 20 to 30 minutes with 100 mL of normal saline so that it can be easily examined visually for clotting, and so that proteins and clotting factors will be moved away from the dialyzer membrane surface. Before the start of dialysis this extra volume is calculated into the required fluid loss in order to achieve the planned fluid removal goal. The risk of clotting the dialyzer, resulting in an average blood loss of 150 mL, must be weighed against the risk of administering an anticoagulant to a high-risk patient.

Patients in an intensive care unit are often attached to a cardiac monitor. It is important to watch for arrhythmias during dialysis because these may relate to the dialysis. However, it is not uncommon to see some aberrant beats or premature ventricular beats during dialysis.

What measures may be taken during acute dialysis to counteract hypotension?

Abnormalities causing hypotension must be identified and corrected as much as possible. These usually involve intravascular volume, cardiac output, and/or vasomotor tone. Although patients are often overhydrated and edematous, some may have hypotension from low intravascular volume and need infusion of normal saline or dextrose and water. Patients who do not respond to normal saline infusion may require colloid or hyperosmolar products such as human plasma protein fraction (Plasmanate) or albumin. These colloids will increase the oncotic pressure and attract fluid from the extracellular space into the vascular space. Hypotension resulting from decreased red cell mass from hemorrhage or other causes may require transfusion of red blood cells. When hypotension is caused by low cardiac output, cardiotonic drugs, particularly inotropic (dopamine) and antiarrhythmic (lidocaine) agents may be helpful. It may be appropriate to reduce the blood flow rate to between 150 and 200 mL/min for an apparent decrease in cardiac output. The physician will need accurate assessment data on duration of dialysis, blood flow rate, ultrafiltration estimate (or weight), blood pressure (BP) readings, and all medications administered to determine the most appropriate treatment. NOTE: When the blood flow is lowered, dialysis efficiency is reduced; that is, there is a decrease in urea reduction, Kt/V and creatinine clearance. If hypotension is caused by poor vasomotor tone, patients may be maintained above their ideal weight to promote vascular filling and normotensive blood pressure.

What measures are appropriate for hypertension?

Most hypertension in acute dialysis patients is related to fluid excess and responds to ultrafiltration. If it is not controlled with fluid removal, the physician may prescribe an antihypertensive medication. Patients on antihypertensive agents may be subject to hypotensive episodes. Administration of antihypertensive agents may need to be deferred prior to hemodialysis if ordered accordingly by the physician.

What is disequilibrium syndrome?

This is a complex of signs and symptoms ranging from headache, restlessness, and impaired mental concentration to confusion, twitching, jerking, and occasionally culminating in a grand mal seizure. It may occur during or soon after dialysis.

What causes dialysis disequilibrium?

Disequilibrium is believed to be related to cerebral edema. The blood-brain barrier has a selective effect on the transfer of solute and of water between the plasma and the brain. During dialysis, plasma solute concentration is lowered faster than brain solute, and the plasma becomes hypotonic in relation to the brain cell water, causing water to shift from the plasma to the brain.

When should disequilibrium be anticipated?

Disequilibrium is most common in the more severely catabolic patient or in those in whom azotemia is severe (BUN greater than 200 mg/100 mL).

What are ways to prevent or minimize disequilibrium?

Prevention is best. Care must be taken not to lower the urea level too rapidly; it is best to do short (2- to 3-hour) dialysis at 24-hour intervals for the first few treatments. A reduced blood flow rate of 150 to 200 mL/min may lessen the risk of dialysis disequilibrium by slowing the rate of solute shift. Using a small dialyzer with lower clearance properties will help. Configuring the extracorporeal blood circuit with the dialysate flow concurrent— rather than countercurrent—to the blood flow is an easy means of decreasing the rapid removal of urea by lowering clearance throughout the treatment. Decreasing the dialysate flow rate also will lead to decreased removal of urea. The physician may also prescribe a high osmotic solution such as 25% mannitol intravenously at the beginning of treatment. Disequilibrium manifested by seizures and coma is unusual with frequent and less aggressive dialysis. Early detection of the potential for severe neurologic changes must be promptly reported to the physician.

PROCEDURES
What is isolated ultrafiltration (UF)?

Isolated UF is a process by which excess fluid is removed with little or no change in solute concentrations of the blood. Very small amounts of urea and creatinine are removed from the patient's serum passively along with the ultrafiltrate. The rate and amount at which the fluid can be removed depend in part on the amount of excess extracellular fluid present, the patient's intravascular volume, and cardiovascular stability.

What are the indications for using isolated UF?

Isolated UF is indicated to remove fluid when the removal of solute is not a priority. Isolated UF can be performed immediately before, after, or independently of hemodialysis treatment.

What equipment is needed for UF?

Isolated UF is performed with the same dialyzer and tubing used for hemodialysis. The dialysate flow is turned off, or placed in bypass mode. The dialyzer membrane does not come into contact with the dialysate solution. With conventional equipment, the total of the negative pressure applied to the dialysate side of the membrane plus the venous pressure represents the transmembrane pressure and determines the amount of UF. With volumetric equipment, the set value for UF determines the fluid to be removed. A blood pump, air detector, blood leak detector, and pressure monitors are standard equipment to perform the procedure safely.

Are there complications with isolated UF?

Rapid removal of fluid can cause hypotension and muscle cramps.

Continuous Renal Replacement Therapy (CRRT)?

CRRT is used primarily to treat patients in acute renal failure, particularly those with multiple organ failure. Such individuals tend to be hemodynamically unstable, to have cardiac insufficiency, and to tolerate hemodialysis poorly. Various hemofilters are available, hollow fiber or plate design, and characterized by small contained blood volume and low resistance to flow. There is increasing evidence that CRRT is improving patient survival in acute renal failure.

What treatments besides hemodialysis are available to treat ARF?

There are many alternatives to conventional hemodialysis. CRRT is the umbrella acronym for the five approaches for this treatment, such as slow continuous ultrafiltration (SCUF), continuous arteriovenous hemofiltration (CAVH), continuous arteriovenous hemodialysis (CAVHD), continuous venovenous hemofiltration (CVVH), and continuous venovenous hemodialysis (CVVHD). Originally SCUF, CAVH, and CAVHD were very popular because they do not require special equipment or the constant attention of nephrology personnel. Now CVVH and CVVHD are being prescribed more. The principles of CRRT are the same, but special equipment is necessary for CVVH or CVVHD. The procedures are limited to the critical care setting for the treatment of ARF. A collaborative approach utilizing the collective expertise of critical care and nephrology personnel is strongly recommended.

CAVH requires both arterial and venous access, but does not use a blood pump. If solute removal by convective transport is not sufficient, diffusive transport is added by also using hemodialysis. CVVH and CVVHD do not require arterial access with its attending problems, but instead use double-lumen catheters in major venous sites. In each person, flow is controlled with a blood pump (Fig. 15-1).

What are problems in the use of CRRT?

For those procedures requiring arterial access, such as CAVH and CAVHD, there is risk of damage to the artery itself, as well as danger of hemorrhage if a connection is faulty or a leak develops in the blood circuit. Critically ill patients are often hypotensive, with the blood flow rate inadequate for effective filtration. In addition, correction of

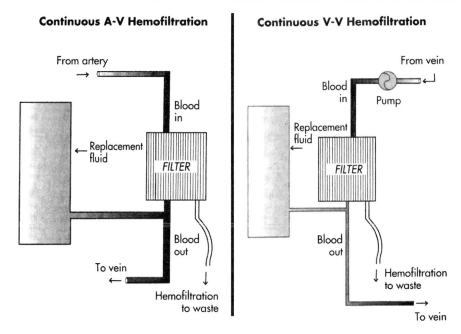

Fig. 15-1 Continuous renal replacement therapy (CRRT) using hemofiltration. *Left:* Continuous arteriovenous hemofiltration (CAVH). *Right:* Continuous venovenous hemofiltration (CVVH).

electrolyte imbalance and/or fluid overload may be slower than desired. Clotting problems are frequent.

For systems utilizing venovenous flow, a blood pump is needed. Monitoring is required to avert air being drawn into the blood circuit and to watch for bleeding from a loose connection in the downstream side.

What is SCUF?

SCUF is a method of gradual fluid removal. As with isolated ultrafiltration, little solute removal takes place; therefore, intermittent hemodialysis may be needed to treat azotemia and maintain electrolyte balance. The amount of fluid removed is usually 2 to 6 L in a 24-hour period.

What are the indications for SCUF?

Many patients with ARF have a high rate of protein breakdown and require large volumes of total parenteral nutrition (TPN) fluid. A few hours of hemodialysis may be inadequate to remove such large volumes of fluid, particularly in the patient with hypotension and hemodynamic instability. SCUF allows for the slow continuous removal of fluid, alleviating the large volume administered.

What equipment is used in SCUF?

A highly permeable hemofilter, similar to a dialyzer, is used. SCUF can be performed without blood pump assistance, relying on the patient's cardiac output and mean arterial pressure (MAP) to provide adequate blood flow through the filter. The hydrostatic pressure of the blood forces the ultrafiltrate across the membrane, and it is collected in a drainage bag for disposal. The length of tubing from the hemofilter to the fluid collection device creates a negative pressure that supports the UF rate. SCUF may also be performed with blood pump assistance from the Prisma machine.

Do patients require heparin during the procedure?

Usually an initial bolus of 500 to 2000 units of heparin is injected, followed by a continuous drip of 250 to 500 units/hr, or 5 to 10 units/kg/hr. Clotting times are monitored. The procedure can be used without heparin by using normal saline flushes, but the chances of clotting the hemofilter are greatly increased.

What problems are associated with SCUF?

The most common problem is failure to obtain the desired quantity of ultrafiltrate. The reasons are usually clotting of the hemofilter or decrease in blood flow through the circuit. A problem with the patient's access, a kink in the tubing, or a drop in the patient's arterial pressure can also result in a low ultrafiltration rate.

What is CAVH?

CAVH is the continuous flow of blood through an extracorporeal circuit to remove excess fluid and solutes over an extended period. Specific hemofilters in different sizes are available to perform CAVH. Product specifications, membrane properties, and hemofilter sizes vary considerably.

What are the indications for CAVH?

CAVH is indicated when large volumes of fluid must be removed from hemodynamically unstable patients. Fluid loss is generally 8 to 15 L a day for adult patients. The large amount of fluid loss allows the removal of solutes from the blood. The solutes are removed by convection in proportion to their plasma water concentration.

What equipment is used during CAVH?

CAVH (Fig. 15-2) is also performed without blood pump assistance, and is dependent on the adequacy of the patient's blood pressure to push the blood through the circuit. As with SCUF, the patient's MAP must be maintained at greater than 60 mm Hg, or ideally 70 mm Hg. A drainage bag is attached to a port on the filter to collect the ultrafiltrate. Ultrafiltrate is replaced before the hemofilter (pre-dilution) or after the hemofilter (post-dilution).

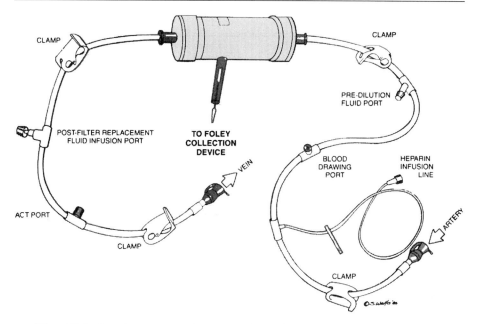

Fig. 15-2 Continuous arteriovenous hemofiltration (CAVH) schematic.

What is CAVHD?

CAVHD (Fig. 15-3) is a modification of CAVH, with the addition of dialysate flowing through the filter at a slow rate, for combined removal of fluid and solutes by diffusion (dialysis) and by convection (ultrafiltration).

What are the indications for CAVHD?

When CAVH does not provide adequate waste product removal, CAVHD becomes the preferred treatment option. CAVHD may be more appropriate for patients who are anuric, hyperkalemic, or severely acidotic.

How is the procedure different from CAVH?

The procedures are similar except that dialysate is circulated around the hemofilter membrane in CAVHD for more efficient clearance of urea and creatinine. The dialysate used may be standard peritoneal dialysis solution containing 1.5% to 2.5% dextrose, which is infused into the hemofilter via one of the ultrafiltrate ports at a rate of 15 to 40 mL/min, or 1 to 4 L/hour. Custom dialysate fluid may be necessary to avoid hyperglycemia and lactic acidosis, or for patients with liver failure. The increased solute removal reduces uremia, acidosis, and potential electrolyte imbalance so that replacement fluid may not be necessary.

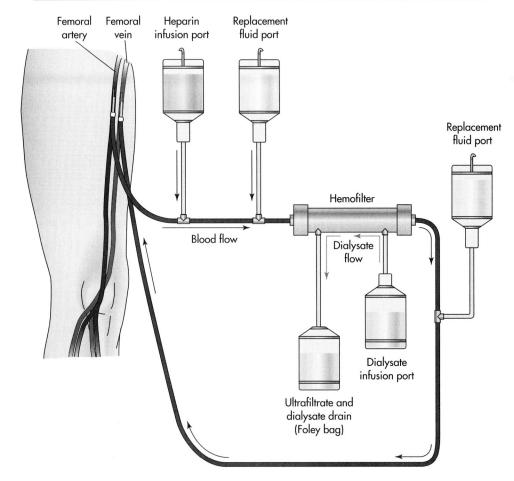

Fig. 15-3 Continuous arteriovenous hemodialysis (CAVHD). *(From Lewis SM, Heitkemper, MM, Dirksen SR:* Medical-Surgical Nursing, *ed 6, St Louis, 2004, Mosby.)*

What type of access is required for these treatments?

Access to the arterial circulation is necessary because no blood pump is used. Generally, a single-lumen catheter is inserted into the femoral artery, with the blood returning to the femoral vein via another catheter. The subclavian vein can also be used for the return of the blood.

What is continuous venovenous hemofiltration (CVVH)?

CVVH (Fig. 15-4) is a form of continuous therapy, similar to its predecessor, CAVH, but a blood pump is used to control the blood flow through the hemofilter. CVVH is a

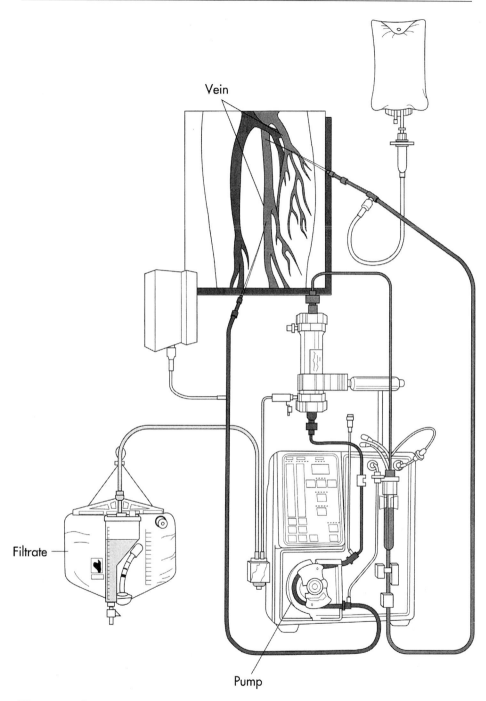

Fig. 15-4 Continuous venovenous hemofiltration (CVVH). *(Courtesy Baxter Healthcare, Renal Division, McGraw Park, Ill.)*

venous therapy so the accesses used for this therapy are the subclavian, internal jugular, or femoral veins. Solute removal is through convection and fluid removal is achieved using ultrafiltration with replacement fluid administered. The replacement fluid composition may vary and can be infused pre- or post-filter to maintain intravascular volume.

What is the objective of CVVH?

The objective of CVVH is to provide continuous renal replacement therapy, allowing the removal of solutes, balance of fluid and electrolytes, and stabilization of azotemia. Because this occurs evenly over time, this is a therapy of choice for those patients who are unable to tolerate rapid fluid and solute concentration shifts similar to that which occurs with hemodialysis.

What are the indications for CVVH?

CVVH is indicated when large volumes of fluid must be removed from hemodynamically unstable patients. CVVH is a recommended therapy to treat acute renal failure patients who exhibit cardiovascular instability. Other indications include **fluid removal** (carcinogenic shock), **increased intracranial pressure** (subarachnoid hemorrhage, hepatorenal syndrome), **shock** (sepsis, adult respiratory distress syndrome), **and nutrition** (burns). CVVH is also indicated for multi-organ failure, non-oliguric patients who require large volumes of intravenous fluids. CVVH is frequently employed in the care of critically ill and unstable pediatric patients.

What equipment is used during CVVH?

The blood pump equipment includes an arterial pressure monitor, a venous pressure monitor, and a venous drip chamber with an air alert detector. The use of a blood pump replaces the patient's MAP as the driving force for the extracorporeal system, which is a significant advantage when treating a patient with decreased blood pressure.

What are some other advantages of CVVH?

Because a blood pump is used with this therapy, higher blood flow rates can be achieved, permitting higher ultrafiltration rates and urea clearance. The increased blood flow also helps to decrease clotting of the hemofilter. CVVH has the ability to remove larger molecular weight solutes because of the more porous nature of the hemofilter used in this treatment.

What is CVVHD?

CVVHD (Fig. 15-5) is similar to CAVHD in principle, but like CVVH, a blood pump is employed to control the blood flow rate. Unlike CVVH, CVVHD requires the use of dialysate running countercurrent to the blood flow through the extracorporeal circuit. The indications for CVVHD are the same as for CAVHD. Intermittent hemodialysis would be insufficient therapy for these patients, plus they may be too unstable to tolerate aggressive hemodialysis.

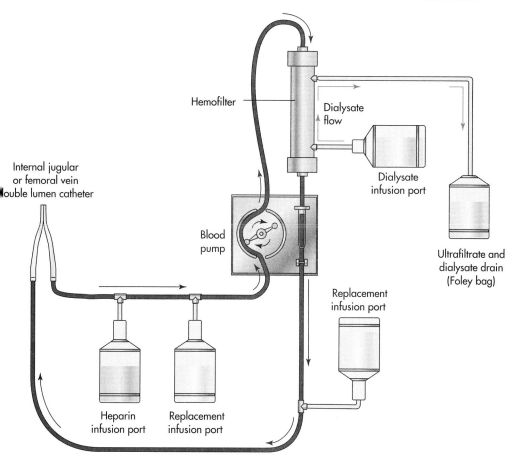

Fig. 15-5 Continuous venovenous hemodialysis (CVVHD). *(From Lewis SM, Heitkemper MM, Dirksen SR: Medical-Surgical Nursing, ed 6, St Louis, 2004, Mosby.)*

What are the primary advantages of CVVH/CVVHD over CAVH/CAVHD?

Arteriovenous extracorporeal circuit requires the prolonged cannulation of an artery. This can lead to compromised blood flow to the extremity, infection, and impaired ability to move the patient. Venovenous extracorporeal circuits do not require use of an artery. A single dual-lumen catheter can be used. Preferred sites are the subclavian or internal jugular vein. Blood flow through the hemofilter is consistent and controlled by the nurse, generally between 100 to 200 mL/min.

What are the disadvantages of venovenous access?

CVVH and CVVHD require more bedside equipment that must be monitored by the critical care nurse. Inservice education must be provided to assist the critical care nurses to be comfortable with the system.

Is the anticoagulation the same for CAVH/CAVHD and CAVVH/CVVHD?

Heparin is the priamry anticoagulation used with all approaches of CRRT. Generally a bolus of 500 to 2000 units is administered into the blood circuit upon initiation of therapy followed by a heparin infusion of 5 to 10 units/kg/hr. If ACTs are permitted in the institution, an apropriate range for CRRT would be 150 to 200 seconds. An alternative or adjunct therapy is to routinely flush the hemofilter and blood circuit with normal saline. This may prolong the life of the hemofilter. Trisodium citrate anticoagulation has been used successfully but requires additional monitoring of serum sodium, calcium and bicarbonate to avoid compromising the patient. Venovenous circuits have fewer clotting problems because of the consistent blood flow.

What are the complications associated with CRRT?

Patient complications include hypotension, cardiac dysrhythmias, dehydration, electrolyte imbalance, blood loss, infection, and air embolism. There are technical complications that include blood leak, membrane rupture, clotted hemofilter, disconnection of the arterial or venous tubing, equipment malfunction, position of catheters, kinked tubing, and inexperienced personnel.

Who is responsible for CRRT?

The ideal situation is for the critical care and nephrology professionals to work collaboratively. Generally the nephrologist prescribes the therapy and then shares the monitoring and appropriate interventions with the intensivists. The nephrology nurses set up the system, provide inservice teaching, assist with nursing interventions such as catheter dressing changes, and remain available on-call for troubleshooting or problem solving. The critical care nurses are responsible for the 24-hour monitoring, documentation of intake and output, replacement fluids, heparinization, and discontinuing a clotted circuit. CRRT offers an approach that focuses on providing the patient with 24-hour renal replacement, rather than attempting to correct a multitude of problems in a 3- or 4-hour hemodialysis treatment. The delineation of clinical responsibilities must be decided upon before initiating a CRRT program for critically ill patients.

What is sustained low efficiency dialysis (SLED)?

SLED is an acute renal failure modality choice that is becoming increasingly popular, particularly in the intensive care unit (ICU) setting. It is an acceptable compromise between intermittent hemodialysis and CRRT. It is also known as extended daily dialysis (EDD).

This form of treatment employs dialysis over a prolonged duration (8 to 12 hours) with modified blood and dialysate flow rates ($\leqq$200 mL/min blood flow rate (BFR) and 100 to 300 mL/min dialysate flow rate (DFR). Conventional dialysis machines preclude the need for costly CRRT machines, filters and tubing. Hemodynamic stability is a benefit of SLED, allowing the patient to achieve the desired ultrafiltration goal. SLED is an alternative for the critically ill patient who has had poor outcomes on intermittent hemodialysis therapy.

Other Extracorporeal Treatment Modalities

There are techniques other than dialysis for removing metabolic wastes, toxic materials, and/or excess water. Some of these are very useful in the ICU for the patient with complex problems and/or multiple organ failure.

What are some of these techniques?

There are three basic modalities in use clinically:
- Hemofiltration
- Hemoperfusion
- Apheresis

HEMOFILTRATION
What is hemofiltration?

In conventional hemodialysis, diffusion or conductive transfer accounts for the major portion of solute movement across the membrane. The natural kidney in its process of glomerular filtration actually uses ultrafiltration, or convective transfer. Convective transfer across a synthetic membrane is also used to remove uremic wastes from blood. This is the process of hemofiltration, or diafiltration.

How effective is hemofiltration?

Using membrane or hollow fibers of polyacrylonitrile (PAN), polyamide, polysulfone, or polycarbonate, UF of more than 100 mL/min is possible at blood flow rates of 200 to 350 mL/min. If the blood urea nitrogen were 50 mg/dL, that amount of BUN would also be removed in 1 minute. The removal of creatinine, middle and large molecules, such as β_2-microglobulin, far exceeds that of conventional hemodialysis.

What problems may occur with hemofiltration?
- The infusion of replacement fluid must be carefully and continually monitored to avoid under- or overhydration.
- Blood leak can be a serious hazard when negative pressure is applied to the filtrate bag to enhance ultrafiltration.
- The serum level of various beneficial medications (antibiotics, cardiac drugs, anticonvulsants) may be adversely altered.
- The essential sterile replacement fluids are expensive.

What are clinical advantages of hemofiltration?

Several low-flow modalities of hemofiltration are useful for critically ill individuals needing multisystem support.

- Hypotension is less of a problem than with hemodialysis, even though a large volume of fluid is removed.
- Disequilibrium and other systems/findings of intracellular osmolar shift are rare.
- Large volumes of parenteral nutrition may be given; fluid balance is maintained at a stable level.
- Improved blood pressure control in hypertensive individuals during periods between treatments has been attributed to better sodium and volume control, and improved autonomic stability.
- Hemofiltration allows removal of harmful substances of large molecular size, such as myocardial depressant factor (MDF).

These positive attributes of hemofiltration have resulted in the development of CRRT

HEMOPERFUSION

In hemoperfusion blood is brought in direct contact with a sorbent material, packaged in a cartridge or column. Most devices use 70 to 300 g of activated charcoal coated with a polymer film to reduce embolism by tiny carbon particles and to decrease platelet and cellular element buildup.

What are the indications for using hemoperfusion?

Hemoperfusion is used primarily for drug overdose or toxic exposure of great severity. Activated charcoal binds most chemicals in the range of 100 to 20,000 Da. Most medications have molecular weights of 500 to 2000 Da. Hemoperfusion is more effective than hemodialysis for removal of most sedatives, theophylline, digoxin, and some pesticides and herbicides.

In association with deferoxamine (DFO) chelation, charcoal may be used to remove excess aluminum or iron from body tissue.

What are the adverse effects of hemoperfusion?

A transient decrease in platelets is frequent; it corrects within 24 hours in most instances. Some patients have a fall in white cell count. Hemolysis or red cell damage is unusual. Hypotension is frequent; the poisoned patient is already very brittle. Heavy anticoagulation is needed, and postprocedure bleeding may be prolonged.

Is there a limit to the capacity of the cartridges?

Yes. Adsorptive capacity is limited and is difficult to determine in advance. The kinetics of adsorption are complex. Overall mass transfer relates to a fluid transfer rate and an intraparticle transfer rate, which depend on microcapillary size and solute diffusion. Clearance of some solutes may decrease gradually over time until the sorbent is filled; for others, clearance may fall off rapidly even though considerable sorbent capacity remains.

Apheresis

The term *apheresis* is a Greek expression for "taking something away." Plasmapheresis has been conducted for a number of years to separate plasma protein components using special centrifuges. Synthetic hollow-fiber technology produces filters of selectively permeable capability to remove specific blood constituents, e.g., antibodies and immunoglobulins.

Plasmapheresis has been used experimentally for a variety of conditions, including transplant rejection by reducing antibody titer. The technique is of definite value in hyperviscosity syndrome, cryoglobulinemia, thrombotic thrombocytopenic purpura, myasthenia gravis crisis, Guillain-Barré syndrome, refractory idiopathic—or autoimmune—hemolytic anemia, multiple myeloma with renal failure, and Goodpasture syndrome.

What substances can be removed either by dialysis or hemoperfusion?

As a general rule, substances completely or almost completely excreted by the normal kidney will be removed by dialysis. Substances metabolized by the liver, or their by-products, may not be removed by hemodialysis. Information about the site of metabolism and excretion of most drugs is often obtainable from the package insert or from pharmacology texts. The *Physicians' Desk Reference (PDR)* is another quick resource. A computerized textbook of treatment options for drug overdoses and poisonings, or *Poisindex,* should be available. Information on this system can be very useful because it is updated regularly. Regional poison centers have information on drugs or poisons. The intoxicating substance(s) should be identified and quantified as soon as possible. Often quantitative results may take several hours and are not available when most urgently needed.

What if the substance is not known or cannot be readily verified?

The decision to treat or not, and by what modality, becomes a clinical one, to be made by the physician. If the patient is severely ill and the circumstances suggest one or more of the substances ingested is likely to be removable by hemoperfusion or dialysis, treatment should be started. This is because the duration of coma, morbidity, and mortality may be reduced by early initiation of treatment.

For what toxic agents is dialysis recommended as specific treatment of choice?

Alcohols, such as methyl alcohol and ethylene or propylene glycol (antifreeze), are easily dialyzed. Salicylates (aspirin), lithium carbonate, and aminophylline dialyze well. Certain mushrooms *(Amanita phalloides)* call for immediate hemodialysis therapy. Early removal of toxins may prevent the blindness, liver necrosis, renal failure, or death that can result from such poisons. Accidental therapeutic intravenous drug overdose from such agents as theophylline, antibiotics, or mannitol may require emergent dialysis to decrease the risk of serious complications.

Is there any particular type of dialyzer preferable for poisonings?

In poisoning, the objective is to remove as much of the offending agent as rapidly as possible. Therefore a dialyzer with the largest surface area the patient will tolerate should be used. High-middle molecule clearance devices (i.e., 500 to 20,000 Da) may be the dialyzer of choice.

What poisonings are best treated by charcoal hemoperfusion?

Sedatives, including barbiturates, ethchlorvynol, and glutethimide, and many insecticides and herbicides have better removal by hemoperfusion than by hemodialysis.

What about bloodstream access for dialysis of poisons?

The most appropriate access, if the patient does not already have a permanent vascular access, is a temporary catheter placed in a large vein, such as femoral, subclavian, or internal jugular. The greater the blood flow, the greater the removal of toxins.

Does peritoneal dialysis have any place in the treatment of poisoning?

It is rarely appropriate, and only if hemodialysis is not available or will be delayed. Peritoneal dialysis has low clearance rates and takes longer in removing drugs than hemodialysis and hemoperfusion. However, if preparation for hemodialysis will be delayed, and peritoneal dialysis can be instituted at once, it can be a temporary treatment option.

Should hemodialysis and charcoal hemoperfusion be used together?

Hemoperfusion has a greater affinity and faster clearance for many toxins than does hemodialysis. However, hemoperfusion does not provide the ultrafiltration that may be needed for hypervolemia or pulmonary edema. Perfusion alone does not correct acid-base imbalance or electrolyte abnormalities, which may be very important in the acidosis associated with many intoxications. Sometimes sequential use of hemodialysis and hemoperfusion is recommended. The appropriate treatment is dictated by the properties of the poison or drug that needs to be removed.

What special patient problems may be encountered in dialysis or hemoperfusion of ingested or intravenous poisons or drug overdoses?

Such patients are generally critically ill, possibly with multisystem failure. Most are hemodynamically unstable. Specific problems may include the following:

Hypotension. This responds poorly to volume replacement; infusion of a pressor agent such as dopamine is frequently necessary; however, the pressor agent's effect may be reduced by the dialysis or hemoperfusion.

Respiratory depression or apnea. The patient may have an endotracheal tube or tracheostomy and may require ventilatory assistance equipment.

Severe acid-base imbalance. Patients who have an alkalosis from the drug intoxication may experience worsening of the condition with the dialysis treatment. The amount of bicarbonate in the dialysate may have to be adjusted. Often custom dialysate is required with changes during the treatment.

DIALYSIS IN RELATION TO TRANSPLANT

Many patients receive dialysis as part of the plan for kidney transplant (see Chapter 16). Dialysis may be initiated immediately pretransplant as preparation for surgery, during surgery, or following transplantation as support because of technical complications or complications during rejection episodes. Patients who require dialysis during posttransplant dysfunction or acute rejection require special treatment considerations.

What is posttransplant kidney dysfunction?

This is a form of acute renal failure seen occasionally with living donor kidneys and more often with deceased donor kidneys. It is usually related to the length of the "warm and cold ischemia time." This is the time measured from the kidney removal to its revascularization in the transplanted patient. The mechanism is similar to that of acute tubular necrosis. The kidney usually begins to function in about 10 days, occasionally going as long as 3 to 4 weeks before producing quality urine (see Chapter 16).

DIALYSIS PATIENTS WITH TRANSPLANT REJECTION
What are special problems in the dialysis of posttransplant patients?

Maintenance of fluid balance is essential to the function of the transplanted kidney. Care must be taken not to be overly aggressive with fluid removal; the resulting hypotension could cause hypoperfusion of the new organ and lead to renal dysfunction. In the early postoperative period, such patients have all the problems of recent major surgery. "No heparin dialysis" should be used to prevent bleeding at the operative site. Because of steroids, patients may be intensely catabolic, with BUN disproportionately high in relation to serum creatinine. Hypertension may be aggravated by steroid treatment. Wound healing may be slow, and some drainage is common. Patients who have lost a transplant to severe rejection usually have been treated with steroids. Their tissues are often edematous and extremely friable. Patients with infections and rejection are almost always catabolic, edematous, and hypoproteinemic. Their cardiopulmonary and cardiovascular systems are often labile, and hypotension or cardiac dysrhythmias and pulmonary congestion should be anticipated.

16 Transplantation

Nephrology nurses who primarily care for patients undergoing dialysis treatment have several roles involving transplantation. They educate and counsel patients regarding the option of transplantation, and they may assist patients undergoing the pretransplant evaluation. They may also need to provide dialysis treatments for transplant recipients experiencing temporary loss of renal function from acute tubular necrosis (ATN) or a rejection episode and patients with permanent loss of a transplanted kidney. Nephrology nurses and technicians may also provide dialysis for recipients of transplanted nonrenal organs (such as liver or heart), who are experiencing acute or chronic renal failure.

What are the advantages of renal transplantation?

The most important advantage of renal transplantation is improved quality of life. Patients with a successful kidney transplant report a higher quality of life compared to patients receiving other forms of renal replacement therapy. With no need for dialysis treatment and more complete resolution of uremic symptoms, successful transplant recipients can experience a more "normal" lifestyle including family, social, and vocational activities. Another benefit is cost. Although the initial year of transplantation is more costly than dialysis treatment, the subsequent years' costs are significantly less. Finally, although the long-term survival rate for patients undergoing dialytic therapies has vastly improved, transplantation may offer patients an opportunity for a longer survival. Since the introduction of cyclosporine, survival rates for transplant recipients are longer than for dialysis patients. This difference is most pronounced in individuals with diabetes mellitus.

What are the disadvantages of renal transplantation?

The disadvantages of transplantation stem from the need for lifelong immunosuppression to prevent the body from rejecting the organ. The necessity for daily medication compliance is a minor nuisance for some patients and an insurmountable hurdle for others. Especially in the initial postoperative period, family support can be crucial in ensuring adherence to what is often a daunting medication regimen.

Probably a more important disadvantage to transplantation is the vast potential complications of immunosuppression. Direct consequences of suppressing the immune system are increased risk of infection and of some malignancies. The medications also carry the potential for some nonimmunologic complications such as bone disease, cataracts, diabetes mellitus, hyperlipidemia, hypertension, and gastrointestinal complications such as ulcers, hyperuricemia, and hyperkalemia. Obesity as well as more cosmetic side effects such as hirsutism and gingival hyperplasia may also occur.

Another major hurdle for many patients is the difficulty paying for the costly immunosuppressive medications. Although Centers for Medicare and Medicaid Services (CMS) provides 80% coverage for the first 36 months after transplantation, many patients do not have other insurance coverage. Nephrology nurses practicing in transplantation, along with social workers, assist transplant recipients in finding solutions to this problem.

The process of transplantation—from evaluation and waiting for a donor organ to the surgical hospitalization and threatened or actual rejection—places a great deal of stress on both the patient and family members. Again, strong social support is a crucial component of successfully coping with the stress of transplantation. Table 16-1 summarizes the risks and benefits of transplantation.

What are the risks and benefits of combined kidney-pancreas transplantation?

Dialysis patients who also suffer from diabetes mellitus may want to consider a combined kidney-pancreas transplant. The major benefits of this procedure are:
- Euglycemia, which may halt or slow the progression of diabetic sequelae
- Freedom from frequent insulin injections and fingersticks for glucose measurement

Table 16-1	The Transplant Trade-Off
Improved quality of life vs.	**Lifelong immunosuppression**
Freedom from dialysis	Necessity for daily medication
More normal lifestyle	Increased risk of infection
Longer survival rate	Increased risk of malignancy
Increased ability to pursue normal activities—work, home, school	Loss of sick role
	Steroid bone disease
More complete resolution of uremic symptoms:	*Potential medication side effects:*
	Hypertension
Normal calcium/phos	Ulcers/dyspepsia/other gastrointestinal effects
Improved cardiac function	
Improved appetite	Hyperkalemia, hyperlipidemia, obesity
Less restrictive diet	Body image changes; hirsutism, gingival hyperplasia
Improved sexual function	
Increased feeling of wellness	Diabetes mellitus, gout, cataracts, tremor
Increased mental acuity	Psychologic stress
Less costly than dialysis	Difficulty paying for costly medications

- For those individuals with hypoglycemic unawareness, the combined procedure is a lifesaver.

The combined kidney-pancreas transplant procedure is more complicated and has more risks than kidney transplantation alone. These risks are associated with:

- Longer surgery
- Exocrine drainage of the pancreas. Many transplant surgeons choose to drain amylase, a digestive enzyme made by the pancreas, to the urinary bladder using a piece of donor duodenum as a conduit. Although this procedure allows for monitoring of pancreatic function by measuring urinary amylase, the amylase may cause acute or chronic cystitis or urethritis. In addition, the patients lose a great deal of bicarbonate and fluid and thus have a tendency to develop acidosis and dehydration.
- Increased immunosuppression-associated risks. The transplanted pancreas is much more prone to stimulate the body's immune system than is a transplanted kidney, thus greater amounts of immunosuppression are required.

Who should be considered as a transplant candidate?

In general, all patients should be offered the option of consultation with a transplant team to determine their eligibility. Box 16-1 summarizes absolute and relative contraindications to transplantation.

Can patients who are human immunodeficiency virus (HIV) positive receive a kidney transplant?

In the past, HIV was an absolute contraindication to transplant because of concerns that the immunosuppressant therapy used in transplants might exacerbate the patient's HIV

Box 16-1
ABSOLUTE AND RELATIVE CONTRAINDICATIONS TO TRANSPLANTATION

Absolute Contraindications

Active infection

Active malignancy

Active substance abuse

Inability to comply with medication regimen

Relative Contraindications

Age: Very young or older than 65 years

Severe comorbidities

Lack of family support

Mental/psychologic problems

infection. Today, most transplant centers do not transplant HIV-positive patients; however, new findings suggest that it may be safe to transplant some HIV-positive patients. The University of Pittsburgh is one of 10 transplant centers participating in a study to determine the safety of liver and kidney transplants in patients infected with HIV. This study is being funded by the National Institutes of Health. There currently is no policy that states that patients with HIV cannot receive transplants.

What is the immunologic basis of transplantation?

The immune system protects the body from foreign invasion by identifying the invaders and then destroying them. Anything that produces this response is called an antigen. The basis of immunology in transplantation is to identify how the body recognizes foreign antigens. Transplant immunologists have identified two main antigen systems that affect the acceptance or rejection of a transplanted organ or tissue. These two systems are blood groups and the human leukocyte antigen (HLA). Blood groups are the first determinant of compatibility for solid organ transplantation. In general, an organ must be ABO compatible with the recipient to be transplanted. For this reason, transplant recipient waiting lists are arranged by ABO group. The rhesus (Rh) factor is not applicable to solid organ transplantation.

The HLA system is composed of a group of genes found on the sixth chromosome. Three main sites or loci on this chromosome—A, B, and DR—have been identified as influencing the recognition of foreign tissue. Because each individual has two of each chromosome, one donated by each parent, six loci are identified for each person. When tissue is introduced to the body with different HLA genes, the immune system is triggered and the rejection process begins.

The components of the immune system that are most important in transplantation are the T-cell and B-cell lymphocytes. T-cell lymphocytes recognize the foreign tissue and initiate the rejection process. B-cell lymphocytes recognize the foreign antigen and produce antibodies to destroy the invader. Once presented, both T and B cells will remember a foreign antigen and attack it more quickly in subsequent presentations. Humans develop immunologic memory to HLA antigens through exposure via blood transfusions, pregnancy, and transplantation.

What is tissue typing?

Tissue typing refers to blood tests designed to identify the HLA genetic markers. Although HLA matching is used to distribute organs objectively, modern immunosuppressive medications have made HLA matching increasingly less important in successful outcomes. Many centers transplant organs with no HLA similarities (zero matched organs), as long as the crossmatch is negative, with excellent results. When the body recognizes and forms immunity to one HLA antigen, it often forms immunity to other related antigens, even though these antigens were not presented to the body. This crossover immunity has been recognized by the development of cross-reactive antigen groups (CREG) tests. CREG matching may improve outcomes in minority groups. The

United Network for Organ Sharing (UNOS) began pilot studies with CREG matching in 1997.

What is crossmatching?

Monthly serum samples from potential recipients are used to perform crossmatching tests. Crossmatching tests are blood tests that determine whether a recipient has acquired immunity to a given donor organ tissue. The tests are performed when a donor organ becomes available. Serum from all eligible recipients is tested with donor lymph cells. A positive crossmatch means that the recipient has memory or acquired immunity to the donor and therefore cannot receive the organ. The routine test is the Amos and antiglobulin test, which takes about 6 hours to complete, although more sophisticated and time-consuming tests, such as flow cytometry crossmatches, may sometimes be performed. In living donor transplantation, an additional test called a mixed leukocyte reaction (MLR) may be ordered, although this takes several days to complete and has not proven to be of great value.

What are PRA levels?

Another important crossmatching test is called panel reactive antibody (PRA). The potential recipient's serum is tested against a panel of random donors. The number of positive reactions to donor panel is expressed as a percentage. This percentage represents the risk of a positive crossmatch and thus incompatibility with any random donor. Therefore, the higher a potential recipient's PRA, the less likely that any given organ will be compatible. For this reason, patients with high PRAs are given preference in the distribution of organs from deceased donors.

What is the purpose of the monthly serum samples? Why send them in every month?

The numbers of sensitized lymphocytes that constitute preformed immunity to any particular antigen may wax and wane over time. Sometimes the number may be so low that the PRA may fall. Because of this phenomenon, sometimes a specific crossmatch using current serum will be negative even though the crossmatch using older or historic serum is positive. Because immunosuppression will be applied to block the memory response, a current negative crossmatch may indicate a window of opportunity for a potential recipient. On the other hand, immunity provoked by a blood transfusion after the most current serum sample was obtained could give a falsely negative crossmatch. The variability of immune status necessitates monthly serum samples for potential recipients.

What does the recipient workup entail?

The evaluation process for a kidney or other organ transplant begins with referral to the transplant center. The potential recipient and family meet members of the transplant team. This team usually consists of transplant nurse coordinators, transplant surgeons, transplant nephrologists, and social workers. Once the team has determined the initial eligibility of a candidate, the transplant nurse coordinator works with the patient, dialysis healthcare team, and primary healthcare provider to facilitate the evaluation. Although the evaluation may find that transplantation is not a viable option for some potential recipients, the ultimate goal of the pretransplant workup is to find out as much about the patient as possible in order to perform a successful transplant.

The evaluation generally consists of blood, urine, and other diagnostic tests such as chest x-ray and electrocardiogram, as well as careful review of the patient's records. Special attention is given to the following areas:

- Cardiovascular assessment, which may include cardiac arteriogram, echocardiogram, and stress testing
- Infection surveillance, which usually includes a dental examination
- Malignancy detection
- Genitourinary tract assessment
- Psychosocial evaluation, which may include screening for illicit drugs

What are the possible sources for organs?

Two main sources of kidneys for transplantation are living donors or deceased donors. Living donors can be related to the recipient by blood, such as a parent or sibling, or emotionally such as a spouse, close friend, or adopted child. The key requirements for living donation are voluntary informed consent and a completely healthy donor.

Deceased donors are individuals who have died from irreversible brain death. Their bodies are kept functioning by artificial ventilation and medications. With the consent of next of kin, the organs and tissues are procured by the organ recovery team and distributed by the regional organ and tissue bank in accordance with national guidelines. There is no expense to the donor family and usual funeral arrangements are not affected by organ and tissue donation. There is currently a shortage in the United States of organs from deceased donors.

What happens after a patient is placed on the deceased donor waiting list?

After a candidate is considered eligible for transplantation and no living donors are available, the transplant center places the candidate's name on the deceased donor waiting list. Kidneys are distributed by a point system. Points are given for length of time on the waiting list and degree of HLA match. Because of the difficulty in finding suitable kidneys for these patients, additional points are given to patients with high PRAs. In general, kidneys from deceased donors in one blood group are only offered to recipients in that same blood group; therefore, the waiting list is divided by blood group. When deceased donor kidneys are procured, the organ bank offers them to transplant centers in this order:

1. Any potential recipient anywhere in the country that matches with the donor at all six HLA loci
2. Locally according to the point system
3. Regionally and then nationally according to the point system

Most kidneys are used locally. Other organs are also distributed in an equitable, objective manner, locally first, with medical need as the main determinant.

What is the responsibility of the dialysis team while the patient waits for a kidney?

Many patients wait 1 to 2 years before receiving their organ. It is important for the dialysis health care team to keep the transplant center informed regarding the health status of potential recipients and make certain that no recipient misses his or her chance at an organ because of missing serum samples.

Where are transplant kidneys placed? How long is the surgery?

The transplanted kidney is usually placed extraperitoneally in the right or left iliac fossa of the recipient. The incision extends from above the iliac crest to just above the symphysis pubis. Although the right iliac fossa is generally preferred for primary transplantation, either side may be used. If the recipient has had a previous transplant, the transplant surgeon will generally select the side not previously used. The donor renal artery is anastomosed end-to-end with the recipient internal iliac (hypogastric) artery or end-to-side with the external iliac artery. The venous anastomosis is generally end-to-side to the recipient's external iliac vein. The donor ureter is attached to the recipient's bladder or rarely, the recipient's ureter (Fig. 16-1). If a pancreas is also being transplanted, it will be placed in the opposite iliac fossa (Fig. 16-2). The kidney transplantation procedure generally lasts $2\frac{1}{2}$ to 4 hours.

The iliac fossae are preferred placement sites even when the patient has had two or more transplants. Occasionally, adhesions and scarring from multiple transplantation or other surgical procedures or severe atherosclerotic disease preclude the use of these sites. In these extremely rare cases, the surgeon may place the kidney intraperitoneally and use other vasculature including the abdominal aorta.

How long do patients stay in the hospital after transplantation?

Transplant recipients are usually discharged at 3 to 5 days after the transplantation procedure. Of course, surgical or medical complications may delay discharge, but the hospital stay may also be prolonged if the transplant team has concerns about the patient's or the patient's family's ability to provide adequate postoperative care.

Why do some transplant recipients require dialysis?

Like other individuals, organ transplant recipients may require dialysis treatment for fluid removal, electrolyte imbalance, uremia, or a combination of these reasons. Renal—as well as extrarenal (such as liver and heart)—transplant recipients often need hemofiltration after surgery because of the vast amounts of fluids used to maintain cardiovascular stability during the procedure. The patient's new kidney may be slow to respond to this fluid load. Kidney transplant recipients with ATN or an acute rejection attempt may

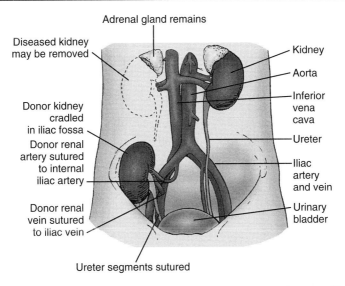

Adrenal gland remains

Diseased kidney may be removed

Donor kidney cradled in iliac fossa

Donor renal artery sutured to internal iliac artery

Donor renal vein sutured to iliac vein

Ureter segments sutured

Kidney

Aorta

Inferior vena cava

Ureter

Iliac artery and vein

Urinary bladder

Fig. 16-1 Transplanted kidney placement in the right iliac fossa. *(From Black JM, Hawks JH, Keene AM:* Medical-Surgical Nursing: Clinical Management for Positive Outcomes, *ed 7, Philadelphia, 2005, Saunders.)*

require temporary dialysis. Recipients of extrarenal organs often have concomitant renal disease or acute renal failure. Uremia and/or electrolyte imbalances may occur in these patients as well. Fluid and solute removal via traditional hemodialysis, peritoneal dialysis, or methods such as slow, continuous ultrafiltration (SCUF) or continuous venovenous hemofiltration (CVVH) may be employed.

What is ATN?

ATN occurs in up to 45% of all deceased donor kidney transplantations and rarely in living donor transplantations. ATN is characterized by oliguria (although high urine output ATN is occasionally seen) and failure of the serum creatinine to fall after a technically successful transplantation procedure. Its etiology is not well described, but it is probably due to a combination of factors including preservation injury, prolonged cold storage time, vascular instability of the donor or recipient during the harvest or transplant procedure, or reperfusion injury. Cyclosporine may exacerbate or prolong ATN and thus the initiation of cyclosporine therapy may be delayed in recipients with ATN. These individuals may require dialysis until the kidney begins to function, which is generally in several days to 2 weeks. ATN can last for several months with a good eventual outcome; however, oliguria and uremia that extend beyond two weeks may also be caused from rejection or drug-induced nephrotoxicity. A percutaneous biopsy of the kidney is usually performed to establish a diagnosis. Patients with ATN need reassurance and support from their caregivers. It is helpful to allow them to ventilate their

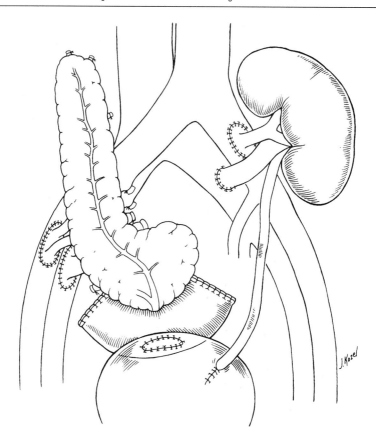

Fig. 16-2 Technique of combined kidney-pancreas transplantation with the duodenal segment bladder drainage technique. *(From Sollinger HW, et al: Experience with simultaneous pancreas-kidney transplantation, Ann Surg 208(4):475-483, 1988.)*

feelings about still requiring dialysis and to inform them that most transplanted kidneys with ATN eventually function well.

What special precautions should be taken when dialyzing a transplant recipient?

The following precautions are most notable:

- During the initial 24 hours after surgery, internal bleeding is a concern, so hypotension should be carefully monitored and brought to the attention of the physician.
- Because of the susceptibility of the transplanted kidney to ischemia, avoid hypotension, even at the cost of decreased fluid removal.
- The integrity of the surgical incision must be maintained.

- Anticoagulation is also a concern in transplant recipients. Heparin-free or minimal anticoagulation is preferred, especially in the immediate postoperative period or if they have undergone a diagnostic percutaneous renal biopsy.
- Electrolyte imbalances are common after transplantation. The most common is hyperkalemia. Hyperkalemia is common in patients with impaired graft function but is also caused by medications such as cyclosporine and tacrolimus. Other electrolyte abnormalities are outlined in Table 16-2.

Is there an increased risk of infection after transplantation?

Increased risk of infection is an inevitable consequence of immunosuppression. In the immediate postoperative period, bacterial infections in sites such as the wound, urinary tract, and lungs are more common, whereas viral infections such as cytomegalovirus (CMV), herpes simplex, and herpes zoster are more prevalent after the first several weeks following transplantation. CMV is a major cause of morbidity and mortality in transplant recipients. Many centers employ prophylactic medications such as ganciclovir or hyperimmune gamma globulin to prevent CMV infection or reactivation. Strict adherence to standard precautions should reduce the number of infectious complications in these patients. Isolation is rarely required, and transplant recipients pose no special risk to other patients or staff.

Does any one immunosuppressive medication place the transplant recipient at higher risk for malignancy?

Transplant recipients have demonstrated a higher risk for lymphoma, Kaposi's sarcoma, cervical cancer, vulvar and perineal cancer, hepatobiliary cancers, sarcomas, and lip cancers than the general population. No one immunosuppressant has been found to increase the risk; rather, the risk increases as the total amount of immunosuppression increases. When detected early, many of these cancers respond well to treatment.

What are the most commonly used immunosuppressive medications?

Immunosuppressive medications can be classified into five groups: steroids, calcineurin inhibitors, antimetabolites, antilymphocyte agents, and chimeric monoclonal antibodies. Table 16-3 outlines the major immunosuppressive medications used in organ transplantation. Most centers employ triple drug maintenance immunosuppressant therapy consisting of steroids, a calcineurin inhibitor, and an antimetabolite. Antilymphocyte preparations are used for a short time as rejection prophylaxis or treatment. All immunosuppressive medications carry the risk of infection and malignancy.

Steroids

Oral prednisone and intravenous methylprednisolone sodium (Solumedrol) are the most commonly used steroids. Steroids are used to both prevent and treat rejection.

Table 16-2	Electrolyte Abnormalities after Transplantation	
Abnormality	Predisposing factors	Treatment
Hyperkalemia	ATN Cyclosporine Tacrolimus Trimethoprim- sulfamethoxazole Blood transfusions	Dialysis IV 50% dextrose/insulin Kayexalate Diuretics Diet
Hypokalemia	Rapid post-treatment diuresis Diuretics	K^+ supplements Diet

Hypocalcemia (often w/
   hyperphosphatemia)
	Parathyroidectomy
	Hyperparathyroidism +
	   ATN
		Calcium supplements
		Increased calcium dialysate
		   calcitriol (Rocaltrol)
		Phosphorus binders

Hypercalcemia (often w/
   hypophosphatemia)
	Hyperparathyroidism +
	   functioning kidney
		Diet
		Phosphorus supplement
		   calcitriol to suppress
		   PTH (if calcium <11)

Hypomagnesemia	Diuresis Cyclosporine	Magnesium supplement
Acidosis	ATN Rejection Cyclosporine Pancreas transplant w/bladder drainage	Sodium bicarbonate Dialysis Sodium citrate

ATN, Acute tubular necrosis; *PTH,* parathyroid hormone.

Steroids, although easy to use and inexpensive, have the potential for a vast number of side effects that can be minimized by using the lowest possible dose.

Calcineurin Inhibitors

Cyclosporine (Sandimmune, Neoral) and tacrolimus (FK 506, Prograf) are immuno-suppressant drugs derived from fungi. These drugs block T-cell action by blocking the chemical signal calcineurin. Cyclosporine and tacrolimus have similar side effect

Table 16-3	Immunosuppressant Medications		
Medication	Action	Side effects	Dialysis of drug
Steroids (prednisone, Solumedrol)	Blocks interleukin-1	Cushingoid appearance, glucose intolerance, hyperlipidemia, bone disease, muscle wasting, cataracts, gastric ulcers, sodium retention, increased appetite, night sweats, skin thinning, delayed healing, psychosis, pancreatitis	HD-Y PD-U
Cyclosporine (Sandimmune, Neoral)	Blocks interleukin-2	Nephrotoxicity, hypertension, hyperlipidemia, tremors, numbness or burning in hands and feet, headaches, nervousness, gingival hyperplasia, hirsutism, hyperuricemia	HD-N PD-N
Tacrolimus (Prograf)	Blocks interleukin-2	Nephrotoxicity, headaches, tremor, gastric distress, glucose intolerance, neurotoxicity	HD-N PD-U
Azathioprine (Imuran)	Prevents lymphocyte proliferation	Myelotoxicity: leucopenia, thrombocytopenia, anemia; hepatotoxicity	HD-Y PD-NA
Mycophenolate mofetil (CellCept)	Prevents lymphocyte proliferation	Gastrointestinal distress, gastric ulcers including perforation and hemorrhage, constipation, leucopenia, anemia, albuminuria	HD-N PD-N
ATGAM	Blocks action of T cells	Thrombocytopenia, neutropenia, anemia, anaphylactic reaction	HD-U PD-U
Daclizumab (Zenapax)	Blocks interleukin-2 receptors of T and B cells	Uncommon: nausea, vomiting, other gastrointestinal effects; headache, fever, hypotension, hypertension	HD-U PD-U

HD, Hemodialysis; *N,* no; *NA,* data not available; *PD,* peritoneal dialysis; *U,* unlikely; *Y,* yes.

Continued

Table 16-3	Immunosuppressant Medications—cont'd		
Medication	Action	Side effects	Dialysis of drug
Basilizimab (Simulect)	Block interleukin-2 receptors of activated T cells	Uncommon: nausea, vomiting, other gastrointestinal effects; headache, fever, hypotension, hypertension	HD-U PD-U
Muromonab-CD3 (OKT3, Orthoclone)	Blocks action of CD3 T cells	First dose: pulmonary edema, fever chills Note: Prevented by premedication and avoiding fluid overload Subsequent doses: flulike symptoms: fever, chills, headache, arthralgias, myalgias; aseptic meningitis	HD-U PD-U

profiles. Nephrotoxicity is a major problem with both medications, complicating the diagnosis of rejection. Tacrolimus offers the advantage of not sharing the cyclosporine effects of hirsutism, or gingival hyperplasia, and may not have as deleterious an effect on serum lipids as does cyclosporine, but is more likely than cyclosporine to cause diabetes and gastrointestinal symptoms. Tacrolimus is a more powerful immunosuppressant than cyclosporine, and thus the doses used are much smaller. The doses of both medications are based on blood levels obtained 12 hours after the last dose of medication. In most cases, these drugs are not used in combination but used interchangeably. A change of medication is usually precipitated by a severe rejection episode or intolerable side effects while receiving one of these medications. Cyclosporine—either as Sandimmune or Neoral, the more readily absorbed microemulsion form—is the primary drug used in kidney and heart transplantation. At many centers, tacrolimus is the primary agent employed in pancreas, liver, and small bowel transplantation.

Antimetabolites

Azathioprine (Imuran) and mycophenolate mofetil (CellCept) are both antimetabolites. Mycophenolate mofetil is rapidly replacing azathioprine in transplantation because it appears to have an improved immunosuppressive effect, including action against B cells. This B-cell-blocking action makes mycophenolate mofetil the only immunosuppressant that may treat chronic rejection.

Antilymphocyte Preparations

ATGAM and OKT3 (Orthoclone) are the primary antilymphocyte agents used as prophylaxis against, or to treat, rejection. These powerful immunosuppressants are made by immunizing an animal with human lymphocytes and using the resultant antibodies. These antibodies block the function of T cells in the recipient. ATGAM is a polyclonal preparation, which means it has antibodies against a host of human blood cells, including platelets and red blood cells. It is administered in a manner similar to that used for other serum products, using a central vein catheter. OKT3 is a product of genetic engineering; the only specific antibodies present are those that block the function of certain T cells known as CD3 cells. This monoclonal preparation is given as an intravenous push medication via a peripheral vein. The most serious side effects from OKT3 occur after the first one or two doses and thus special precautions, including avoiding fluid overload, are observed.

Chimeric Monoclonal Antibodies

Several new monoclonal antibodies have been developed for use in transplantation. Basiliximab (Simulect) and daclizumab (Zenapax) are similar drugs developed to prevent transplant rejection. They are both humanized or chimeric antibodies, that is, the majority of the antibody is partial human immunoglobulin with only a small portion being murine antibody. This humanization means that the body is less likely to recognize it as a foreign protein, and thus first-dose side effects are minimized, and the drug enjoys a prolonged half-life. Both drugs prevent rejection by interfering with interleukin-2 binding of lymphocytes. They are given intravenously in the first weeks after transplant. Baciliximab is given in two doses (2 hours before transplant and on postoperative day 4); the recommended course of daclizumab is five doses beginning immediately before surgery and then every other week. Both drugs appear to be similar in efficacy and safety.

Mammalian Target of Rapamycin (mTOR)

Sirolimus (Rapamune) was approved for use by the U.S. Food and Drug Administration (FDA) in 2000 for the prevention of organ rejection in patients receiving a kidney transplant. Sirolimus inhibits T-lymphocyte activation and proliferation as well as antibody production, which makes it unique. This medication is initially taken in combination with cyclosporine and steroids. Cyclosporine can later be withdrawn from some patients with a low immunologic risk while increasing the dose of sirolimus. Side effects associated with this medication include increased serum cholesterol and triglycerides, hypertension, acne, fever, diarrhea, and rash. Increased creatinine levels may also be seen.

What is meant by rejection?

When the body's immune system recognizes the transplanted organ as foreign, it will attempt to destroy it. This phenomenon is called rejection. Rejection is carried out in two ways: cellular or humoral. Cellular rejection is initiated by T cells, and humoral rejection refers to destruction of the transplanted organ by specific antibodies.

What are the different kinds of transplant rejections?

There are basically three types of rejection processes: hyperacute rejection, acute rejection, and chronic rejection. Rejection episodes represent a great amount of stress to the recipient and his or her family.

Hyperacute Rejection

Hyperacute rejection is a humoral rejection process primarily caused by preformed antibodies to the transplanted tissue HLA or ABO antigens. This type of rejection occurs within minutes to hours of the transplantation procedure. The onslaught of specific antibodies causes massive intravascular coagulation and cell death. There is no treatment for hyperacute rejection. It is prevented by careful crossmatching.

Acute Rejection

When helper T cells recognize tissue cells as foreign, they initiate the cascade of events known as acute rejection. Acute rejection usually occurs weeks to months after transplantation. This form of cellular rejection generally occurs the first time the immune system is presented with a specific foreign tissue cell or antigen. The majority of immunosuppression is directed at preventing and treating acute rejection.

Chronic Rejection

In humoral rejection, B cells, stimulated by nonself-antigens produce antibodies to destroy the transplanted organ. Chronic rejection is a slow humoral rejection process that occurs months to years after transplantation. The hallmark of chronic rejection is slow gradual loss of function caused by fibrosis in the organ's blood vessels. Chronic rejection of the kidney may be difficult to distinguish from chronic cyclosporine toxicity.

How is rejection diagnosed and treated?

Increased serum creatinine, in the absence of other causes, is most commonly used as the diagnostic indicator of rejection. A percutaneous biopsy may be used to confirm the diagnosis.

Hyperacute Rejection

Hyperacute rejection is often diagnosed as soon as the vascular anastomoses are completed and the clamps released. The kidney will rapidly turn black and fail to produce urine, or the recipient may suffer severe symptoms of oliguria, fever, and pain soon after the transplant procedure. There is no treatment; the organ must be surgically removed.

Acute Rejection

Oliguria, fever, edema, weight gain, and graft tenderness are the cardinal physical symptoms of acute renal transplant rejection. However, modern immunosuppression blocks these symptoms, causing transplant clinicians to rely on biochemical markers. A rapid rise in the serum creatinine over several days with or without physical symptoms may indicate acute rejection. Nephrotoxicity is also a possible diagnosis, especially if drug levels are high.

Many rejection attempts can be treated by increased steroids. The steroids are delivered by intravenous boluses or "pulses" of methylprednisolone and/or increased oral prednisone that is rapidly tapered over several days back to baseline dose. If the rejection is severe or does not respond to steroids, antilymphocyte preparations (ATGAM, OKT3) are used. Most acute cellular rejections are successfully treated.

Chronic Rejection

Patients with chronic rejection often do not experience symptoms until the rejection has progressed to serious renal compromise. The serum creatinine slowly increases over months to years until the kidney ceases to function. Definitive diagnosis is made by biopsy. Traditionally, there has been no treatment for chronic rejection; however, mycophenolate mofetil (CellCept), which has action against antibody-inducing B cells, has demonstrated some success in treatment. Because it probably begins as very mild acute rejection, chronic rejection is best prevented by adequate immunosuppression and regular laboratory follow-up.

Who should provide long-term care/health maintenance after transplant?

A variety of healthcare providers are qualified to provide long-term care to successful transplant recipients. These care providers include transplant physicians, nephrologists, internists, family practice physicians, and nurse practitioners. The goal of long-term care is to assist the patient in achieving his/her maximum health potential. This goal is achieved by routine health maintenance, as well as a focus on the prevention, early detection, and treatment of the consequences of immunosuppression. As cardiovascular disease remains the number one cause of death in the first decade after successful renal transplantation, particular attention is paid to this area. Cancer and infection surveillance are also focus areas. The degree of rehabilitation to career, family, and social life is assessed and interventions implemented if necessary.

What happens when the transplanted kidney irreversibly fails?

When the transplant team has determined that the transplanted kidney has irreversibly failed and that further treatment would be unsuccessful or detrimental, the patient returns to maintenance dialysis treatment. Except in the cases of hyperacute rejection, early vascular catastrophe, or untreated acute rejection, the transplanted kidney usually slowly scars and shrinks as function ceases, thus surgical removal is not necessary. Failed transplanted kidneys are removed for severe hematuria, infection, or malignant hypertension. Immunosuppression is discontinued gradually to prevent superimposed acute rejection and to allow the adrenal glands to regain function.

These individuals require special nursing care. In addition to the effects of immunosuppression, which may remain for several months, the failed transplant represents a crisis for the patient and family. The loss of the transplanted kidney may provoke depression, feelings of hopelessness, anger, and worthlessness. Individuals may experience the grieving process similar to the process described for those experiencing death and dying. Emotional support is essential for these patients. The dialysis staff should encourage the individual to seek another transplant, if appropriate.

17 Peritoneal Dialysis and Home Dialysis Therapies

Peritoneal dialysis (PD) is an alternative dialytic modality for the patient with end-stage renal disease (ESRD). From 1997 to 2001, the incident rates for hemodialysis rose 3.3% while the rates for PD fell almost 4%. The U.S. Renal Data System (US RDS) reports that only 7% of the prevalent ESRD population is on PD. It is primarily a home dialysis therapy for chronic renal failure, but it can also be a treatment option for the patient with acute renal failure in the hospital setting. The range of home therapies for the ESRD patient includes PD and home hemodialysis. Home therapy allows patients to remain somewhat independent in their own care and have greater control over their schedules. Of all the home therapies, PD is the most commonly used.

What is PD and how does it work?

PD is a process during which the peritoneal cavity acts as the reservoir for the dialysate and the peritoneum serves as the semipermeable membrane across which excess body fluid and solutes, including uremic toxins, are removed (ultrafiltrate). The peritoneal membrane surface area is approximately equal to the body surface area (1.73 m^2). The peritoneum consists of the lining of the inner surface of the abdominal and pelvic walls, including the diaphragm (parietal peritoneum) as well as the covering of the abdominal organs (visceral peritoneum). In males the peritoneum is a closed cavity, but in females the fallopian tubes and ovaries open into the peritoneal cavity.

The peritoneal membrane is in contact with the rich blood supply to the abdominal organs. Dialysate is infused into the peritoneal cavity via a catheter, allowed to dwell for a predetermined amount of time, and then drained (effluent). This process is called an exchange. Dextrose is used in the dialysate to create an osmotic gradient that causes water to be moved into the peritoneal cavity. The excess fluid is removed when the effluent is drained. Electrolytes and uremic toxins are removed by diffusion from an area of higher concentration (bloodstream) to an area of lower concentration (peritoneal cavity). Solute removal is further enhanced by "solute drag," created when hyper-tonic dialysate is used, which increases ultrafiltration (UF) and causes additional low-molecular-weight solutes to be "dragged" along with the UF by convective transport.

What solutions are used for peritoneal dialysis?

Commercially available solutions approximate the composition of extracellular body water except for potassium because many patients tend to be hyperkalemic. Potassium may be added (2 to 4 mEq/L) if necessary to correct hypokalemia. Oral potassium supplementation may also be prescribed. Dextrose provides the osmotic gradient between the plasma and the dialysate that leads to fluid and solute removal. The more hypertonic the dialysate (i.e., 2.5% and 4.25% dextrose) the greater the UF. After a 2-L exchange has been dwelling for 4 hours, an average of 200 mL of ultrafiltrate will be obtained with a 1.5% exchange and 600 to 1000 mL with a 4.25% exchange. Table 17-1 highlights some commercially available solutions.

What is Icodextrin?

Icodextrin (Extraneal) is a newer peritoneal dialysis solution that differs from standard dialysis solutions in that it does not contain dextrose. In standard PD dialysate, glucose is the osmotic agent. Icodextrin is a starch derived osmotic agent made from a mixture of glucose polymers. This solution allows for increased fluid removal from the bloodstream during peritoneal dialysis as well as reduced net negative UF and increased small solute clearance. Icodextrin is intended to be used for once daily, long dwell exchanges lasting 8 to 16 hours. The dialysate solution should be used for no more than one exchange in a 24-hour period. Icodextrin is contraindicated for those with glycogen storage diseases or an allergy to cornstarch. The most common adverse effect from the use of icodextrin is a skin rash. Sterile peritonitis, hypertension, cold, headache, flulike symptoms, and abdominal pain are other possible side effects.

Are there different ways to perform peritoneal dialysis?

PD can be done either manually or automatically with a cycler. The manual form of PD is called continuous ambulatory peritoneal dialysis (CAPD). In CAPD, four or more exchanges are performed each day. The patient connects to a tubing system, drains the effluent, and infuses new dialysate to dwell for a prescribed amount of time. Most patients do "bagless" CAPD; they disconnect from the tubing system at the end of the exchange, leaving a short transfer set or the capped catheter. Most CAPD tubing systems involve a Y configuration that enables the patient to "flush" any contaminants that might have been introduced while connecting to the system. Spiking the bag has been eliminated from most systems thus reducing the potential for contamination by as much as 50%.

What is automated peritoneal dialysis (APD)?

APD is performed with a cycler, usually at night while the patient sleeps. Cyclers are programmed according to the physician's prescription to perform the following functions automatically: (1) measure the volume of dialysate to be infused; (2) warm the dialysate to body temperature before infusion; (3) time the frequency of exchanges; (4) count the

Table 17-1	Commercially Available Peritoneal Dialysis Solutions							
				(mEq/L)				
Solution	Vol (mL)	% Dextrose	Na	Cl	Ca	Mg	Lactate
Dianeal PD-2 (Baxter Healthcare, Deerfield, Ill)	250, 500, 750, 1000, 1500, 2000, 2500, 3000, 5000, 6000	1.5 2.5 4.25	132	96	3.5	0.5	40
Dianeal PD-1 (Baxter Healthcare, Deerfield, Ill)	2000, 5000	1.5 2.5 4.25	132	102	3.5	1.5	35
Dianeal Low Ca (Baxter Healthcare, Deerfield, Ill)	1500, 2000, 2500, 3000, 5000, 6000	1.5 2.5 4.25	132	95	2.5	0.5	40
Icodextrin (Baxter Healthcare, Deerfield, Ill)	1500, 2000, 2500	N/A	132	96	3.5	0.5	40
Delflex (Fresenius, USA)	1000, 1500, 2000, 3000, 5000	1.5 2.5 4.25	132 132	102 96	3.5 2.5	1.5 0.5	40 40
Delflex (Fresenius, USA)	1500, 2000, 2500, 3000, 5000	1.5 2.5 4.25	132	95		0.5	40

N/A, Not applicable.

number of exchanges; and (5) measure UF. Cyclers can be programmed for volumes from 50 to 3000 mL per exchange, have a last bag option to accommodate a unique diurnal (day) dwell (volume, percentage, additives), and have the ability to program one or more exchanges during the daytime hours. All machines can be programmed to perform tidal PD. APD enables the patient to mix dextrose concentrations to achieve the desired UF, e.g., 2.5% mixed with 4.25% to get 3.3%.

What are the different forms of APD?

Continuous cycling peritoneal dialysis (CCPD). Three to five exchanges are performed
   nightly with a full diurnal dwell. The diurnal dwell improves the clearance of
   middle molecules.
Nocturnal intermittent peritoneal dialysis (NIPD). Three to five exchanges are
   performed nightly, but there is a minimal or no diurnal dwell. NIPD is indicated in
   patients who are unable to tolerate a diurnal dwell (e.g., those with
   hyperpermeability of the peritoneum to dextrose, resulting in absorption of diurnal
   dwell) and those with problems exacerbated by increased intraabdominal pressure,
   including hernias, low back pain, cardiopulmonary compromise, etc.
Intermittent peritoneal dialysis (IPD). Several frequent exchanges are performed three
   or four times a week, and the peritoneum is left "dry" between treatments. IPD is
   appropriate for patients with residual renal function or institutionalized patients.
   Also, it is used in economically underdeveloped countries because of the financial
   constraints imposed by daily peritoneal dialysis.
Tidal peritoneal dialysis (TPD). An initial volume of dialysate is infused, followed
   by partial drainage of effluent at the end of each exchange (leaving a constant
   reserve volume); finally a "tidal" volume of fresh dialysate is infused. TPD is
   intended to enhance clearance by maintaining continuous contact of dialysate
   with the peritoneum and maintenance of the dialysate/plasma gradient. TPD may
   improve clearances by 20% but increases costs because of the need for additional
   dialysate.
TPD may also be used for patients who experience discomfort or "drain pain" at the
   end of the drain cycle because of the position of tip of the PD catheter. By always
   having a reserve of fluid, the tip is allowed to float, thus alleviating discomfort in
   sensitive individuals.

What kinds of catheters are used for peritoneal dialysis?

Catheters for both acute and chronic PD must transport fluid into and out of the peritoneal cavity as rapidly as possible as well as be biocompatible (maintain normal structure and function of the tissues near the catheter tract). Catheters manufactured for both acute and chronic PD come in sizes to accommodate neonates to adults.

Catheters for acute PD are usually placed at the patient's bedside and include rigid catheters or soft silicone catheters. The patient should have an empty bladder and the rectum should be free of stool at the time of insertion to minimize the risk of organ perforation. Placement may be by direct insertion with a trocar or guidewire or by use of a peritoneoscope. Dialysis may be initiated immediately after insertion. Risks with the rigid catheter include bowel or organ perforation, dialysate leaks, peritonitis, discomfort, and inadvertent catheter loss. Silicone catheters, used for acute dialysis, are more comfortable and may be used for chronic dialysis if necessary. When an acute PD catheter is used immediately, the patient should be kept supine whenever dialysate is in the peritoneal cavity to minimize the occurrence of leaking of dialysate around the catheter.

Catheters used for chronic PD are usually placed surgically during a laparotomy or laparoscopically. The exit site should be directed in a downward or lateral direction and located in the right or left midquadrant area avoiding the belt line, scars, and skinfolds. Catheters are made of silicone or polyurethane with a radiopaque stripe for x-ray visualization. Catheters may be straight or coiled and have one or two cuffs. Coiled catheters are believed to minimize catheter migration out of the pelvis and have fewer outflow problems than straight catheters. The coiled catheter is also thought to improve patient comfort by keeping the tip of the catheter away from direct contact with the peritoneal membrane.

Cuffs are made of Dacron polyester or velour and provide for tissue ingrowth to stabilize the catheter. Cuffs are also intended to prevent migration of bacteria along the subcutaneous tunnel into the peritoneum. When placing double-cuffed catheters, the internal cuff is placed in the rectus muscle, and the external cuff is placed in the subcutaneous tissue proximal to the exit site. Implanted catheters (Fig. 17-1) consist of the following: an intraperitoneal segment containing side holes and an open tip for fluid flow; a subcutaneous segment that passes through the peritoneal membrane, muscles, and subcutaneous tissues; and an external segment that extends from the external cuff out to the exit site. There are several versions of chronic catheters including the Tenckhoff, column disk, Toronto Western, swan neck, Cruz, and Moncrief catheters (Fig. 17-2). All include features intended to improve dialysate flow and decrease catheter complications.

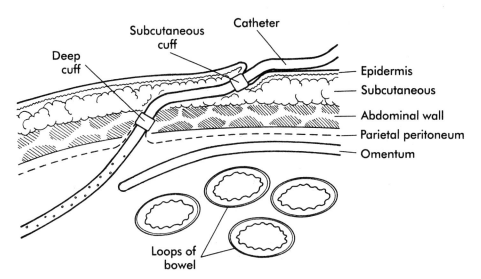

Fig. 17-1 Placement of double-cuffed Tenckhoff catheter. *(From Ash SR, Carr DJ, Diaz-Buxo JA: Peritoneal access devices. In Nissenson AR, Fine RN, Gentile DE, editors:* Clinical Dialysis, *ed 2, Norwalk, CT, 1990, Appleton & Lange.)*

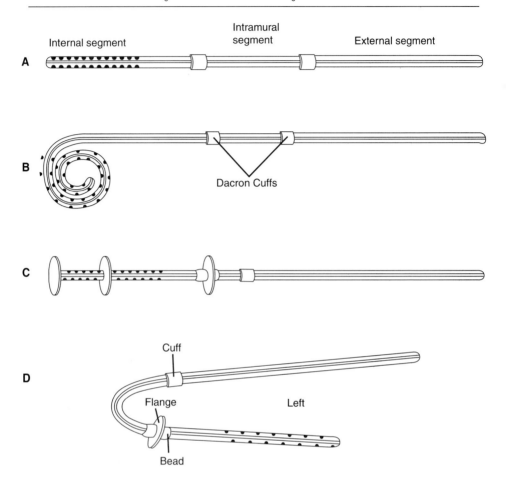

Fig. 17-2 Chronic catheters. **A,** Straight Tenckhoff catheter. **B,** Curled Tenckhoff catheter. **C,** Toronto Western catheter. **D,** Swan-neck (Missouri) catheter. *(From Smith T, editor:* Renal Nursing, *Philadelphia, 1998, Harcourt Brace & Co., Ltd., Bailliere Tindall.)*

What is meant by catheter break-in?

Catheter break-in is the period after the chronic catheter is placed, during which there is healing and tissue ingrowth into the cuff(s). The goals are to promote healing and prevent complications such as dialysate leaks, infections, or catheter obstruction. Healing may take up to 6 weeks and includes scab formation, granulation of tissue at the exit site, and epithelialization of the sinus tract. Full-volume dialysis, especially CAPD, should be avoided for at least 10 to 14 days to allow healing to occur. This healing period may necessitate the placement of a temporary hemodialysis access if the patient is severely uremic, or is fluid overloaded and in need of immediate dialysis. Postoperatively the patient should remain supine when possible and avoid activities that increase intraabdominal pressure such as straining to defecate, excessive coughing, crying, and lifting. Treatment options during the postoperative period include:

- Infusion of heparinized saline solution (1 to 10 units heparin/mL saline), 25 to 100 mL every 4 to 8 hours for 1 to 3 days postoperatively. This protocol will not detect catheter malposition or outflow problems.
- Low volume in and out exchanges with heparinized saline or dialysate done several times a day until the effluent is no longer bloody, then daily for 1 to 2 weeks and weekly thereafter until the patient is on PD. A small volume of heparinized solution should remain in the peritoneum to inhibit the formation of fibrin (whitish protein formed in response to bleeding, inflammation, or infection) and prevent the development of adhesions. There is no systemic anticoagulation from the administration of low-dose intraperitoneal heparin.
- Low-volume dialysis in the patient who needs immediate dialysis but who is unable to undergo hemodialysis. Frequent, low-volume exchanges (500 to 1000 mL) are performed using a cycler with the patient in the supine position. The volume is gradually increased to eliminate the signs and symptoms of uremia.

How is exit site care performed?

The goals in the immediate postoperative period are to stabilize the catheter, promote healing, and prevent infection. The exit site dressing should not be changed for 5 to 7 days postoperatively unless there is excessive drainage under the dressing (blood, exudate, dialysate). The first dressing change should be performed by trained dialysis personnel and may then be taught to the patient. It is recommended that masks be worn during dressing changes to avoid contamination with oral or nasal flora. The skin around the exit site may be pink, similar to a healing scar, or it may have a brownish or purplish discoloration. During dressing changes, the exit site should be assessed for signs of infection (erythema, exudate, induration, tenderness); the subcutaneous tunnel should be palpated for tenderness; and the catheter and connections should be inspected for integrity. The exit site should be cleansed with an antibacterial soap and water and covered with a sterile nonocclusive dressing such as gauze and tape or an air-permeable adhesive sheet. Cytotoxic agents such as 1% povidone-iodine, 3% hydrogen peroxide, and 0.5% sodium hypochlorite may interfere with wound epithelialization during the postoperative period. The catheter should be secured to the patient's skin with tape or an immobilization device to avoid tension on the catheter and trauma to the exit site.

The goal of chronic exit site care is the prevention of infection. Exit site care is usually performed in the shower and consists of daily cleansing with an antibacterial soap with careful rinsing and drying. An antibacterial solution (e.g., 1% povidone-iodine, 3% hydrogen peroxide, 0.5% sodium hypochlorite) is then applied in a circular motion to the skin around the exit site. The exit site should not be submerged in bathwater or hot tubs. Many programs allow swimming in chlorinated pools and the ocean. After the healing period (4 to 6 weeks), a dressing may or may not be worn, according to patient or unit preference. It is extremely important to secure the catheter to the skin with tape or an immobilizing device to avoid trauma and infection should the catheter be accidentally tugged.

How is the adequacy of PD determined?

The clinical condition of the patient should be paramount when evaluating the adequacy of PD. Important elements of the evaluation includes careful attention to both overt signs of uremia—laboratory values, fluid overload—and covert signs, such as sleep and concentration disturbances, anorexia, and nutritional indices. Because PD is primarily a home therapy, patient compliance with the prescribed regimen must also be assessed in the evaluation of dialysis adequacy.

The efficiency of PD depends on the ability of the peritoneal membrane to ultrafiltrate fluid and solutes. Peritoneal clearance of solutes is determined by diffusion, which is driven by the concentration gradient between dialysate and plasma and by the "solute drag" created by hypertonic dialysate. Solutes and fluid may move from the intravascular compartment to the peritoneal cavity or from the peritoneal cavity to the intravascular compartment. Other substances lost in the effluent include protein (8.8 to 12.9 g/day), amino acids, water-soluble vitamins, trace minerals, and certain hormones.

UF and solute clearance in PD are influenced by (1) permeability of the peritoneal membrane, (2) volume of the exchange, (3) dialysate glucose concentration, (4) dwell time, and (5) molecular size of the solute. Clearance of solutes is expressed as the dialysate/plasma (D/P) ratio at a given point in time during the exchange. Equilibration is achieved when the D/P ratio approaches one. Small solutes such as urea (molecular weight = 60 Da) are highly diffusible and approach equilibration at 4 hours. Creatinine (molecular weight = 113 Da) moves more slowly toward equilibration, never reaching it during the typical 4-hour CAPD exchange. Table 17-2 demonstrates solute clearances that can be achieved with different types of peritoneal dialysis.

The peritoneal equilibration test (PET) is a standardized test of peritoneal membrane permeability used to determine solute transport characteristics, glucose absorption, and net UF. The PET assists in prescribing therapy and in making changes based on the current transport characteristics of the peritoneum. The PET involves giving the patient an exchange of 2.5% dialysate and obtaining a serum sample at hour 2 and dialysate samples at hours 0, 2, and 4. Samples are analyzed for urea, creatinine, and glucose. Urea and creatinine are also analyzed from the long dwell (12 hours) obtained when the patient arrives for the PET.

The D/P ratios are calculated and plotted on the graphs (Fig. 17-3). Decisions are made as to the best dialytic therapy according to Table 17-3, based on the solute transport characteristics of the patient.

Although the PET helps determine the transport characteristics of the peritoneum, a 24-hour collection of urine (residual renal function) and effluent (dialysis clearance)

Table 17-2	Solute Clearances with Various Peritoneal Dialysis (PD) Modalities				
	CLEARANCE (L/DAY)		SCHEDULE		
Modality	Urea	Creatinine	n Exchanges	Volume	Duration (Hr)
Acute PD	24	16	24	2	24
CAPD	8.1	6.2	4	2	24
CCPD	8.0	6.0	Nocturnal 4	2	10
NIPD	7.7	5.3	Diurnal 1	2	14
TPD	10.4	6.3	12	2	8
			—	TV* 1.5	8
				RV† 1.5	
				Total‡ 27	

From Diaz-Buxo JA: Clinical use of peritoneal dialysis. In Nissenson AR, Fine RN, Gentile DE, editors: *Clinical dialysis,* ed 2, Norwalk, CT, 1990, Appleton & Lange.
CAPD, Continuous ambulatory peritoneal dialysis; *CCPD,* continuous cycling peritoneal dialysis; *NIPD,* nightly intermittent peritoneal dialysis; *TPD,* tidal peritoneal dialysis.
*TV, Tidal volume.
†RV, Residual volume.
‡Total, Total dialysis volume/8 hr.

must be obtained at regular intervals to determine whether adequacy targets are being met. These collections are analyzed for urea and creatinine and the weekly Kt/V and creatinine clearance are determined. The current adequacy targets recommended by the Kidney Dialysis Outcomes Quality Initiative (K/DOQI) of the National Kidney Foundation (NKF) are summarized in Table 17-4.

What complications are encountered in PD?

Table 17-5 summarizes the common complications encountered in PD, including the causes, signs, symptoms, and interventions.

Can diabetics be treated with PD?

PD offers many advantages to the diabetic patient. In PD there is a steady physiologic state without the drastic biochemical or fluid fluctuations seen with hemodialysis in the diabetic patient with cardiovascular instability or autonomic neuropathy. There is no need for a vascular access. Blood sugar is well controlled with intraperitoneal administration of regular insulin because the peritoneal cavity containing insulin provides a steady,

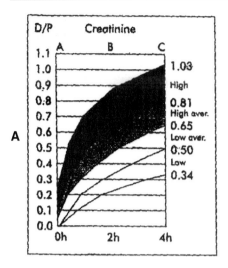
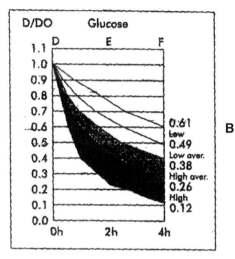

Calculate D/P and D/DO as follows:

$$D/P = \frac{\text{dialysate concentration of corrected creatinine}}{\text{serum concentration of corrected creatinine}}$$

at 0, 2 and 4 hours

$$D/DO = \frac{\text{dialysate concentration of glucose at 2 and 4 hours}}{\text{dialysate concentration of glucose at 0 hrs}}$$

Fig. 17-3 Plotting graphs for PET. *(Redrawn from Twardowski ZJ, et al: Peritoneal Dial Bull 7:138, 1987.)*

gradual, and prolonged appearance of insulin in the peripheral circulation. The total daily intraperitoneal (IP) dose of insulin may need to be much higher than the previous subcutaneous dose because of any or all of the following factors: its slow absorption from the peritoneal cavity; the effect of dilution in the dialysate on insulin absorption; extra insulin needed because of the dextrose in dialysate; binding of insulin to the plastic bags and tubing (10%); and hepatic degradation of insulin. Although IP insulin requires the daily addition of medication to the dialysis bags, the incidence of peritonitis is no higher than in other PD patients. There are numerous protocols for the IP administration of insulin.

Table 17-3	Baseline Peritoneal Equilibration Testing (PET) Prognostic Value		
	PREDICTED RESPONSE TO CAPD		
Solute transport	**UF**	**Dialysis**	**Preferred dialysis prescription**
High	Poor	Adequate	NIPD, DAPD†
High average	Adequate	Adequate	Standard dose PD*
Low average	Good	Adequate	Standard dose PD*
		Inadequate‡	High-dose PD§
Low	Excellent	Inadequate‡	High-dose PD§ or hemodialysis¶

*Standard-dose PD, standard-dose CAPD with 7.5-9.0 L of dialysis solution used per 24 hours or standard-dose continuous cycling peritoneal dialysis (CCPD), 6-8 L of dialysis solution used overnight and 2 L daytime.

†NIPD, IPD performed every night for 8 to 12 hours using 10-20 L of dialysis solution. DAPD, Ambulatory peritoneal dialysis performed only during daytime using 3 or 4 exchanges.

‡Inadequate dialysis likely in patients with body surface area >2.00 m^2.

§High-dose PD. CAPD with >9.0 L of dialysis solution used per 24 hours or CCPD with >8 L of dialysis solution used overnight or >2 L daytime.

¶Hemodialysis may be needed in patients with body surface area >2.00 m^2.

CAPD, Continuous ambulatory peritoneal dialysis; *DAPD*, daytime ambulatory peritoneal dialysis; *IPD*, intermittent peritoneal dialysis; *NIPD*, nightly intermittent peritoneal dialysis, *PD*, peritoneal dialysis; *UF*, ultrafiltration.

From Twardowski ZJ: *Blood Purification,* vol 7, Berlin, New York, 1989, S. Karger.

Table 17-4	DOQI Peritoneal Dialysis Adequacy Targets	
	Kt/V	**Creatinine clearance (1/wk/1.73 m^2)**
CAPD	2.0	60
CCPD	2.1	63
NIPD	2.2	66

CAPD, Continuous ambulatory peritoneal dialysis; *CCPD*, continuous cycling peritoneal dialysis; *NIPD*, nightly intermittent peritoneal dialysis.

From Clinical practice guidelines for peritoneal dialysis adequacy, DOQI. Medical Education Institute, Madison, WI, 1997.

Table 17-5	Complications of Peritoneal Dialysis		
Complication	Cause	Signs/symptoms	Interventions
Peritonitis Infections of the peritoneal cavity	Invasion of peritoneal cavity with microorganisms, usually due to break in closed system; may also enter along outer surface of catheter and through bowel wall	Cloudy effluent; abdominal pain; nausea/vomiting/peritoneal fluid cell count with greater than 100 WBC and greater than 50% neutrophils Culture results: Gram + Gram – Multiple organisms Fungi Other No growth No culture done	Prompt diagnosis and treatment; flushes with 1.5% dialysate; IP antibiotics are as effective as IV; coverage for gram + and gram – until organism identified; heparin added (0.5-1.0 unit/mL dialysate) to combat fibrin and adhesions PERITONITIS TREATMENT DECISION TREE (Fig. 17-4)
Exit Site Infection Purulent drainage and erythema of the skin at catheter exit point through the skin	Microorganisms in epidermal area; may be related to trauma, *Staphylococcus aureus* nasal carriage Causative organisms: *Staphylococcus epidermidis,* *S. aureus, Pseudomonas*	Erythema: purulent drainage; positive culture; induration; pain	Oral/IV/IP antibiotics; exit site care increased to bid; duration of therapy unknown; may lead to peritonitis; catheter removal may be necessary for recurrent or resistant infection *S. aureus* nasal carriages Mupirocin ointment Intranasally bid × 5d qn or rifampin 200 mg bid × 5d q 3 mo

Tunnel Infection			
Inflammation along the subcutaneous tunnel-catheter tract	Migration of microorganisms along the tunnel	Erythema or thickening along the tunnel—"sausage" appearance; pain; may or may not be exit site drainage	IV/IP antibiotics; often leads to peritonitis; often results in catheter removal
Fibrin Formation	Formed in response to inflammation due to decreased fibrinolysis of fibrinogen; increased during peritonitis	Whitish strands/clots seen in effluent or catheter; may lead to catheter obstruction if untreated	Heparin added to dialysate to prevent fibrin production and adhesion formation (500–1000 units/L)
Hemoperitoneum	Menstruating women (retrograde menstruation); trauma; ovarian cysts; ovulation; peritonitis; postcolonoscopy or enema	Blood effluent; 2 mL blood/L will result in blood-tinged effluent; effluent hematocrit greater than 5%, indicative of major bleeding; usually resolves spontaneously	In-and-out flushes with room-temperature dialysate (vasoconstriction); addition of heparin to prevent obstruction

Continued

Table 17-5	Complications of Peritoneal Dialysis—cont'd		
Complication	Cause	Signs/symptoms	Interventions
Inflow/Outflow Problems	Obstruction of catheter with fibrin, blood, omentum; catheter migration out of pelvis; loculation of fluid in abdominal cavity due to adhesions; constipation	Dialysate will not inflow or outflow; resistance when catheter irrigated	Relief of constipation; x-ray for internal kink, catheter position; inspect catheter for external kinks; irrigation of catheter with heparinized saline; irrigation with a thrombolytic reposition/replace catheter; peritoneogram with contrast medium to identify loculation
Air in Peritoneum	Air entering peritoneal cavity due to air in system/loose connections	Shoulder pain; peritoneal eosinophilia	Drain patient in knee-chest position or Trendelenburg; may need to resolve over time; tighten connections
Dialysate Leak Around exit site or into subcutaneous tissue	Increased intraabdominal pressure; delayed healing after catheter placement	Clear fluid from exit site; abdominal, penile, scrotal edema	Dextrostick to document glucose; resuture exit site of acute catheter; stop PD for 2 or more weeks to allow healing; decrease volume with APD in supine position if unable to stop PD; stabilize catheter; catheter replacement

| Hernias | Increased intraabdominal pressure caused by presence of dialysate in peritoneum, seen in patients with congenital or acquired defects or previous abdominal surgeries | Swelling in inguinal, ventral, incisional, umbilical area, nonpainful, reducible | APD with minimal or no diurnal dwell; decreased exchange volume; surgical repair |
| **Pain on Inflow** | Migration of catheter; catheter resting against pelvic wall; rapid infusion of dialysate; hyperosmolarity of dialysate; acidity of dialysate | Pain when dialysate is entering peritoneum | Slower infusion of dialysate; addition of $NaHCO_3$ to increase pH; local anesthetic (2% lidocaine, 3-5 mL/L dialysate IP); surgical revision/replacement of catheter |

APD, Automated peritoneal dialysis; *bid,* twice per day; *IP,* intraperitoneal; *PD,* peritoneal dialysis; *WBC,* white blood cell.

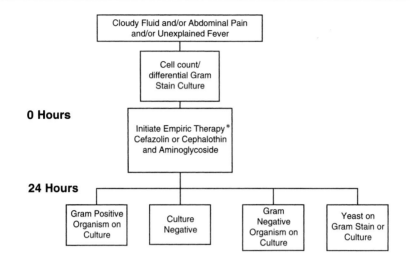

0 Hours

24 Hours

A

* *Empiric Therapy*

Agent	Continuous Dose	Intermittant Dose (in 1 exchange/day)	
		Residual urine output (mL/day)	
		Anuria (< 500)	Non-anuria (> 500)
cefazolin or cephalothin	500 mg/L load, then 125 mg/L in each exchange	500 mg/L (or 15 mg/kg)	Increase dose by 25%
gentamicin netilmicin tobramycin	8 mg/L load, then 4 mg/L in each exchange	0.6 mg/kg body weight	1.5 mg/kg initial loading dose. See footnote for maintenance dose recommendations
amikacin	25 mg/L load, then 12 mg/L in each exchange	2 mg/kg body weight	5 mg/kg initial loading dose. See footnote for maintenance dose recommendations

Fig. 17-4 Peritonitis treatment tree. *(From Keane WF, et al: Peritoneal dialysis-related peritonitis treatment recommendation: 1996 update, Peritoneal Dial Int 16[6]:557-573, 1996.)*

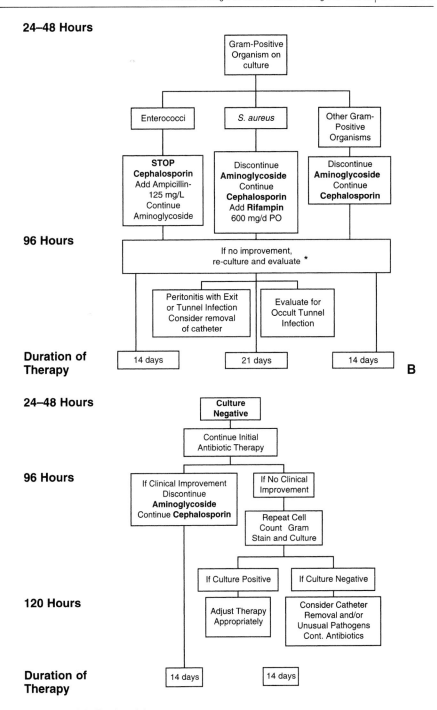

Fig. 17-4, cont'd. Peritonitis treatment tree.
*If methicillin-resistant S. aureus is cultured and the patient is not responding clinically, clindamycin or vancomycin should be used.

Continued

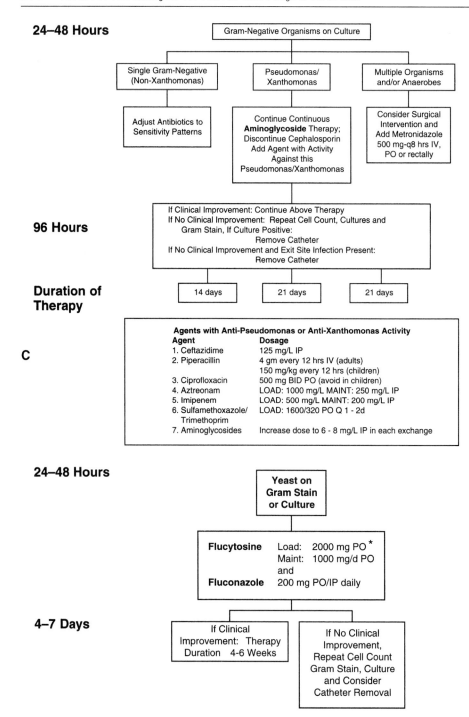

Fig. 17-4, cont'd. Peritonitis treatment tree.

*Pediatric doses: Flucytosine 50–100 mg/kg load PO, 25–50 mg/kg maintenance PO; fluconazole 1–3 mg/kg IP every 2 days.

HOME DIALYSIS THERAPY: PERITONEAL
How are patients selected for PD as a home dialysis therapy?

Before a person is selected as a home PD patient, there must be a thorough evaluation by the interdisciplinary dialysis team. The following areas need to be assessed:

1. Relative medical contraindications for PD such as:
   - Abdominal adhesions
   - Concurrent abdominal disease such as neoplasms
   - History of ruptured diverticulum
   - History of recurrent hernias
   - Documented inability of peritoneal membrane to ultrafiltrate or diffuse solutes (PET results)
   - Opening between the peritoneal and pleural cavities
   - Patients weighing more than 70 kg without residual renal function
2. Psychosocial evaluation including:
   - Patient motivation for self-care
   - Lifestyle (job, school)
   - Educational background
   - Health beliefs
   - Support system within the family/community
   - Patient's decision-making abilities
   - History of compliance with medical treatment
   - Distance from a dialysis center
   - Characteristics of the home (cleanliness; availability of water, electricity, and telephone; space for storage of supplies, etc.)
   - Availability of alternate caregiver (spouse, sibling, parent, friend, etc.)
3. Physical characteristics/limitations of the patient including:
   - Vision
   - Strength
   - Dexterity
   - Fine motor coordination

PD may be medically indicated in the patient with cardiovascular difficulties.

Home PD is particularly well suited to the pediatric patient because it allows for the "normalization" of the child's and the family's life (normal school attendance, fewer dietary restrictions than hemodialysis, fewer needlesticks, steady state of body fluid and electrolyte status, independence, etc.).

How is a patient trained for home PD?

If possible, training is delayed for at least 2 weeks after the catheter is inserted to allow time for healing to occur and for the patient to recover physically and psychologically from surgery. Another family member should train with the patient for support and backup. It is important that the patient be trained by a primary nurse who establishes a trusting relationship with the patient and family and subsequently acts as the liaison between the patient and the dialysis team. Training is performed primarily on an outpatient basis. Medicare will fund 15 outpatient training sessions and up to 18 sessions with written medical justification.

Content and method of presentation must be individualized to the patient's learning abilities. Content of training includes normal kidney function and the effects renal failure has on body homeostasis; mechanism of PD; performance of aseptic technique; catheter and exit site care; monitoring of weight and blood pressure (BP); dialysis record keeping with weight, BP, and dialysis treatments performed; CAPD exchange procedure; use of cycler if on APD; decision making regarding dialysate to be used to maintain dry weight and normalize BP; recognition of the signs and symptoms of infections (e.g., exit site, tunnel, peritonitis); importance of adequate PD treatment of peritonitis; medications; dietary counseling by the dietitian; ordering dialysis supplies; and management of complications. There must be ample time for return demonstration of dialysis techniques and attainment of all training objectives before the patient is allowed to perform PD independently at home. At the completion of training, a home visit should be made by the primary nurse. Additional support is provided by having a PD nurse on call to assist the patient with problems encountered during the off hours.

How is quality of care monitored in peritoneal dialysis?

Quality assurance programs are mandated by the Joint Commission on the Accreditation of Healthcare Organizations (JCAHO) and by the Centers for Medicare and Medicaid Services (CMS) whose mandates are administered by the regional end-stage renal disease (ESRD) networks (see Chapter 23). The focus of quality assurance should be continuous improvement in the quality of care patients receive.

The following are examples of quality assurance indicators:
- Incidence of infections such as peritonitis, exit site/tunnel infections
- Incidence of catheter complications such as pericatheter leaks, migration, obstruction necessitating catheter replacement, holes/cracks in the catheter, etc.
- Patient morbidity (number of hospital days/year and causes for hospitalization) and mortality
- Attainment of adequacy targets
- Revision of policies and procedures to improve patient care

PD is a viable dialytic modality for both the acute or chronic patient. Acute PD is appropriate in the patient who cannot tolerate hemodialysis. Care must be taken in the selection of patients for chronic home PD to optimize the chances for success. Ongoing evaluation of patient satisfaction and compliance with the treatment, incidence of complications, and adequacy of PD in removing uremic toxins and excess fluid must be undertaken and adjustments made to ensure quality patient care.

What are the drawbacks to PD?

Recently, concern has grown about the frequency of malnutrition and inadequate dialysis in PD patients. Protein malnutrition is frequent as a result of the loss of amino acids and protein in the dialysate, and because of appetite suppression resulting from inadequate dialysis and the glucose load absorbed from the dialysate. The latter often causes hypertriglyceridemia, and the increased calorie intake results in weight gain, especially in patients already overweight when they started on PD. The other major concern is adequacy of dialysis. In the past, most CAPD patients used four exchanges of 2 to 2.5 L daily, but it has become clear that many PD patients are getting inadequate dialysis once they lose their residual renal function.

The number of hospital days has declined 17% and 21% for patients on hemodialysis and PD, respectively. Although patients on hemodialysis and PD are admitted with approximately the same frequency, patients on PD have more hospital days. Admissions for peritonitis in the PD population have decreased 47% since 1991 (US RDS, 2003).

The *Clinical Practice Guidelines for Peritoneal Dialysis Adequacy,* developed by the NKF-K/DOQI, state that adequate dialysis with CAPD requires a Kt/V of at least 2.0 per week and a creatinine clearance of at least 60 L/1.73 m^2 per week (see Appendix A for additional information on K/DOQI). Corresponding figures for CCPD are a Kt/V of 2.1 and a weekly creatinine clearance of 63 L/m^2. For patients who are malnourished, even more dialysis is recommended. As a result, more CAPD patients are now using five exchanges daily, often with larger volumes of up to 3 L, and/or supplementing this with cycler dialysis overnight. This may increase the patient time required for carrying out the procedure, as well as increased discomfort.

What are the implications of these findings?

One implication of these findings is that the use of PD in the United States may have peaked. Continuous ambulatory PD and cycler dialysis are good initial treatments for many patients, allowing them to experience the advantages of home dialysis after only a few days of training. However, as their residual renal function declines, many patients will become inadequately dialyzed on PD. They will then need to change to hemodialysis, and unfortunately at present, home hemodialysis is not likely to be available to many of them.

After peaking in 1998, the decline in the PD population has slowed (US RDS, 2003). A significant proportion of PD patients have always transferred to hemodialysis each year. There are many reasons for this, including inadequate dialysis or inadequate ultrafiltration once residual renal function has been lost, repeated episodes of peritonitis, and inability to do the dialysis. Some patients put on hemodialysis while treating a catheter infection or peritonitis may elect to stay on this treatment permanently.

HOME DIALYSIS THERAPY: HEMODIALYSIS

Home hemodialysis is an excellent but underutilized alternative to dialysis in a center for many patients with ESRD. Of the 287,494 patients in the United States with ESRD receiving dialysis, only 1122 are on home hemodialysis (US RDS, 2003). This section briefly recounts the history of home dialysis in the United States, describes the use of home hemodialysis today, and discusses its advantages in comparison with PD.

What is the history of home hemodialysis?

Dialysis for the treatment of ESRD became possible with development of the Teflon arteriovenous shunt by Belding Scribner and coworkers at the University of Washington in 1960. For the first time, it was possible to get repeated access to the bloodstream for long-term hemodialysis. Clyde Shields, the first patient so treated, lived for some 11 years on home hemodialysis, and died from a myocardial infarction.

In 1963, home hemodialysis programs were started in Boston, London, and Seattle, the prime reason for this being financial. At that time, there was no funding for long-term dialysis from insurance or government sources other than research funds, and so this expensive treatment was paid for by patients themselves or from public donations. It soon became obvious that suitably trained and supported patients could do hemodialysis safely themselves at home for a fraction of the cost of staff-assisted dialysis in a hospital or dialysis unit. Furthermore, these patients were better rehabilitated and had a better quality of life than those treated as outpatients in a dialysis center. For the next 10 years, until introduction of the Medicare ESRD program in 1973, funds for dialysis in the United States remained in very short supply. In consequence, in 1973 some 42% of the 10,000 or so dialysis patients in the United States were on home dialysis, almost all of them on home hemodialysis for 6 to 8 hours three times weekly.

Intermittent peritoneal dialysis (IPD) for the treatment of ESRD patients also was developed in the 1960s and early 1970s. This was usually done at home, overnight for 12 hours, 3 nights weekly, using sterile dialysate from plastic bags or bottles or prepared by a machine. However, this was a time-consuming and inconvenient treatment and, because survival was not as good as with hemodialysis, it did not become widely used.

What was the effect of the Medicare ESRD program on home dialysis?

The Medicare ESRD program in 1973 provided almost universal entitlement to dialysis and transplantation for ESRD patients, and as a result the picture changed radically. Funding was readily available for outpatient hemodialysis, resulting in rapid proliferation of dialysis units across the United States. Many of these were for-profit units that were often reluctant to present home hemodialysis as a treatment option, and most were directed by nephrologists lacking personal experience with a home hemodialysis program. At the same time, the patient population treated changed rapidly to include many more diabetics, minorities, and elderly patients. As a result, the use of home hemodialysis declined rapidly. By 1995, less than 1% of all dialysis patients in the United States were treated by home hemodialysis, although a few programs still persist in providing this. In contrast, in 1995 in Australia, 14% of patients were on home hemodialysis.

The next home dialysis innovation occurred in the late 1970s with development of CAPD by Moncrieff and Popovich. This simple technique, coming at a time when access to home hemodialysis training programs was declining rapidly, gave more patients the opportunity to experience the benefits of self-care dialysis at home. Following the success of CAPD, other varieties of peritoneal dialysis were developed, and two of these now account for about 15% of peritoneal dialysis patients in the United States. CCPD uses a cycler for treatment overnight with one or more exchanges during the day, and NIPD uses a cycler for nightly overnight peritoneal dialysis. In the United States in 2001, about 27,000 patients (9.3% of all dialysis patients) used some form of PD, which remains the principal mode of home dialysis.

Recently, interest in home hemodialysis has revived. New dialysis machines are being developed to allow patients to dialyze themselves at home without the need for an assistant. At the same time, there have been reports from Toronto and elsewhere of very impressive results with daily home hemodialysis.

What is daily nocturnal hemodialysis (DNHD)?

DNHD is an alternate home dialysis therapy in which the patient dialyzes at home, at night, while sleeping. The patient on daily nocturnal generally dialyzes for 7 to 10 hours six or seven times a week. DNHD allows patients to dialyze for longer periods and with greater frequency. Because of this, the blood flows are usually reduced to about 200 mL/min and dialysate flows to 300 mL/minute. Some patients are monitored at home by way of an Internet connection, by trained staff, at a remote location. This monitoring allows the dialysis staff to be alerted via the Internet when a machine alarm occurs. If the patient does not respond to the alarm within the established protocol time frame, the staff monitoring the patient will call the patient's home. If no response is received from the home, the staff will call the emergency medical service. A benefit of monitoring by trained dialysis staff is that the patient and caregiver have a greater sense of comfort and confidence in performing the nocturnal dialysis treatment. Patients dialyzing daily reportedly have an increased sense of well-being, are hospitalized less, and take fewer medications. Of all the treatment options, nightly nocturnal dialysis is the best at removing larger-molecular-weight particles. This is related to the long amount of time that it takes these larger molecules to move from the intracellular space into the plasma (Curtis, 2004). Because there are fewer hours between dialysis treatments, the removal of fluid and waste products more closely resembles normal kidney function.

What is short daily dialysis?

Short daily dialysis is performed over 2 hours in a highly efficient manner, six or seven times a week. This method of treatment resembles in-center hemodialysis in that it is intense and rapid. Patients on this modality report taking fewer medications and feeling better than in-center patients. Short daily dialysis allows the patient to have fewer dietary and fluid restrictions, and helps to reduce the number of medications they must take.

Why is frequent dialysis desirable?

Changes in the fluid and biochemical state of the body affect total body function by the extent of such changes and by the rate of change. A large accumulation of wastes or fluid makes the patient ill. However, rapid reduction of the accumulation can also make the patient ill because of the shifts between intracellular and extracellular compartments. Frequent hemodialysis reduces the interval for accumulation of metabolic wastes and fluid. Total accumulation is less, and rate of reduction during dialysis is less.

Why not dialyze every day?

Equipment and supplies are expensive. The dialysis procedure takes time, which the patient would prefer to spend elsewhere. The duration and frequency of most dialysis prescriptions are a compromise between what is best for the patient's health and the practical limitations of money and time.

What is intermittent nocturnal dialysis?

Intermittent nocturnal dialysis is another option for the ESRD patient. Nocturnal in-center dialysis allows the patient to dialyze at an in-center facility three nights a week. The patient runs on lower blood and dialysate flow rates for approximately 8 hours each treatment. Less hypotensive episodes and other dialytic complications are seen as the patient is dialyzed more gently. This is becoming a popular modality for some patients because they can sleep at night and carry on their normal daytime activities. Better clearances are observed, and these patients report a better sense of well-being because of the less intensive treatment.

How does home hemodialysis compare with in-center hemodialysis?

Home hemodialysis does not differ essentially from outpatient hemodialysis in a facility, except that it is done by the patient, aided by a family member or other helper. There are fewer than 2000 home hemodialysis patients in the United States; nevertheless, this is an important treatment because of its advantages for patients. Also, with the promise of new technology and growing concern about the long-term adequacy of PD, home hemodialysis could be poised for a comeback in the not-too-distant future.

What is the patient selection process for home hemodialysis?

Suitably trained and supported patients of all ages, including children and the elderly, can do hemodialysis at home. Contraindications include serious cardiovascular or other problems during dialysis, lack of good blood access, documented noncompliance, lack of an assistant, lack of a suitable home, inability to learn, excessive anxiety on the part of patient or family, and lack of patient motivation and willingness to undertake treatment at home. All other patients should be regarded as potential candidates for self-care and should be given information on the advantages of home dialysis, both home hemodialysis and PD, when they are selecting a modality of treatment. A multidisciplinary team, working with the patient and family and the patient's nephrologist, should assess the patient's suitability for home hemodialysis, looking at medical, psychosocial, and vocational factors that might affect choice of treatment modality.

Inspection of the home itself is important. There must be suitable plumbing, water and electricity, and space to store the equipment and supplies. Many homes and apartments require only minor modifications to allow for home hemodialysis.

How would you train a home hemodialysis patient?

Home hemodialysis training is best done in a separate area using specialized staff, and, because of its specialized nature, consideration should be given to establishing regional training units. Training should begin as soon as possible once a patient has made the decision to be treated at home and is well enough to absorb information. The most difficult task for most patients is learning to do needle insertion, but this is something patients do best for themselves. From the beginning, they must be reassured that home hemodialysis is a relatively simple and safe procedure, and that when any problems occur at home, support and advice are always available from the training staff by telephone. In addition to the technique of dialysis, the patient must learn about diet, the disease and its complications, and the medical regimen. He or she should meet with a social worker, a financial counselor, a nutritionist, and an exercise coach and, when appropriate, a vocational counselor.

Training usually takes between 3 and 8 weeks once the patient becomes proficient with fistula puncture, and progress should be assessed at regular intervals. The training schedule should be arranged to allow the patient maximum opportunity to continue to work or to have access to vocational and other rehabilitation services as required.

What are the qualifications of home hemodialysis training staff?

Selection of home hemodialysis training staff is most important. They should be experienced in dialysis, have good teaching skills, be committed to encouraging independence and self-care, and be willing to allow patients to learn by making mistakes. Written materials, videotapes, films, posters, models, and other educational aids can facilitate training.

What patient support services are required?

Provision of support services for home hemodialysis patients is most important. These should include follow-up visits to the physician's office at least once a month, monthly routine laboratory testing, review of dialysis records, provision of supplies, equipment maintenance and repair, availability of on-call advice from a training nurse at all times, regular follow-up visits to the home by a training nurse, and access to social, nutritional and other services as required. Patients can take their own blood samples for laboratory tests and mail these to the laboratory. The results of these are shared with the nephrologist, the patient, and the home dialysis training program.

Back-up dialysis in a facility must be available for when a patient develops medical, technical, or social problems that make dialysis at home difficult. Patients are able to take vacations, either by arranging to dialyze at a center elsewhere, or by using portable equipment. Back-up dialysis should also be available to give the opportunity for the family member or other helper to have a vacation.

What are the advantages of home hemodialysis?

Although home dialysis was first introduced for financial reasons, its other advantages for the patients soon became obvious. These included the increased patient independence, a feeling of accomplishment, opportunity to schedule dialysis into daily life, better quality of life, greater opportunity for rehabilitation, and a reduced risk of exposure to hepatitis and other infections. In contrast, patients treated in a dialysis unit have a fixed schedule and very easily become dependent on nursing and technical staff. Interestingly, very similar advantages have been reported with other treatment technologies that have been moved into the home. As Scribner pointed out many years ago, with any chronic disease, the more patients understand about the illness, and the more responsibility and control taken for their own care, the greater the opportunity for adjustment and rehabilitation. A major aim in treating ESRD patients should be to maximize quality of life and encourage rehabilitation to the greatest extent possible. Studies have shown that the quality of life of home hemodialysis patients is better than that of CAPD patients, and in turn, that the quality of life of CAPD patients is better than that of patients dialyzing at a center.

Recently revived interest in more frequent hemodialysis also has implications for home hemodialysis as it is much easier for patients to treat themselves six times weekly at home than to have to come to a center. Reports from Canada, Italy, and elsewhere have shown that with such a regimen, much more dialysis can be provided. This results in remarkable improvements in blood chemistry, patient well-being, quality of life, and rehabilitation. As a result, knowledgeable patients are likely to be demanding home dialysis in the future.

In summary, CAPD and CCPD are relatively short-term but very effective initial treatments for many ESRD patients. When treatment becomes inadequate, these patients usually transfer to outpatient hemodialysis because they do not have access to home hemodialysis. Fortunately, attention is again being paid to improving home hemodialysis, and with the advent of safe, effective, and easily used equipment, patients will have the opportunity for better and more frequent dialysis and improved quality of life. Those patients, physicians, and nurses with experience of home hemodialysis continue to believe that this provides, by far, the greatest benefits for patients who can undertake it. Consequently, now is the time to pursue home hemodialysis again as a readily available treatment option for all ESRD patients.

18 Diabetes and Hemodialysis

More than 18.2 million people, or 6.3% of the population, in the United States have diabetes (National Diabetes Information Clearinghouse, 2002). Diabetes mellitus continues to be the leading cause of end-stage renal disease (ESRD) in this country; however, the rate has slowed considerably since the mid-1990s. The most recent data show that in 2001, 96,295 new patients entered the ESRD program, and 406,081 were under treatment on December 31. Medicare was providing renal replacement therapy (RRT) for 42,813 diabetic patients, 44% of the ESRD patient population (US Renal Data Systems [RDS], 2001). In 2001, a total of 142,963 people with ESRD due to diabetes were living on chronic dialysis or with a kidney transplant. The percentage of new cases of ESRD caused by diabetes is the highest for Native Americans. In 2001, the rate per million population for whites was 112, compared with 193 in Asians, 294 in Latinos, 437 in African Americans, and 503 in Native Americans (US RDS, 2003).

What is diabetes mellitus?

Diabetes mellitus is a disease process that prevents proper metabolism of glucose because of insufficient production or inefficient use of the hormone insulin. Insulin is produced by the β-cells of the pancreas. The function of insulin is to regulate blood sugar (blood glucose). Glucose is "food" for the cells of the body, and insulin facilitates the diffusion of glucose from the bloodstream to the cells. If there is a deficiency of insulin, or if the insulin cannot effect transport of glucose into the cells, the cells will "starve."

What are the two types of diabetes?

Type 1, formerly called juvenile diabetes or insulin-dependent diabetes mellitus (IDDM), is caused by the destruction of the β-cells of the pancreas. The susceptibility to the disease is inherited, but the actual onset of the disease is due to some environmental trigger such as a virus or allergen. The resulting autoimmune response leads to β-cell dysfunction.

Type 2, previously known as adult-onset diabetes or non–insulin-dependent diabetes mellitus (NIDDM), accounts for more than 90% of diabetes in the United States. This number is increasing because of the growth in the more susceptible minority populations. In this condition, insulin requirements are greater than the supply, or the patient's cells are insulin resistant and require help using insulin. Dietary control, exercise, and weight loss are important factors in lowering insulin requirements and increasing insulin utilization. Family history, obesity, hypertension, and smoking are major risk factors for this type of diabetes.

How is diabetes treated?

Diabetes is best managed with a multidisciplinary approach, in which the physician, nurse, and dietitian plan and implement a comprehensive plan of care. Often these professionals specialize in diabetic care and work with the primary care physician. The diabetologist (physician) determines the severity of the disease and assesses its effects. Other specialists such as nephrologists and ophthalmologists are consulted periodically for assessment of organ damage and for treatment. Annual visits to the ophthalmologist are necessary for all diabetic patients. A podiatrist should be consulted early to treat existing foot problems, assess risk of future problems, and recommend appropriate footwear. The medical goal is to arrest tissue and organ damage by normalizing the blood sugar. Among adults with diagnosed diabetes, 12% take both insulin and oral medications, 19% take only insulin. Oral medications alone are taken by 53% of those diagnosed with diabetes, and 15% take either insulin or oral hypoglycemics. (National Diabetes Information Clearinghouse, 2004). In the type 1 patient, glycemic control is achieved through diet, exercise, and insulin administration via subcutaneous injection or insulin pump. For the type 2 patient, the treatment varies and can be diet and exercise alone, or include an oral hypoglycemic agent and/or insulin injections. Monitoring of blood glucose values dictates the need for medication or dosage adjustments (Table 18-1). The dietitian creates a meal plan based on the American Diabetes Association guidelines and the individual's lifestyle preferences. In addition, the dietitian teaches and counsels the patient about the vital role that diet and exercise play in the patient's long-term outcomes. The nurse coordinates care, educates the patient and family about all aspects of care, and assesses all parameters of the patient's health, including psychosocial adjustments, response to medication, diet and exercise, foot care, and other follow-up assessments as needed.

How is blood sugar measured and what is normal?

There are four blood sugar tests used for diagnosing and monitoring diabetes.
- A fasting blood glucose is measured after an 8-hour fast. For a nondiabetic patient, the range is 60 to115 mg/dL. A value greater than 126 mg/dL on repeated studies may indicate diabetes.
- A random blood glucose greater than or equal to 200 mg/dL is diagnostic if accompanied by classic signs and symptoms.
- The glucose tolerance test measures both the blood and urine glucose after the patient drinks a 75-g glucose solution. Normal blood values are less than 200 mg/dL after 2 hours.
- Nurses teach patients or family to perform a fingerstick blood sugar for ongoing monitoring and evaluation. It is not used to diagnose diabetes. As implied by the

Table 18-1	Medication Monitoring in Diabetes Mellitus		
Drug	**Action and duration of drug**	**Dialyzability**	**Dosing in renal failure**
Insulin agents	Direct glucose metabolism		As per blood glucose and hemoglobin A_{1c}
Humulin (human insulin)	Short and long acting	No	Reduced
Humalog (Lispro)	Rapid acting	No	Reduced
Iletin (beef/pork insulin)	Short and long acting	No	Reduced
Oral hypoglycemics Sulfonylureas	Increased insulin secretion and utilization		
Acetohexamide (Dymelor)	Moderate to long acting	Unlikely	No change
Chlorpropamide (Diabinese)	Long acting	Yes	Avoid
Glipizide (Glucotrol)	Moderate to long acting	Unlikely	No change
Glyburide (DiaBeta, Micronase)	Moderate to long acting	No	Avoid
Glimepiride (Amaryl)	Long acting	Unknown	Unknown
Biguanides Metformin (Glucophage)	Reduces insulin resistance	Yes	Strictly avoid

Continued

Table 18-1	Medication Monitoring in Diabetes Mellitus—cont'd		
Drug	Action and duration of drug	Dialyzability	Dosing in renal failure
Other			
Acarbose (Precose)	Blocks gastrointestinal glucose absorption	Unknown	Unknown
Pioglitazone (Actos)	Decreases insulin resistance; long acting	Unlikely— conventional No data—high flux	No dose adjustments necessary
Repaglinide (Prandin)	Stimulates the release of insulin from the pancreas; fast acting	Unlikely— conventional Supplemental dosing not required	Reduced with severe renal impairment
Rosiglitazone (Avandia)	Increases insulin sensitivity; long acting	No—conventional No data—high flux No data available	No adjustments necessary

name of the test, blood is obtained from a fingerstick, and the amount of glucose is measured by a handheld device called a glucometer.

What is hyperglycemia?

Hyperglycemia means high blood glucose. Signs and symptoms include frequent urination, excessive thirst, nausea and vomiting, weakness, confusion, and dehydration. If hyperglycemia is confirmed by a fingerstick test, the episode is treated with insulin and fluids (if dehydrated).

What is hypoglycemia?

Hypoglycemia means low blood sugar. Signs and symptoms include anxiety, confusion, tachycardia, diaphoresis, and tremors. The blood sugar will usually be less than 70 mg/dL, although some patients become symptomatic at higher values. The treatment is to return the blood sugar value to normal by giving glucose-containing liquids either orally or intravenously.

Both hyper- and hypoglycemia can lead to coma, a life-threatening emergency. Prior to becoming comatose the patient may appear to be very drunk.

Is there a cure for diabetes?

Not at this time. Prevention of diabetes is being studied by identifying people at risk and instituting treatments designed to delay or prevent damage to the pancreas in type 1 or the insulin receptors on the patient's cells in type 2. A successful pancreas transplant can restore normal insulin production, but as with any organ transplant, the patient is immunosuppressed and at risk for adverse effects of those medicines.

What is diabetic nephropathy?

Diabetic nephropathy is kidney disease caused by diabetes. The pathology seen is glomerulosclerosis, a fibrotic thickening of the glomeruli. It is thought to be caused by hyperfiltration and accumulation of glycosylated, or "caramelized," proteins. As the disease progresses, the glomeruli lose their ability to filter blood effectively, resulting in the accumulation of waste products such as urea and creatinine in the body.

Diabetic nephropathy occurs in five stages:

Stage 1. Increased blood flow through the kidney (hyperfiltration) results in enlarged kidneys (renal hypertrophy).

Stage 2. This hyperfiltration of the glomeruli damages the membrane, causing it to leak larger molecules that would normally not pass across. The leak of albumin from the blood into the urine is known as microalbuminuria. As the loss of this and other proteins increase, the clearance of waste products such as urea and creatinine decreases.

Stage 3. Microalbuminuria exceeds 200 mcg/min.

Stage 4. Glomerular filtration rate has dropped to 75 mL/min or less, proteinuria is significantly increased, and the patient has become hypertensive. This stage is called advanced clinical nephropathy.

Stage 5. ESRD.

Can diabetic nephropathy and progression to ESRD be prevented?

Diabetic nephropathy does not occur in all diabetic patients and is more likely in type 1 than in type 2. Studies show that tight glycemic control can significantly reduce the development and rate of progression of diabetic nephropathy. With an intensive regimen of blood glucose monitoring, insulin and/or oral hypoglycemic agent administration, and adherence to a program of diet and exercise, the majority of patients can maintain normal blood glucose levels.

Progression of diabetic nephropathy can be delayed by the use of an angiotensin-converting enzyme (ACE) inhibitor medication. This class of drugs is usually prescribed to control hypertension but is useful for both purposes in the patient with diabetic nephropathy. It is given in stage 1 to control hyperfiltration.

When should a diabetic patient who has nephropathy start dialysis?

Initiation of dialysis depends on the individual needs and condition of the patient, but a clear indicator is a low creatinine clearance combined with symptomatic edema. Patients with diabetes suffer symptoms of uremia earlier than their nondiabetic counterparts. For this reason, it is usual to begin dialysis when the creatinine clearance is between 10 to 15 mL/min, but it may be started with a clearance of up to 20 mL/min. Hypertension is very difficult to manage in patients with a clearance less than 10 mL/min. Blood pressure control is important in the management of diabetic retinopathy, as well as cardiovascular and peripheral vascular disease.

For a patient with diabetes, is hemodialysis better than peritoneal dialysis?

There are advantages and disadvantages to both modalities of treatment. The healthcare team and the patient must choose the treatment that best suits his or her lifestyle, taking into consideration comorbidities and medical history.

Advantages for the in-center hemodialysis include frequent medical surveillance and smaller loss of protein into the dialysate. Disadvantages are a higher risk of vascular access complications, risk of predialysis hyperkalemia, and an increased incidence of hypotension during dialysis.

Peritoneal dialysis may offer better glycemic control, especially if intraperitoneal insulin is used; it also offers better cardiovascular tolerance and potassium control and does not require vascular access. Contraindications are all the usual problems of peritoneal dialysis magnified. Examples include more episodes of peritonitis due to reduced immune response to infection, protein loss, and increased intraabdominal pressure complications, such as gastroparesis.

Finally, inability to do peritoneal dialysis because of poor eyesight or fine motor control requires the patient to be dialyzed in-center if he or she does not have an assistant at home.

Can a patient with diabetes receive a transplant?

Yes. Living related donor transplantation is the treatment of choice for these patients because it offers a higher rate of survival than dialysis. Many younger patients with type 1 diabetes receive combined kidney-pancreas transplants that offer the additional benefit of normal insulin production. However, many are not considered transplant candidates because of advanced age and/or atherosclerosis. A thorough evaluation is required and cardiac surgery is often necessary before listing the patient for a deceased donor transplant. A higher percentage of transplanted patients with diabetes undergo limb amputation than their dialysis counterparts. Infection and peripheral vascular disease are exacerbated by steroids. However, the increased length of survival posttransplant probably accounts for the development of these complications in this patient population.

Why do diabetic patients need more dialysis than those without diabetes?

Diabetes affects every cell, tissue, and organ of the body, as does uremia. Patients with diabetes who also have ESRD offer a unique challenge. According to current mortality data, only one in five such patients who begin dialysis will be alive in 5 years. In order to have better survival prospects, patients with diabetes need to achieve higher urea clearance rates than other patients. Some sources say they need a Kt/V (delivered dose of dialysis) of 1.4 or greater, but with multisystem organ involvement this may be difficult to achieve. Patients with diabetes and autonomic neuropathy are at risk for underdialysis because of hypotension in the first hour of dialysis. A diseased cardiovascular and autonomic nervous system cannot adequately respond to intravascular volume changes that occur with ultrafiltration. Dialysis blood flow is frequently lowered to treat this hypotension along with administration of extra saline. Symptomatic hypotension sometimes leads to early termination of treatment, affecting the adequacy of dialysis and leaving the patient fluid-overloaded, thus further stressing the cardiovascular system. Peripheral vascular disease contributes to vascular access problems with subsequent inadequacy of dialysis. Because of steal syndrome and previous graft failures, many patients with diabetes can only dialyze with catheter access.

Why do some dialysis patients say that they are "no longer diabetic" after they start dialysis?

Kidney failure due to diabetes has the paradoxic outcome of making the insulin that is available last longer because it cannot be broken down and excreted as efficiently. Patients with uremia frequently eat a lot less, and so need less insulin. Patients with type 1 diabetes will always need some insulin injected unless they have a successful pancreas transplant. Type 2 patients, however, frequently no longer need additional insulin or oral medication. If they lose weight, their own insulin will be better utilized. Oral hypoglycemics, especially the long-acting ones, can cause severe hypoglycemia in the hemodialysis patient. These drugs are excreted by healthy kidneys and are not dialyzable.

How does hemodialysis affect the patient with diabetes?

The chemical composition of the dialysate is designed to be compatible with normal blood values. For all patients it has been determined that a dextrose level of 200 mg/dL is optimal. For those with diabetes, this level prevents hypoglycemia and improves hyperglycemia.

Should the diabetic patient with retinopathy get standard-dose heparin?

No. Definitive evidence has been presented to show that heparinization during dialysis puts the diabetic patient at increased risk for progression of retinopathy. But heparin requirements should be carefully monitored and dosages adjusted accordingly.

Is insulin or the oral hypoglycemic agents dialyzable?

Insulin is the most common hypoglycemic agent for patients with diabetes on hemodialysis. Insulin and most oral agents are not dialyzable. Exceptions are metformin (Glucophage) and chlorpropamide (Diabinese). These drugs are contraindicated for use in the ESRD patient.

How is hypoglycemia managed during hemodialysis?

Hypoglycemia must be verified with a glucometer. The signs and symptoms of hypoglycemia can be confused with hypotension. Some patients require a snack or some apple juice. However, blood volume diverted to the gut for digestion may increase a patient's risk for hypotension. Profound hypoglycemia may require a physician's order for an intravenous dextrose infusion.

How is hyperglycemia managed during hemodialysis?

If hyperglycemia is verified with a glucometer, the physician may order some regular insulin. Hyperglycemia can be a sign of infection, and the patient must be assessed and treated if an infection is present. Heparin doses may need to be increased if unusual incidences of clotting occur associated with hyperglycemia.

Are diabetic patients more difficult to keep healthy than nondiabetic hemodialysis patients?

Yes. Statistics show a higher mortality rate for patients with diabetes on dialysis. Cardiovascular disease is the leading cause of death, followed by sepsis and voluntary withdrawal from dialysis. The progression of atherosclerosis is accelerated in diabetic patients on hemodialysis, making them more prone to cardiovascular complications such as hypertension, angina, gangrene, and myocardial infarction. Hyperglycemia coupled with uremia delays wound healing and compromises immunity. Gastrointestinal neuropathy resulting in constipation as well as sudden, uncontrollable diarrhea can be a source of great distress to the patient with diabetes. Gastroparesis may cause regurgitation and aspiration.

What is gastroparesis?

Gastroparesis occurs as a consequence of autonomic neuropathy. Delay of gastric emptying is evidenced by difficulty swallowing, heartburn, nausea and vomiting, abdominal pain, and erratic blood glucose values. Treatment includes small low-fat, low-fiber meals; the use of drugs to improve gastric motility, such as metoclopramide (Reglan) and cisapride (Propulsid); and improved glycemic control.

Do individuals with diabetes have more vascular access problems than nondiabetic patients?

Along with atherosclerotic peripheral vascular disease, calcification of the vascular tree further limits the quantity and quality of blood vessels normally used to create a vascular access. Diabetic patients on dialysis do not experience more episodes of sepsis with their vascular access, but do require more hospitalization and have a poor prognosis. These patients do have a higher rate of graft thrombosis.

How should diabetic patients modify their diets once they are on hemodialysis?

Patients with diabetes already know about diet modification necessitated by errors of glucose metabolism. Now they must further modify their diets to accommodate renal failure and hemodialysis. Some patients hear about restrictions in the renal diet and feel there is nothing left to eat. Not so! Although they must make new adjustments to avoid the dangers of hyperkalemia and bone disease, it is imperative that they eat well to keep up with the demands of hemodialysis, which increases the risk for malnutrition. Hemodialysis removes nutrients by depleting amino acids at the rate of 1 to 2 g/hr during treatment. Blood loss in the dialyzer and lines also contributes to protein loss. Dietary protein replacement should be at a minimum of 1.2 g/kg/day. A caloric intake of 35 kcal/kg is required to prevent the body from burning protein stores for energy. Generally, protein should make up about 20% of the diet with 30% fat (preferably monounsaturated), and 50% carbohydrate. Diets should be tailored to patient preferences and customs. The dietary goal is to make eating pleasurable while meeting nutritional needs. Highly refined carbohydrates such as candy, cake, and pie can be incorporated into the diabetic renal diet as long as they are factored into the overall dietary plan. High-calorie, low-nutrient foods must be limited, but are not forbidden. The goal is to maintain good glycemic control.

If diabetic patients on dialysis no longer need medication for blood sugar control, should their blood sugar still be checked?

Yes. Daily checks are important to confirm good glycemic control with more frequent checks if the patient is not feeling well. An elevated blood sugar may indicate the presence of infection.

What is glycosylated hemoglobin?

A glycosylated hemoglobin value is the measurement of glucose bound to the hemoglobin of the red blood cells. Elevated blood sugar levels cause the hemoglobin to become saturated with glucose in the form of glycohemoglobin. Glycohemoglobin is present for the 120-day life span of the red blood cell. An average of the measurement of the glycolated part of the hemoglobin is called hemoglobin A_1. It can be measured as subunits designated as hemoglobin A_{1a}, hemoglobin A_{1b}, and hemoglobin A_{1c}. In most laboratories, only hemoglobin A_{1c} is measured because it is the most prevalent form. Other laboratories measure the total glycohemoglobin as A_1. Glycohemoglobin A_1 values are 2% to 4% higher than hemoglobin A_{1c} values, so it is imperative to know which standard of measurement is being used by the laboratories serving the hemodialysis facility. This test is a good indicator of compliance with the prescribed diet and medication regimen because it measures long-term glycemic control. However, studies have

Table 18-2	Values for Hemoglobin A_{1c} and Glycosylated Hemoglobin	
Values for hemoglobin A_{1c}		**Values for glycosylated hemoglobin**
2.2% to 4.8%	Nondiabetic adult	
1.8% to 4.0%	Nondiabetic child	
2.5% to 5.9%	Good glycemic control	<7.6%
6.0% to 8.0%	Fair glycemic control	7.6% to 8.9%
>8.0%	Poor glycemic control	≥9.0%

not been done to demonstrate that Hgb A_{1c} values are a reliable measurement for evaluating diabetic patients with uremia. The values and interpretations for both tests in the general population, as presented in Table 18-2, allow healthcare professionals to recommend changes in the patient's diet and medications and to educate the patient on the importance of compliance.

What assessments of diabetic patients on dialysis are critically important?

Though diabetic patients make up only 6.3% of the US population, 60% of all lower limb amputations are performed on this population (National Diabetes Information Clearinghouse, 2004). Frequent and careful assessment of the feet and legs of diabetic patients on dialysis should be done to identify potential problems of skin breakdown or infection. Early detection and prompt treatment may prevent serious complications.

Can diabetic foot problems be prevented?

Absolutely! Regular foot inspections should be done by the nephrology nurse with referrals to the podiatrist for attention to potential problem areas such as toenails, corns, bunions, and so on. Patients should never cut their own corns or calluses and should be warned never to use heating pads, hot water bottles, or unsupervised hot water soaks. Patients and caregivers must be educated in the basics of good foot hygiene. Prosthetic footwear to protect insensitive feet from trauma is a necessity. Medicare now reimburses for prescribed shoes.

19 Infection Control

Infection control is used in the dialysis setting to prevent patients and staff from acquiring infections specific to the dialysis unit. Infection control incorporates policies and procedures that include surveillance and monitoring activities for water treatment, dialyzer reuse, bacterial contamination, and transmission of blood-borne and other infectious diseases.

The Centers for Disease Control and Prevention (CDC) have issued and updated blood-borne infection control strategies and precautions (including standard precautions) over the years for dialysis centers as well as for other healthcare agencies. The Occupational Safety and Health Administration (OSHA) has issued regulations that enforce the use of standard precautions and other infection control strategies for all healthcare agencies. The OSHA blood-borne pathogen regulations provide specific measures that healthcare workers and their employers can do together to substantially reduce the risk of healthcare workers contracting a blood-borne disease while on the job. The CDC has also issued recommendations for preventing the spread of drug-resistant organisms and other potentially infectious diseases such as tuberculosis.

This chapter reviews information that personnel are required to know to help prevent the spread of infectious diseases in dialysis facilities. It also includes a review of blood-borne diseases and standard precautions, as published by the CDC, as well as strategies to prevent the spread of methicillin-resistant *Staphylococcus aureus* (MRSA), vancomycin-resistant enterococcus (VRE), and tuberculosis (TB). Questions commonly asked by dialysis personnel regarding water treatment, bacterial contamination, dialyzer reuse, and infection control issues are addressed in the specific chapters dealing with those subjects.

The CDC has issued specific recommendations for the prevention of blood-borne pathogens in dialysis facilities. Box 19-1 outlines these guidelines.

What are standard precautions?

A recommendation that blood and body fluid precautions be used consistently for all patients, regardless of their blood-borne infection status, is the basic tenet of standard precautions. Blood-borne pathogens, such as the human immunodeficiency virus (HIV) and hepatitis B virus (HBV) infect people of all ages, socioeconomic classes, and from all geographic areas. Healthcare workers may not be able to identify patients who harbor a

Box 19-1

COMPONENTS OF A COMPREHENSIVE INFECTION CONTROL PROGRAM TO PREVENT TRANSMISSION OF INFECTIONS AMONG CHRONIC HEMODIALYSIS PATIENTS

Infection control practices for hemodialysis units:

1. Infection control precautions specifically designed to prevent the transmission of blood-borne viruses and pathogenic bacteria among patients
2. Routine serologic testing for hepatitis B virus and hepatitis C virus infections
3. Vaccination of susceptible patients against hepatitis B
4. Isolation of patients who test positive for hepatitis B surface antigen.

Surveillance for infections and other adverse events

Infection control training and education

From Centers for Disease Control Recommendations for Preventing Transmission of Infections among Chronic Hemodialysis Patients, April 27, 2001.

virus or who may transmit infection. The application of "standard precautions" assumes all patients are infectious.

Reducing exposure to and transmission of blood-borne pathogens through the use of standard precautions involves appropriate work practices such as the use of barrier precautions. Appropriate barrier precautions are to be used to prevent skin and mucous membrane exposure in contact with blood or any other body fluid of any patient. Barrier precautions also known as personal protective equipment (PPE) include the use of the following:

- Gloves
- Face shields/masks/protective eyewear
- Gowns

Gloves are to be worn for touching blood and body fluids, mucous membranes, or nonintact skin of all patients; for handling items or surfaces soiled with blood or body fluids; and for performing vascular access procedures where blood spill is likely. Gloves are to be changed and hands washed after contact with each patient, whenever the gloves are blood stained, and after handling infectious waste containers.

Masks and protective eyewear or face shields shall be worn during any procedure likely to generate droplets, blood splashes, or body fluids near the face. Initiating and terminating dialysis and troubleshooting the vascular access are examples of procedures that may increase a healthcare worker's risk of exposure to blood-borne pathogens if barrier precautions, such as gloves, face shield, and impervious gowns/aprons are not used.

Impervious gowns or aprons are to be worn during procedures likely to generate droplets, blood splashes, or body fluids near the body. Before leaving the work area, all PPE should be removed and placed in a designated area or container for washing, decontamination, or disposal. Hands should be thoroughly washed after the removal of PPE and before leaving the work area. In addition to barrier precautions, employee work practices, such as diligent handwashing, are essential in order to reduce risk of exposure to and transmission of blood-borne pathogens.

Employee work practices include precautions that healthcare workers should take to prevent injuries caused by needles, scalpels, and other sharp instruments that may be responsible for the transmission of blood-borne diseases.

Precautions should be taken in the following situations: when cleaning used instruments; during disposal of used needles; and when handling sharp instruments after procedures. Needles should not be recapped, purposely bent, or broken by hand, removed from disposable syringes, or otherwise manipulated by hand. After use, disposable syringes and needles, scalpel blades, and other sharp items must be placed in puncture-resistant containers located as close as practical to the use area.

Sharps containers should not be mounted too high, but should be easily accessible. They also should not be allowed to overfill.

To minimize the need for emergency mouth-to-mouth resuscitation, mouthpieces, pocket masks, resuscitation bags, or other ventilation devices should be available for use in areas where the need for resuscitation is predictable.

Healthcare workers with exudative lesions or weeping dermatitis should refrain from direct patient care and from handling patient equipment until the condition resolves. All skin defects (cuts, abrasions, ulcers, etc.) must be covered with an occlusive bandage.

Pregnant healthcare workers are not known to be at greater risk of contracting HBV or HIV infection than healthcare workers who are not pregnant; however, if a healthcare worker develops HBV or HIV infection during pregnancy, the infant is at risk of infection resulting from perinatal transmission. Therefore, pregnant healthcare workers should be especially familiar with and strictly adhere to precautions to minimize the risk of HBV or HIV transmission.

Why is handwashing so important?

The most common method of transferring pathogen from patient to patient or staff to patient is by the hands. Handwashing reduces the risk of transferring contamination from hands to other individuals, to other areas of the body, or the other surfaces the healthcare worker may later contact. Hands should be washed when entering or leaving patient care areas, before gloving and after gloves are removed, and after touching an environmental surface such as the dialysis machine, without having gloved first.

It is important to remember that gloves should never be used as a replacement to handwashing.

Adherence to handwashing guidelines is essential to provide safe patient care. The CDC has issued guidelines on the use of alcohol-based handrubs as an alternative to using traditional soap and water when providing patient care: before patient contact, after contact with a patient's intact skin, contact with body fluids or excretions, nonintact skin or wound dressings, and after removing gloves. The traditional method of handwashing with soap and water is indicated when hands are visibly dirty, contaminated, or soiled.

When handwashing with soap and water, the hands should be rubbed together for at least 15 seconds followed by a rinse. When decontaminating with an alcohol-based handrub, the product should be applied to the palm of the hand and the hands rubbed together until dry. Some dispensers can be set to deliver the exact amount of soap or handrub recommended by the manufacturer.

The length of fingernails should be considered because studies have documented long fingernails (>$1/4$ inch) may harbor high concentrations of bacteria. Even after careful washing, long fingernails may harbor significant numbers of pathogens in the subungual space, such as gram-negative rods, corynebacteria, and yeasts. Artificial fingernails also contribute to the spread of certain gram-negative pathogens and should not be worn when providing care to patients who have compromised immune systems. This is extremely important to keep in mind when caring for those with a high risk of developing infections.

What are specific examples of standard precautions in a dialysis unit?

Standard precautions in a dialysis unit can be summarized into four main categories:
- Barrier precautions/personal protective equipment such as gloves, face shield masks, protective eyewear, gowns, and aprons
- Protection against penetration caused by sharps
- Good personal hygiene
- Good environmental control/avoidance of environmental contamination

During initiation and termination of dialysis, or any time there is a risk of exposure to blood-borne pathogens, a mask, protective eyewear (glasses or face shield), and gloves must be worn. An impervious gown or plastic apron should be worn if there is likely to be blood splashed. A sharps container should be positioned within reach of the patient caregiver so that the needle can be disposed of immediately without having to be placed down and picked up a second time. Hands must be washed after removing gloves and before touching any environmental surfaces such as machine knobs, charts, phones, or other equipment. Eating, smoking, applying cosmetics or handling contact lenses in the treatment room must be prohibited. Good environmental controls include maintaining separate areas for clean and soiled areas, as well as adequately cleaning and disinfecting the treatment area and equipment in contact with the patient, such as chair and blood pressure cuff.

What is the Needlestick Safety and Prevention Act?

The Needlestick Safety and Prevention Act went into effect on April 18, 2001, with a goal of protecting healthcare workers from accidental exposure to blood-borne diseases. The CDC estimates that each year 385,000 needlesticks and other sharps-related injuries are sustained by hospital personnel. This does not include needlesticks sustained in other settings such as long-term or home healthcare, or private offices.

This law applies to any facility that is bound by federal OSHA regulations where an employee may be exposed to blood or other potentially infectious material. This act requires healthcare employers to provide their employees with safety-engineered sharp devices. Employers must also maintain a log of injuries from contaminated needlesticks. Information to be collected must solicit exposure information on type and brand of device causing the injury, department where the injury occurred, and an account of how the injury was sustained. Employers are required to obtain employee input when choosing safer needle devices, and staff must be properly trained in the appropriate use of safe needle devices used in their facility.

What are the most significant blood-borne pathogens?

A blood-borne pathogen simply means a microorganism (usually a virus) transmitted in the blood or body fluids. The two most significant blood-borne pathogens are HBV and HIV. Other blood-borne pathogens include non-A, non-B (NANB) hepatitis, delta hepatitis, hepatitis C, syphilis, malaria, and cytomegalovirus (CMV). Efficiency of transmission varies among the viruses because of the number of viruses present in the blood.

What is hepatitis?

Hepatitis is an inflammation of the liver caused by infectious agents, medications, or toxins. There are several types of infectious hepatitis (A, B, C, non-A, non-B, and delta), but hepatitis B presents the greatest risk to dialysis personnel. The CDC estimated that 12,000 HBV infections occurred in healthcare personnel in 1985. The number has declined to an estimated 500 in 1997, largely because of the widespread immunization of healthcare workers and the use of standard precautions.

How infectious is HBV?

Hepatitis B is a highly transmissible virus because of the high concentration of the virus in the blood of infected people (1 mL of HB_sAg-positive blood may contain 100 million infectious doses of virus) and the ability of the virus to survive for several days on environmental surfaces at room temperature.

How is hepatitis B transmitted?

In the dialysis unit, exposure to blood with the possibility of HBV transmission can be either direct or indirect. Direct exposure consists primarily of penetration of the skin (percutaneous) by sharp objects such as needles, scalpels, and broken capillary tubes, or blood on broken skin and on mucous membranes of the eyes, mouth, or nose.

Indirect exposure involves transmission from environmental surfaces such as clamps, control knobs on dialysis machines, and doorknobs.

The most common ways hepatitis B is spread in dialysis units are by penetration of the skin by sharps and by contact of blood with broken skin or mucous membranes.

Are additional precautions necessary to safely dialyze an HB_sAG-positive patient in the dialysis unit?

Patients who are HB_sAg positive should be dialyzed in a separate room designated only for HB_sAg-positive patients. If this is impossible, the positive patient should be separated from hepatitis B seronegative patients in a separate area removed from the mainstream of activity and should be dialyzed on a dedicated machine. The same hemodialysis equipment should not be used for both HB_sAg-positive and seronegative patients. HB_sAg-positive patients should not participate in a dialyzer reuse program. Ideally, dialysis staff members should not care for both HB_sAg-positive and seronegative patients during the same shift, but can care for HB_sAg-positive and anti–HB_s-positive patients during the same shift. Staff members who are HB_sAg positive may be assigned preferentially to care for HB_sAg-positive patients. If, for some reason, staff members must care for both HB_sAg-positive and seronegative patients during the same shift, they must change gowns between patients, wash hands, and change gloves to prevent cross-contamination.

What are the CDC recommendations for hepatitis B serologic screening?

Patients and staff should be screened for HB_sAg and hepatitis B surface antibody (HB_sAb) to determine their serologic status before they first enter the dialysis unit. Patients and staff are each identified as one of the following: infected-Hb_sAg positive; immune-Hb_sAb positive; or susceptible-Hb_sAg negative and Hb_sAb negative. The CDC recommends periodic screening for each of the above categories of serologic status (Tables 19-1 and 19-2).

What about the hepatitis B vaccine?

The CDC strongly recommends the administration of hepatitis B vaccine to susceptible patients and staff as an additional means of preventing HBV in the hemodialysis unit (Table 19-3). In addition, if a healthcare worker has the potential to be exposed to HBV on the job, the employer is required by law to make the hepatitis B vaccination available at no cost.

Today's vaccines are safe and effective. Hepatitis B vaccines now used in the United States are made from yeast and cannot be infected with HIV or blood-borne pathogens. More than 2 million US healthcare workers have already been vaccinated. The complete series of HBV vaccinations is 85% to 97% effective at protecting someone from getting the disease or becoming a carrier.

What if I lose antibody protection after a couple of years?

The Public Health Service Advisory Committee on Immunization Practices states: "Individuals who have initially responded to the hepatitis B vaccine with protective levels of anti-HB_s, and then lose detectable antibodies, do not need to receive booster shots. They are protected and will not develop clinical hepatitis." However, dialysis patients may have less complete vaccine-induced protection that may persist only as long as the antibodies remain at a certain level. Dialysis patients may need a booster dose and should have antibody testing done annually.

What steps should be taken for occupational exposures to blood?

Institutions have in place a plan for occupational exposures that include reporting, evaluating the risk of infection, available treatments, and postexposure monitoring. When

Table 19-1	Schedule for Routine Testing for Hepatitis B Virus (HBV) and Hepatitis C Virus (HCV) Infections			
Patient status	**On admission**	**Monthly**	**Semiannual**	**Annual**
All patients	HB_sAg^* Anti-HB_c^* (total) Anti-HB_s,* anti-HCV, ALT†			
HBV susceptible, including nonresponders to vaccine		HB_sAg		
Anti-HB_s positive (>10 mL/U) anti-HB_c negative				Anti-HB_s
Anti-HB_s and anti-HB_c positive		No additional	HBV testing	Needed
Anti-HCV negative		ALT	Anti-HCV	

*Results of HBV testing should be known before the patient begins dialysis.
ALT, Alanine aminotransferase; *anti-HB_c,* antibody to hepatitis B core antigen; *anti-HB_s,* antibody to hepatitis B surface antigen; *HB_sAg,* hepatitis B surface antigen; *anti-HCV,* antibody to hepatitis C virus.
Source: Morbidity and Mortality Weekly Report (MMWR) April 27, 2001.

exposed to blood, the administration of first aid to the exposed individual is the first step. Needlesticks should be washed with soap and water, and splashes to the mouth, nose, or skin should be flushed with water. Eyes that have been exposed to blood should be irrigated with clean water, saline, or sterile saline solution. The exposure should then be reported to the immediate supervisor so the appropriate evaluation and counseling can take place. Postexposure blood testing of the exposed and source patient should be completed as soon as possible. Postexposure prophylaxis (PEP) will be offered if indicated to reduce the chance of becoming infected with HIV. It is important to be prompt when seeking PEP because the prophylaxis for HIV should be instituted within hours after the exposure. The medications used for PEP have numerous side effects, which is why it is recommended only when the exposure is a risk of transmission. PEP for hepatitis B should begin within 24 hours after exposure, which can significantly reduce the risk of acquiring the virus (Table 19-4). No PEP exists for a hepatitis C virus (HCV) exposure. Baseline testing for anti-HCV and alanine aminotransferase (ALT) is recommended as well as follow-up testing and monitoring for symptoms. Healthcare workers

Table 19-2	Recommendations for Staff Hepatitis B Serologic Surveillance in Chronic Hemodialysis Centers	
Vaccination and serologic status	Staff frequency of HB_sAg screening	Staff frequency of Anti-HB_s screening
Unvaccinated		
Susceptible	Semiannually	Semiannually
HB_sAg carrier	Annually	None
Anti-HB_s positive*	None	None
Vaccinated		
Anti-HB_s positive*	None	None
Low level or no anti-HB_s	Semiannually	Semiannually

Anti-HB_s, Antibody to hepatitis B surface antigen; *HB_sAg*, hepatitis B surface antigen.
*At least 10 miU (milli-international units)/mL. or at least 10 SRUs by RIA or positive EIA.

Table 19-3	Recommended Doses and Schedules of Currently Licensed Hepatitis B Vaccines for Adults	
Group	Vaccine Recombivax HB*	Engerix-B†
Dialysis patients	40 mcg (1 mL)‡	10 mcg (1 mL)
Healthy adults older than 19 yr	40 mcg (2 mL)§	20 mcg (1 mL)

*Usual schedule; three doses at 0, 1, and 6 months; HIB dose 0.06 mL/kg IM.
†Alternative schedule; four doses at 0, 1, 2, and 12 months.
‡Special formulation for dialysis patients.
§Two 1-mL doses given at one site, in a four-dose schedule at 0, 1, 2, and 6 months.
Adequate anti-HB_s is ≥10 SRU by RIA or positive by EIA.

should always protect themselves and their co-workers by using safe needle devices (SNDs) when indicated, using SNDs as the manufacturer suggests, disposing of needles and sharps immediately and into an appropriate container, and reporting all sharps and needlestick exposures.

What is HIV?

HIV attacks the body's immune system, causing the disease known as acquired immunodeficiency syndrome (AIDS). Currently, there is no vaccine to prevent infection. Through December 2001, the CDC had received voluntary reports of 57 documented and 138 possible episodes of HIV transmission to healthcare personnel in the United States.

Table 19-4   Recommended Postexposure Prophylaxis for Exposure to Hepatitis B Virus

Vaccination and antibody response status of exposed workers*	TREATMENT		
	Source Hb$_s$Ag† positive	Source Hb$_s$Ag† negative	Source unknown or not available for testing
Unvaccinated	HBIG‡ × 1 and initiate HB vaccine series§	Initiate HB vaccine series	Initiate HB vaccine series
Previously vaccinated			
Known responder¶	No treatment	No treatment	No treatment
Known nonresponder**	HBIG × 1 and initiate revaccination or HBIG × 2††	No treatment	If known high-risk source, treat as if source were Hb$_s$Ag positive
Antibody response unknown	Test exposed person for anti-HB$_s$‡‡ 1. If adequate,¶ no treatment is necessary 2. If inadequate,** administer HBIG × 1 and vaccine booster	No treatment	Test exposed person for anti-HB$_s$ 1. If adequate,‡‡ no treatment is necessary 2. If inadequate,‡‡ administer vaccine booster and recheck titer in 1-2 months

*Persons who have previously been infected with HBV are immune to reinfection and do not require postexposure prophylaxis.

†Hepatitis B surface antigen.

‡Hepatitis B immune globulin; dose is 0.06 mL/kg intramuscularly.

§Hepatitis B vaccine.

¶A responder is a person with adequate levels of serum antibody to Hb$_s$Ag (i.e., anti-HB$_s$ ≥10 mIU/mL).

**A nonresponder is a person with inadequate response to vaccination (i.e., serum anti-HB$_s$ <0 mIU/mL).

††The option of giving one dose of HBIG and reinitiating the vaccine series is preferred for nonresponders who have not completed a second three-dose vaccine series. For patients who previously completed a second vaccine series but failed to respond, two doses of HBIG are preferred.

‡‡Antibody to HB$_s$Ag.

Updated U.S. Public Health Service Guidelines for the Management of Occupational Exposures to HBV, HCV, and HIV and Recommendations for Postexposure Prophylaxis, June 29, 2001/50(RR11), 45-46.

How infectious is HIV?

The efficiency of HIV transmission in the dialysis setting is much less than HBV because of the lower concentration of HIV in blood when compared with HBV. The concentration of HIV in blood is approximately 10 to 10,000 infectious viruses/mL.

How is HIV transmitted?

Like other blood-borne pathogens, the AIDS virus is present in the blood of infected individuals. HIV is transmitted primarily through sexual contact, but may also be transmitted through contact with blood and body fluids. The virus can also be passed to a newborn infant from an infected mother. Transmission through contact with contaminated environmental surfaces has not been documented. The virus is very sensitive to chemical disinfection and is completely inactivated by a 10% solution of 0.5% sodium hypochlorite (bleach) within 1 minute of exposure.

No airborne transmission of HBV or HIV has been documented. However, splashing, splattering, centrifuge accidents or removal of stoppers from tubes can produce droplet transfer into the mouth or eyes or onto defects in the skin surface.

What HIV precautions are necessary in a dialysis unit?

Standard precautions are the only thing necessary to protect patients and staff from HIV infection in the dialysis setting. Patient isolation is not necessary due to the lack of an environmental route for transmission of the virus and the low number of viruses in the blood. It is not necessary to cohort or group together HIV-positive patients. HIV testing is not recommended as a part of infection control in a dialysis unit. Also, it should not be used as a prerequisite for admission to a dialysis unit, but it may be helpful for optimal medical management and counseling. HIV testing should be part of a transplant workup because a transplant could be contraindicated in someone who is already immunosuppressed because of the HIV virus. If HIV antibody testing is performed, informed consent, appropriate confirmation testing, appropriate professional counseling, and confidentiality of test results must be provided.

How about reuse of dialyzers for known HIV patients?

Although the CDC believes that dialyzer reuse poses no specific threat if done correctly, there are dialysis units that do not reuse dialyzers of known HIV-positive patients.

What if I am exposed to blood of someone known to be positive or test positive for HIV?

As with any blood exposure, you should immediately notify your supervisor. The source patient should be tested for evidence of HIV infection after consent is obtained. The CDC recommends that workers with occupational exposures to HIV should receive follow-up counseling and medical evaluation, including HIV-antibody tests at baseline and periodically for at least 6 months postexposure (e.g., 6 weeks, 12 weeks, and 6 months), and should observe precautions to prevent possible secondary transmission.

In 1996 the Public Health Service published source material and provisional recommendations for chemoprophylaxis (preventive drug therapy) after occupational exposure to HIV, by type of exposure. Though these recommendations are provisional, because they are based on limited data, chemoprophylaxis should be recommended to exposed workers after occupational exposures associated with the highest risk for HIV transmission. For exposure with a lower, but nonnegligible risk, PEP should be offered, balancing the lower risk against the use of drugs having uncertain efficacy and toxicity. For exposures with negligible risk, PEP is not justified. If exposed, you should consult your physician regarding chemoprophylaxis.

What is hepatitis C?

Hepatitis C is the most common form of NANB hepatitis worldwide and accounts for 90% of posttransfusion hepatitis in the United States. Currently, there is no vaccine to prevent infection.

How infectious is hepatitis C?

Hepatitis C is less concentrated in blood than hepatitis B and does not survive long on environmental surfaces. Concentration of infectious virus is thought to be less than 1000 virus organisms per mL. However, outbreaks have occurred in dialysis units and are thought to be due to poor infection control practices. Persons at increased risk of acquiring hepatitis C include IV drug users, healthcare workers with occupational exposure to blood, hemodialysis patients, and transfusion recipients.

How is hepatitis C transmitted?

Like hepatitis B and other blood-borne pathogens, hepatitis C is transmitted through percutaneous exposure to infected blood. HCV transmission within the dialysis environment can be prevented by strict adherence to infection control precautions recommended for all hemodialysis patients.

Are additional precautions necessary to safely dialyze a hepatitis C–positive patient in the dialysis unit?

Patients who are positive for hepatitis C antibody or who have a diagnosis of NANB hepatitis do not have to be isolated or dialyzed separately on dedicated machines. They may participate in dialyzer reuse programs if liver enzyme values are acceptable.

What are the CDC recommendations for hepatitis C serologic screening?

Routine screening of patients or staff for hepatitis C antibody is not necessary for purposes of infection control. However, dialysis centers may wish to conduct serologic surveys of their patient populations to determine the prevalence of the virus in their center, and to determine medical management for patients or staff with a diagnosis of hepatitis C.

Although this test has a sensitivity of about 90%, it does not distinguish between acute and chronic infection. In addition, the test does not distinguish between people who are infectious and those who have completely recovered and cannot pass the disease on to someone else. Although the CDC does not recommend routine screening for hepatitis C, regular monitoring of liver enzymes is recommended for the detection of all types of NANB hepatitis, including hepatitis C.

All patients should be monitored monthly for liver enzymes, ALT, and aspartate aminotransferase (AST), to detect any type of NANB hepatitis, including hepatitis C. Elevations in liver enzymes are currently more sensitive indicators of acute hepatitis C infection than is detection of hepatitis C antibody.

In the absence of unexplained ALT elevations, testing for anti-HCV every 6 months should be sufficient to monitor the occurrence of new HCV infections. If unexplained ALT elevations are observed in patients who are anti-HCV negative, repeat anti-HCV testing is warranted. If unexplained ALT elevations persist in patients who repeatedly test anti-HCV negative, testing for HCV ribonucleic acid (RNA) should be considered (Centers for Disease Control, 2001).

What should be done if exposed to HCV?

Testing for the HCV antibody and liver enzymes should be done immediately after an exposure and repeated 4 to 6 months after the exposure. Anti-HCV tests detect the presence of antibodies to the virus, indicating exposure to HCV. These tests cannot tell if you still have an active viral infection, only that you were exposed to the virus in the past. Testing for HCV RNA 4 to 6 weeks postexposure will detect infection earlier. Unlike antibody tests, HCV RNA tests directly measure for the presence of the hepatitis C virus.

What is tuberculosis (TB)?

TB is an infectious disease caused by the bacterium *Mycobacterium tuberculosis.*

How is TB transmitted?

The bacterium is carried in airborne particles (droplet nuclei) that are generated when people with pulmonary or laryngeal tuberculosis, who are not on effective antituberculosis medication, cough or sneeze. The small droplets can remain suspended in the air for prolonged periods. While airborne on normal room current, these droplet nuclei can infect individuals as soon as the inhaled droplets containing the bacilli become established in the alveoli of the lung.

Two to 10 weeks after initial infection, the healthy immune system usually limits further multiplication, and the person does not become ill. A positive TB skin test is usually the only evidence of infection.

Approximately 10% of these healthy individuals with latent TB will develop active TB months or years later. However, for people infected with HIV, the risk of progression to active infectious disease is markedly increased. The CDC estimates that approximately 10 to 15 million people in the United States are infected with the *M. tuberculosis.*

What is the difference between TB infection and active TB?

Patients who progress to active contagious TB are capable of transmitting the disease. Those who are infected but who have not progressed to active TB will have no symptoms, will not be contagious, and will not know they are infected unless they have a positive Mantoux skin test. It may take months or years before the person progresses into active TB, or the person may never develop active TB at all. Symptoms of active TB include prolonged coughing for 3 weeks or more, fatigue, fever, weight loss and night sweats. Medication and therapy are available.

Is TB a problem in dialysis units?

More than 16,000 cases of TB were reported in 2000 in the United States (Centers for Disease Control, 2002). Outbreaks have been reported in correctional facilities, hospitals, and some dialysis units. The level of risk for transmission varies by the type of healthcare facility. For example, the risk of acquiring TB may be greater in emergency departments, where patients are provided care before screening and diagnosis take place.

Can a patient with active contagious TB be safely dialyzed in the outpatient facility?

Patients with active TB disease should not be dialyzed in ambulatory settings while infectious. These patients must be referred to hospitals with appropriate isolation accommodations (separate room, negative pressure, etc.) as prescribed by CDC guidelines. ESRD program regulations require freestanding dialysis units to have back-up agreements with a hospital. This may provide the mechanism for referring active TB patients for dialysis treatment until no longer infectious.

What are the CDC recommendations for TB screening?

Staff should be screened at the onset of employment. TB screening is often done at least annually. Frequency of TB screening is based on an institution's risk assessment including the community TB profile. If you live and work in an area with a high incidence of TB, the frequency of screening may be more often.

Patients should be screened on or before their first dialysis encounter. New dialysis patients may arrive after a hospitalization and/or extensive workup. If a recent (within past year) chest x-ray or tuberculin skin test was included, initial screening may not be necessary unless risk factors are present.

CDC recommends that the two-step Mantoux be used for baseline screening. The Mantoux technique involves intradermal injection of 0.1 mL of purified protein derivative (PPD) tuberculin containing 5 tuberculin units. The two-step procedure (if initial PPD is negative, PPD is repeated 1 to 3 weeks later) is used for baseline testing in people who periodically receive TB skin tests to reduce the likelihood of mistaking a booster reaction for a new infection.

Nonroutine screening of patients and staff should be conducted as needed in response to clinical symptoms or documented exposure, for example, an active case identified among patients or staff.

What are drug-resistant organisms?

Drug-resistant organisms are bacteria that have mutated to defend themselves against commonly used antibiotics. Resistant strains develop quickly and crossbreed, transferring their resistance to other bacteria. VRE and MRSA are two bacteria known to be resistant to antibiotic therapy. Both have become significant nosocomial pathogens in United States hospitals and healthcare facilities. MRSA and VRE may cause infections in patients who are immunosuppressed, including ESRD patients, cancer and HIV patients, the elderly, newborns, and those being treated with multiple antibiotics. Those at increased risk of acquiring infections due to drug-resistant organisms include the following: nursing home patients; patients with frequent hospital admissions or prolonged hospital stays; patients with chronic illnesses requiring steroid therapy; patients with catheters, such as subclavians; and patients with incisions and other openings into the body.

How are MRSA and VRE transmitted?
MRSA

The main route of transmission of MRSA is by healthcare workers' hands that have become contaminated by contact with a patient who is either infected with or carries the organism. People may carry the organism in their nose or on the skin. Some people are carriers; others can become infected through boils, wound infections, pressure ulcers, and so on. MRSA commonly infects wound, exit sites, and access sites. Environmental surfaces may also be contaminated with MRSA and act as a reservoir for the bacteria.

VRE

Enterococci are normal flora of the gastrointestinal and female genital tracts. Because of this, most infections with these microorganisms have been attributed to sources within the patient. However, recent reports indicate that enterococci, including VRE, can spread by direct person-to-person contact or indirectly via transient carriage on hands of personnel or contaminated environmental surfaces and patient-care equipment.

Can a patient with MRSA and VRE safely dialyze in the outpatient facility?

Standard infection control or standard precautions recommended by CDC should provide sufficient protection against the transmission of MRSA in the dialysis unit.

The CDC standard precautions include the following:
- Wash hands after touching blood, body fluids, excretions, and contaminated items, even when wearing gloves. Also, wash hands after gloves are removed,

between tasks, and between procedures on the same patient to prevent cross-contamination of different body sites.

- Wear gloves when touching blood, body fluids, excretions, and contaminated items. Gloves should be put on before touching mucous membranes and nonintact skin, and they should be removed promptly after use.
- Wear a mask and eye protection or face shield. These will protect the mucous membranes of the eyes, nose, and mouth during procedures that are likely to cause splashing or spraying of body fluids.
- Wear a gown for protection from skin contamination and soiling of clothing during procedures and patient-care activities.
- Handle patient-care equipment that is soiled with body fluids and excretions in a manner that prevents skin exposures and contamination of clothing. Make sure reusable equipment is not used for the care of other patients until it has been sanitized.

In addition to these standard precautions, patients with VRE who have draining wounds not contained by dressings, who have diarrhea or are incontinent, who have poor hygiene, or are confused and are handling their dressings, and so on should be dialyzed in a separate room or area. It is important to dedicate the use of noncritical items, such as stethoscope or sphygmomanometer, to a single patient or group of patients who are infected with or are carriers of VRE. If such devices are to be used on other patients, adequate cleaning and disinfecting must first take place.

What are the sterilization and disinfection procedures in a dialysis unit?

All dialysis units must have written policies and procedures that deal with disinfection of the dialysis fluid pathway of the hemodialysis machine. These procedures are targeted to control bacterial contamination and have nothing to do with preventing blood-borne infections. The procedures generally consist of using sodium hypochlorite (bleach) on a regular basis (according to the manufacturer's instructions) and a sterilant overnight at certain intervals (e.g., every 100 hours of use). Studies have shown that HIV is inactivated rapidly after being exposed to commonly used chemical germicides at concentrations that are much lower than used in practice. The much hardier HBV is also known to be inactivated by common household bleach. Suggested concentrations of sodium hypochlorite prepared daily range from 500 parts per million (ppm) (1:100 dilution of household bleach) to 5000 ppm (1:10 dilution).

How should other surfaces be cleaned?

Machine surfaces, patient chairs, and other surrounding furniture and equipment, such as an infusion pump, should be routinely wiped down with a 1:100 to 1:10 bleach solution following every patient treatment. Environmental surfaces such as walls, floors, and other surfaces should be routinely cleaned consistent with good housekeeping practices. Extraordinary attempts to disinfect or sterilize these surfaces are not necessary. Blood spills should be cleaned immediately. Linen soiled with blood or body fluids should be transported in leakproof bags.

What about waste disposal?

There are two kinds of waste seen in the dialysis unit: regular trash and infectious waste. Regular trash, which is mostly paper and plastic, can be disposed of by the usual practice. Infectious waste, which is usually defined in a dialysis unit as "bloody," must be disposed of in specially labeled red bags. Various states have laws regarding the definition of infectious waste and its disposal.

Has peritoneal dialysis waste tested positive for HIV?

HIV antibody has been detected in the dialysate waste of AIDS patients. To date there are no national guidelines for the disposal of waste dialysate from AIDS patients.

Should additional precautions be taken when caring for the patient on home peritoneal dialysis?

Standard precautions must be observed with all patients when there is a possibility of contact with blood or body fluids. In addition, each renal unit devises its own criteria for safe disposal of waste fluids for the patient both at home and in the unit setting. Patients at home should be instructed to drain their bags into the toilet and then seal the empty bag in a plastic bag before disposal with household garbage. In the continuous ambulatory peritoneal dialysis (CAPD) unit a toilet or sluice should be used whenever possible. Many units use a 1:10 bleach solution following the dialysate. Some units suggest adding 10 mL of bleach to the bag before disposal. If a sink is used for waste disposal, a bleach solution should follow the waste and preferably sit for 30 minutes.

20 Psychosocial Aspects of Dialysis Therapy

Dialysis, as a means of prolonging life for an indefinite period, took on new psychosocial implications on July 1, 1973, when the Medicare End-Stage Renal Disease Program (Public Law 92-603, Section 2991) became effective in the United States. The Medicare act made major financial coverage available to 90% of patients with renal failure, without regard for age or complicating disease processes.

Psychosocial issues were recognized by medical and mental health professionals as impediments to adjustment and satisfactory quality of life for end-stage renal disease (ESRD) patients long before Medicare entered the dialysis picture. This became even more apparent when federally supported dialysis treatment was determined to be the right of all persons with kidney failure. Some of the psychosocial factors include changes in an individual's work and family situation, financial concerns, and the stress of living with a life-challenging illness.

What are the psychologic consequences of long-term dialysis?

Dialysis may have a major impact on a patient's psychosocial status. Some patients have a gradual decline in quality of life, particularly as medical complications become more severe. This can lead to depression and an increased risk of suicide. Other patients experience an excellent quality of life and are highly rehabilitated and productive. What distinguishes these two patient groups remains uncertain. Close attention to psychosocial adaptation, with psychiatric intervention and counseling when needed, can help patients optimize the quality of their lives while on dialysis.

Is it possible to predict how a patient will react to maintenance hemodialysis?

Little work has been done to help healthcare professionals predict how patients will react to the multiple changes and stresses associated with life on dialysis. Most studies have involved small numbers of patients and showed little agreement regarding predictive parameters. An individual's method of coping with past life stresses remains the best single indicator of his or her adaptability to daily life with dialysis. Frustration tolerance, aggression, denial of the sick role, and obsessive-compulsive characteristics are personality traits that can be evaluated and used to help predict a patient's potential adjustment to dialysis.

An evaluation of the patient's coping methods is conducted in part by a mental health professional (usually a clinical social worker) on the dialysis treatment team. An in-depth psychosocial evaluation that includes interviews with both the patient and his or her family is conducted by the social worker at the initiation of chronic dialysis treatment. Based on this evaluation, a treatment plan is formulated to include psychosocial counseling and community resource referrals that can enhance the patient's ability to cope. Often the social worker can provide support and reassurance to patient and family as well as help alleviate pressing resource needs, such as assistance with financial and insurance problems.

What are the stages of adjustment to dialysis that a patient with ESRD may experience?

When the onset of ESRD is gradual, the patient has time to adjust to the idea of dialysis and to make well-informed treatment choices. The initial response to dialysis itself can be one of relief, especially if the patient has been feeling ill for a period of time. Unfortunately, some patients delay beginning dialysis until they are quite ill and then may require the initiation of dialysis on an emergency, hospitalized basis.

When the onset of ESRD is sudden, there can be an acute crisis phase of adjustment, often marked by feelings of shock, disbelief, desperation, and depression. In such cases, a crisis intervention approach by a trained mental health professional is indicated. Three stages of patient adjustment to dialysis have been identified:

- *The "honeymoon" period* is defined as a patient's initial response to dialysis, which can last from a few weeks to 6 months or more. Usually this phase is one of physical and psychologic improvement and is accompanied by renewed feelings of hope and confidence. During the honeymoon period, patients may respond to staff in a positive and grateful manner. This does not mean that patients do not also experience periods of anxiety and depression but rather that they may view dialysis in a more positive way overall because they feel better than they did before the initiation of dialysis.
- *The period of disenchantment and discouragement* is marked by reduced feelings of confidence and hope and can last from 3 to 12 months. This phase is usually triggered when an individual returns to some previous routine or employment and is forced to confront the limitations dialysis places on these activities. During this time, feelings of sadness and helplessness may arise.
- *The period of long-term adaptation* is characterized by the patient's arrival at some degree of acceptance of the limitations, shortcomings, and complications that dialysis brings into his or her life. Patients can experience long periods of contentment alternating with episodes of depression. Adaptation often can be facilitated by a return to some form of meaningful work or by settling down to doing little or no work at all. Incorporation of diet and activity restrictions and the dialysis procedure into the daily lifestyle is part of long-term adaptation.

These periods of adjustment are presented as general guidelines only. Not all researchers and practitioners agree about this sequence of phases. There is not always a linear progression from one stage to another, and for individual patients the various stages may be much briefer or much longer than indicated above. Further, patients may shift back and forth from stage to stage for a variety of reasons, including medical complications.

How can the quality of life of a patient on dialysis be evaluated?

Quality of life is a phrase that is sometimes used interchangeably with such terms as *life satisfaction, well-being,* and *morale.* Usually, quality of life is defined as encompassing major areas of functioning in the physical, psychological, and social realms. Further, feelings about this issue are relative perceptions for each individual, and any attempt to evaluate quality of life must take into account the significance of these highly subjective perceptions. What is an intolerable situation for one patient may not be for another.

Several instruments that measure quality of life for research purposes may be used for clinical assessment as well. In addition to using formal measures, dialysis personnel should provide patients with opportunities to talk about their own feelings and perceptions regarding their quality of life.

What can be done to enhance the quality of life for dialysis patients and their families?

Evaluation and planning for psychosocial intervention should begin before the patient actually needs dialysis. Patients and their families should be educated about dialysis and be encouraged to participate actively in deciding various aspects of the treatment program, including the type of dialysis. Evaluation of the type of dialysis to be used for a patient should include an assessment of the challenges he or she is facing, as well as personal, family, work, and social considerations. It is essential for staff to identify individuals who are at great risk for psychosocial dysfunction because early introduction of vocational and psychotherapeutic counseling (for the individual or family) can increase the patient's rehabilitation potential and improve his or her quality of life.

Once a patient has begun dialysis, the dialysis staff needs to institute interventions to maximize the positive and minimize the negative effects of dialysis on the patient's quality of life. Such interventions might include counseling by the dialysis social worker or other mental health professional that is familiar with the dynamics of ESRD and the dialysis process.

What are common sources of stress for dialysis patients?

Patients with ESRD are confronted with severe limitations and demands on themselves and their families. They must contend with changes in family relationships, such as role reversal and deteriorating sexual responsiveness, and with accompanying feelings of guilt, depression, and loss. The threat of reduced job responsibility or unemployment can contribute to feelings of worthlessness and loss of self-esteem. Many patients experience conflict between the need to be dependent on a machine and on other people and the desire to remain independent. They may feel that they have relinquished control of their lives to the dialysis team. Underlying many of these feelings is the basic fear of dying. The patient's dependence on the dialysis machine can be a constant reminder that he or she has been rescued from death.

How can the dialysis team assist patients and families in coping when dialysis becomes necessary?

Dialysis patients and family members who regard renal failure and the need for dialysis as a loss may grieve over that loss. Dialysis personnel should be familiar with the issues of grief and the grieving process and be prepared to provide appropriate intervention or call upon a resource person, such as a psychiatric nurse, social worker, psychologist, or psychiatrist, as needed. If members of the dialysis team are able to recognize periods of exceptional stress and use appropriate crisis intervention approaches, they can help patients cope with such periods and prevent major adjustment problems.

Patients who are unable to accept the restrictions imposed upon them by dialysis may become depressed and unable or unwilling to adhere to their dialysis regimen. When this occurs, the diminished quality of life and increased potential for death should be addressed by prompt recognition and social work or psychotherapeutic intervention.

What are some psychologic reactions and common coping mechanisms of patients on maintenance dialysis?

Anxiety is the initial reaction for most patients and families faced with the prospect of life on dialysis. Such anxiety is entirely normal, and dialysis staff need to reassure patients that this is the case.

Depression may occur early on during the treatment process. Again, this is a rational reaction to the prospect of a limited and risky life that will require totally different objectives than would have been planned otherwise.

Hostility and anger are frequent reactions of patients on dialysis. Hostility toward dialysis personnel and the medical regimen is actually a reaction to the limitations imposed by the disease, but the anger is displaced to the treatment staff and procedure.

A difference of opinion exists as to the role that the *denial* mechanism plays in patients who have become stabilized on dialysis. To staff involved in the primary care of these patients, denial seems to be a common defense that allows patients to cope with the realities of the situation while regarding them as not a part of their real selves. Denial used in this way can be very useful for the patient because it shuts out negative aspects of the illness. However, denial can be carried to extremes, subverting medical management, and the result can be disastrous.

Do emotional factors affect the patient's long-term survival?

Successful life with a dialysis regimen requires a willingness and ability to adhere to dietary and fluid restrictions, medication regimens, and dialysis procedures. Most people adjust to these restrictions and show great responsibility.

In what ways does nonadherent behavior affect the patient's physical condition?

Nonadherent behavior can be manifested in a number of ways:

- Nonadherence to the prescribed diet is a manifestation of the denial mechanism gone astray. This can contribute to increased morbidity and even mortality.
- Ingestion of excess fluid represents denial of kidney failure with potentially harmful results.
- Inadequate care of vascular or peritoneal access is sometimes a problem. A clotted or infected vascular access may not be discovered until time for a dialysis treatment. With peritoneal dialysis, use of an improper technique may lead to infection.
- Manipulation of treatment time can be another manifestation of nonadherent behavior. Skipping treatments and shortening treatment times are examples of this behavior.

Such behaviors can contribute to malnutrition, neuropathy, bone disease, cardiac failure, and the like. If these behaviors persist, they result in physical deterioration and, in extreme cases, death—a form of passive suicide.

How can such adverse behaviors be countered?

Patients sometimes resent consultation with a psychiatrist. In such cases, the patient may be defensive and unwilling to admit that a problem exists or that problems may have an emotional basis. Even if the psychiatrist is recognized as a member of the treatment team, there is a tendency to avoid such counsel. Group sessions that involve patients as well as family members and are guided by a skilled and accepted social worker or psychiatric nurse (using the psychiatrist as a resource person) may be a more readily accepted form of help. Within such a group setting, ventilation, sharing of problems, and discussions with peers can help resolve many problems. The psychiatrist, psychiatric nurse, or social worker can also help medical and other personnel deal with a patient's resistant behaviors. These professionals can offer reassurance and suggest approaches to help other members of the dialysis team assist the patient in handling the challenges of dialysis.

What emotional problems are commonly seen in family members?

Anxiety is a common and normal response in family members, particularly when the patient first begins dialysis. With the passage of time, other stresses may bring added reactions. The continued drain on financial resources and the need for role changes within the family may create additional problems and resentment. Often, a patient on dialysis may become increasingly dependent, demanding and irascible. Resenting the loss of a positive self-image and self-esteem, either real or imagined, he or she may be antagonistic toward the rest of the family. Family members, in turn, may become hostile toward the patient and then feel guilty for having these feelings.

Nurses and other dialysis personnel can provide opportunities for family members to ventilate hostility and anxiety through the use of active listening techniques. Staff can offer reassurance that these are normal reactions. Furthermore, other team members may act as liaisons with the psychiatrist or social worker in developing a realistic plan to help the patient and family resolve problems that arise.

What are some of the physical problems that can adversely affect the psychosocial adjustment of dialysis patients?

Insomnia, chronic pruritus, neuropathy symptoms, muscle cramps, and bone and joint pain are some of the most commonly identified physical problems that contribute to a diminished quality of life for patients on dialysis. Ongoing assessment of the physiological response to ESRD and dialysis therapy is essential. In many cases, medical management can alleviate the physical problems, enhancing the patient's psychologic adjustment and improving his or her quality of life. Some patients need to be encouraged to report physical symptoms because they may otherwise assume that nothing can be done about them.

How does the dialysis procedure itself affect the psychosocial adjustment of dialysis patients?

The time commitment is probably the single aspect of the dialysis regimen that exercises the largest influence on a patient's adjustment to treatment. The time demand may interfere with the patient's ability to perform activities of daily living, resulting in loss of independence and, ultimately, lowered self-esteem and depression. Dialysis personnel need to work with the patient to design the least restrictive regimen possible. Encouraging the patient to perform self-care activities and to maintain some degree of independence will sustain a more positive psychosocial adjustment.

How does social support influence the psychosocial adjustment of patients on dialysis?

Social support, both in terms of quantity and quality, has been associated with better levels of psychologic adjustment in persons living with any chronic illness. Family members are usually the greatest source of social support for a patient. However, to maintain their ability to be supportive of the patient, family members may need the assistance of dialysis personnel. In addition, patients and family members should be encouraged to continue to participate in social and leisure activities both within and beyond the family. The dialysis social worker can provide referrals to patient and family support groups and community resources for socialization. Caregiver groups, peer support, and senior-citizen centers can be included as appropriate.

What type of relationship should there be between the dialysis patient and the nurse or technician?

It is not uncommon for a dependence to develop between dialysis personnel and patients. This type of relationship may be very satisfying to the nurse or technician and may fulfill a desire to be needed. However, an excessively close relationship may cause the professional to exercise faulty judgment, which can be detrimental to the patient.

Patients need to be encouraged to do things for themselves, whenever possible, to preserve and promote a sense of independence.

It is best if one staff person can be responsible for working with a given patient and his or her family. This helps prevent the problems that can be created by inconsistent responses to questions. In their anxiety, people tend to ask slightly different versions of their questions of everyone. The result can be ambiguity and chaos. Questions should be answered consistently, accurately, and honestly, and this is best accomplished if one team member serves as the primary information source for each patient and his or her family.

What are professional boundaries?

Professional boundaries are the limitations that healthcare providers impose on themselves to maintain a safe and comfortable therapeutic relationship with their patients. The National Council of State Boards of Nursing, Inc. (1996) defines professional boundaries as "the spaces between the nurse's power and the client's vulnerability." The nurse or dialysis technician is in the position of power because they are the individuals who have the ability to perform the life-sustaining treatments that the patient requires for survival. The dialysis staff is involved with the care of the patient 3 days a week over the duration of many years. This type of setting lends itself to the potential development of personal relationships between patients and nurses or patients and technicians. Whereas most relationships are therapeutic, sometimes healthcare personnel become overinvolved with the needs of the patient. These boundary crossings or violations may be interpreted as inappropriate by an employer or state board of nursing.

It is never appropriate to have anything other than a professional relationship with a patient. Neither a business nor a personal relationship should be established between a patient and staff member. Healthcare professionals should not spend time outside of the workplace with patients or socialize with them. Intimate relationships are never appropriate to establish with a patient—any type of sexual relationship with a patient is misconduct and a serious violation of the Nurse Practice Acts of most states. It is the responsibility of the nurse or technician to ensure that professional boundaries are maintained. The patient is always considered vulnerable if litigation should occur as the result of an inappropriate relationship. Gifts, monetary or otherwise, should never be accepted from a patient or family member.

It is the healthcare professional who is responsible to maintain professional boundaries. A good rule to determine the appropriateness of a relationship is to ask if you would establish the same relationship or engage in the same activities or behaviors with every patient in the clinic. If the answer is no, chances are, this would be a boundary violation.

Do patients have unrealistic expectations of dialysis therapy?

It is not uncommon for patients to expect a greater degree of curative capability than dialysis can actually provide. Dialysis provides a lifesaving therapy, but it does not cure uremia. The patient and his or her family still must live and cope with a chronic illness.

What role does pre-ESRD education have for the patient with chronic kidney disease (CKD)?

Education programs are in vogue and can help to ease the CKD patient's transition through all phases of the disease. Pre-ESRD education is known to lower the stress for both the patient and family, improve mortality and morbidity, enhance self-care and decision making, play a role in the continuation of employment, and allow for more informed decision making when replacement therapy must finally be initiated. The American Association of Kidney Patients (AAKP) has developed several predialysis education programs to assist those experiencing CKD. Kidney Options is a program jointly sponsored by AAKP and Fresenius Medical Care North America. Educational materials include a website, newsletters, brochures, and local patient education programs. AAKP has also teamed up with Baxter Healthcare to establish the Stay in Touch program, which offers educational mailings based on a patient's current needs, a toll-free hotline, and an informational website.

How may these problems be countered?

Patients and their families need to be well informed and have a solid understanding of the disease process and the necessary treatment. A well-planned and well-executed patient education program is a vital aspect of the care of any person with ESRD.

Patient and family group meetings, held at regular intervals and guided by a qualified team member, can provide a great deal of support and problem solving of a self-help nature. Patient care conferences involving all members of the dialysis team should be held regularly to keep all personnel current on patient problems and how they are being approached. Otherwise, with a large number of patients, the effort can become fragmented.

Is the sexual dysfunction experienced by many dialysis patients emotional?

Sexual dysfunction in dialysis patients involves both emotional and organic factors. Organic elements that contribute to decreased sexual functioning are thought to include severe anemia, impaired testosterone and other hormonal levels, and increased parathyroid hormone (PTH) levels. These conditions can lead to reduced fertility and libido. Medications, particularly some antihypertensive agents, also may contribute. In addition to these organic causes, depression also seems to be an important element in the sexual dysfunction of dialysis patients. Even with correction of anemia with erythropoietin (EPO), sexual dysfunction is still a major problem.

Both the patient and his or her partner need to be aware of the potential for sexual dysfunction and be provided with a framework for discussion about sexuality. In many cases, the nephrologist or mental health professional will need to initiate the discussion about sex, rather than expect patients to bring the topic up on their own. Together, the physician and social worker can provide a forum for discussion. Counseling may be helpful in some cases, and it should be possible for a couple to work out acceptable alternatives.

What degree of rehabilitation may be anticipated for dialysis patients?

Rehabilitation can be defined in both broad and narrow terms. Using a liberal definition, rehabilitation may be considered successful if an individual is able to fulfill family role responsibilities and occupy him- or herself with meaningful activities.

As defined in the narrow sense, meaning the return to a prior level of functioning, dialysis patients may have limited rehabilitation potential. Homemakers and students frequently are able to resume their customary activity schedules with minor limitations. The growing number of ESRD patients with concurrent illnesses and accompanying sensory and motor deficits has resulted in a decrease in the proportion of patients able to return fully to their previous level of functioning. With improved dialysis techniques and the correction of anemia, it is increasingly realistic for ESRD patients to consider returning to some type of work after commencing dialysis.

How can a dialysis patient's rehabilitation potential be enhanced?

In recent years there has been an increased focus on rehabilitation in the dialysis population. The dialysis social worker can refer patients to state vocational rehabilitation programs that can be helpful in assessing the patient's potential and identifying alternative sources of employment. These programs may include an educational component with referral to job training or educational programs within the community college system or at local universities. In some cases, financial assistance is available to low-income patients.

What is an Advance Directive (AD)?

An AD is a written document that specifies in advance what kind of medical treatments an individual wants or does not want in the event of an incapacitating condition. In 1991, a federal law, the Patient Self-Determination Act (Danforth Bill: Public Law 101-508) went into effect. The law applies to most healthcare organizations and providers. It requires that patients be given information concerning their legal rights to make decisions about the medical care and treatment they are about to receive. An AD can be a durable power of attorney for healthcare or a living will. Requirements for what needs to be specified vary from state to state. This is a hard subject to discuss with anyone but can be particularly difficult to explore with someone who is confronting a life-threatening illness. Often it is the role of the social worker to provide information about AD to patients and their families, but all staff should be familiar with the law and issues surrounding ADs.

What about patients who decide to discontinue dialysis?

In planning the treatment regimen, the staff should include a comprehensive and open discussion about the options available to patients. The right not to begin dialysis and the right to withdraw from dialysis are among these options. Such decisions are based on the specific needs and desires of the individual patient, with consideration of his or her medical condition. A decision to discontinue or not to initiate dialysis is usually made in conjunction with family members, the physician, and other members of the dialysis team, including the chaplain and the psychiatrist. In general, older persons who have complications because of underlying illnesses are more likely to discontinue dialysis than are younger individuals. When a patient has elected to discontinue dialysis, members of the professional team need to provide supportive care with an emphasis on physical and emotional comfort.

In what ways can ESRD patients achieve more control over their own situation?

Patients who previously led independent lives may be at increased risk for psychosocial difficulties with the onset of dialysis treatment. It is especially important that these individuals be given opportunities to participate in their treatment regimens as much as possible. Patients may feel a greater sense of control over their situation if they are encouraged to perform self-care dialysis in the hemodialysis unit or during home hemodialysis. Peritoneal dialysis (PD) can be a positive choice for patients with a need or desire for freedom from dialysis schedules.

What is palliative care?

Palliative care is a bridge of hospice care that treats the patient earlier in the course of the illness or disease process. Palliative care deals with the physical, emotional, social, and spiritual pain associated with incurable, progressive illnesses. Patients' needs are assessed throughout the course of illness and changes are made based on those needs, with a transition to hospice care when indicated. A core belief of hospice and palliative care is that the patient deserves to die pain-free and with dignity. Bereavement support is provided to the family for a period following the death of the patient. Palliative care should be discussed for any ESRD patient who opts to decline dialysis or transplantation, as well as any patient who wishes to discontinue the current dialytic therapy. In order to be referred to the Centers for Medicare and Medicaid Services (CMS) for benefits, the patient must have a life expectancy of less than 6 months. The ESRD benefits will be covered when a patient withdraws from dialytic therapy, or when a terminal disease will result in death in less than 6 months. The patient can continue to receive dialysis in the form of ultrafiltration to ease the symptoms of fluid overload should dialysis be discontinued.

What is HIPAA and how does it affect the dialysis community?

HIPPA stands for the Health Insurance Portability and Accountability Act, which was enabled in 1996. New privacy regulations, which went into effect on April 14, 2003, protect patients' medical records and other health information that might be provided to insurance groups, doctors, hospitals, and other healthcare providers. The new privacy regulations, developed by the Department of Health and Human Services (DHHS), ensure privacy for patients by limiting the ways that health plans, hospitals, and other healthcare providers can use a patient's personal medical information. Any identifiable health information that is on paper, in computers, or orally communicated, is protected under the new law.

21 Pediatric Hemodialysis

Treating children is complicated by the fact that they are still growing and developing, and chronic kidney disease (CKD) interferes with this normal growth and development. Thus pediatric nephrology nurses must have a comprehensive knowledge of pediatric nursing and childhood growth and development.

What is family-centered care in a pediatric patient population?

The concept of family-centered care developed from awareness that young patients' emotional and developmental needs are best met by incorporating their families into the plan of care.

What are the staffing considerations for a pediatric hemodialysis population?

The hybrid of services that a pediatric dialysis facility provides necessitates a good method of matching resources to patient workload activity. The best choice is a time/motion study–based, statistically validated patient-dependency classification system. A patient-dependency system takes into account factors such as developmental age versus chronologic age and matches care requirements with the appropriate numbers of staff at each skill level. The patient-dependency system captures the care requirements of a patient who may be less ill, but is more dependent due to age, developmental level, or cultural requirements or who requires more frequent or different types of interventions than other patients with the same diagnosis. Because of the many pediatric patient-dependency categories, staffing requirements for pediatric care comprise a complex matrix that is most easily implemented with a staffing and scheduling system that targets staffing by skill level. As a patient's dependency level increases, increased caregiver skills are usually required. The system must also recognize the potential for day-to-day variation in an individual child's care requirements and in the staff required to provide that care. Determining staffing by matching caregiver-to-patient ratios with patient ages or sizes can be a disadvantage because ratios presume that all patients with the same age or weight necessarily require the same level of care every day.

How can a pediatric facility maximize operations when it has a small patient base?

Many pediatric dialysis facilities maximize operations by cross training nursing staff in both acute and chronic renal replacement therapy. During orientation the pediatric dialysis nurse learns how to manage all the therapies furnished by a particular facility. Commonly these include the pediatric modalities of hemodialysis, peritoneal dialysis, and continuous renal replacement therapy. Some pediatric dialysis facilities offer additional extracorporeal therapies such as hemoperfusion and plasmapheresis. Orientation can take anywhere from 6 weeks to 3 months, depending on prior experience and learning opportunities. Simulated clinical experiences in a skills laboratory can supplement learning experiences. A broad orientation plan and a gradual progression to independence with a designated preceptor guiding the progress toward acquisition of knowledge and mastery of skills have worked best in our experience.

Is there a place for technical support in the care of children on hemodialysis?

Some programs employ technicians for well-defined tasks, such as preparing equipment for dialysis or assisting registered nurses with children who are not developmentally delayed and who weigh more than 35 kg. A well-defined orientation plan, competency list, and method of documenting progress are important. Some states have specific stipulations for technical support personnel; check with the state department of health for specific state guidelines.

What are the causes of acute renal failure in children?

Acute renal failure in children usually results from hypoperfusion of the kidneys due to septic shock, hypotension, and severe dehydration from gastroenteritis or from acute blood loss from surgery or an accident. The pathology is that of acute tubular necrosis. Acute tubular necrosis can also occur after nephrotoxic drugs, especially aminoglycoside antibiotics and amphotericin B. The most common cause of primary acute renal failure in children in North America is the hemolytic uremic syndrome. Acute poststreptococcal glomerulonephritis, though common in children, rarely leads to acute renal failure severe enough to warrant dialysis.

What are the causes of CKD in children?

The causes of CKD are different for children than for adults. About two thirds of the cases in children are caused by congenital urinary tract anomalies, such as posterior urethral valves, obstructive uropathy, reflux nephropathy, renal dysplasia and neurogenic bladder associated with spina bifida, or hereditary diseases, including cystinosis, hyperoxaluria, and autosomal recessive polycystic kidney disease. The other one third is caused by acquired kinds of glomerulonephropathy, like focal segmental glomerulosclerosis or membranoproliferative glomerulonephritis. Unlike CKD in adults, diabetic nephropathy, chronic hypertension, autosomal dominant polycystic kidney disease, and membranous glomerulonephritis are rarely causes of CKD in childhood and adolescence.

When is hemodialysis the right choice for pediatric patients requiring chronic replacement therapy?

The preferred modality of treatment for end-stage renal disease (ESRD) for most pediatric patients is renal transplantation. If a pediatric patient needs chronic dialysis, home peritoneal dialysis is the usual choice, but may not always be possible. Some family situations are unable to support chronic peritoneal dialysis. Some patients may have lost peritoneal function from previous abdominal surgery or peritonitis. Currently younger children, including infants and toddlers with ESRD, who have failed peritoneal dialysis and who are not yet eligible for transplantation or who are waiting on the deceased donor transplantation list, require chronic hemodialysis. Technical advances in equipment and vascular access catheters have made chronic hemodialysis possible even in small children. Some adolescents may choose hemodialysis because of concerns about body image or their ability to comply with the discipline of chronic peritoneal dialysis and the need for daily treatment.

What is the significance of body surface area to renal function in pediatrics?

Normal serum creatinine concentration increases with age and body mass. The normal serum creatinine level in a 2-year-old is 0.4 mg/dL, whereas in an adult it is about 1.0 mg/dL. If it were 1.0 mg/dL in a 2-year-old, that child would have renal failure with about a 60% reduction in renal function. In order to compare parameters of renal function in different sized pediatric patients from infancy to adolescence, creatinine clearance and other measures of glomerular filtration rate are usually normalized to the average adult body surface area of 1.73 m^2. The normal range for creatinine clearance in a pediatric patient older than 2 years of age is 100 to 120 mL/min/1.73 m^2. When the creatinine clearance decreases less than 10 mL/min/1.73 m^2, the pediatric patient has ESRD.

Is there a preferred measure of weight for children?

The preferred measure of weight in children is metric because most therapies are prescribed per weight in kilograms. Consistent use of the metric system to measure weight in children lessens calculation error. If a kilogram scale is not available, convert pounds to kilograms by dividing by a factor of 2.2.

Are there particular considerations when choosing a hemodialysis station location for the child dialyzing in an integrated pediatric and adult care facility?

Because of the higher dependency of the pediatric hemodialysis patient, especially those weighing less than 35 kg, the station for hemodialysis should be within easy access and centrally visible. In the event of an emergency in another patient, every effort should be made to protect the child from viewing the stressful event.

Do children ever require isolation?

Communicable diseases, such as varicella (chickenpox), are common in childhood. In addition to isolation for blood-borne pathogens, children may need to be isolated during periods when they are at risk of manifesting communicable diseases after recent exposure. Each facility should develop general recommendations for isolation for children exposed to communicable diseases like varicella to avoid exposure of susceptible adult patients.

What is the safe limit for extracorporeal volume for a child?

The safe limit for extracorporeal volume in a child is 10% or less of the child's blood volume (Table 21-1). This blood is returned to the patient at the end of the treatment, unless it is needed for laboratory tests. In this case, no more than 3% to 5% of the child's blood volume should be removed on a given day. Many laboratories have microcontainers for blood sampling for small children or use minimal blood volumes for tests to help avoid excess blood loss in pediatric patients.

How does one calculate extracorporeal volume?

Extracorporeal volume is the total volume of the dialyzer plus the bloodlines. Specific values are available from product manufacturers.

Can hemodialysis treatment be done when the extracorporeal volume exceeds the safe limits?

When extracorporeal volume is 10% to 12.5% of blood volume, the system must be primed with a volume expander such as 5% albuminized saline. When extracorporeal volume exceeds 12.5% of blood volume, reconstituted whole blood may be the safest for priming and is imperative when extracorporeal volume is 15% or more. There are specific dialysis products designed to minimize extracorporeal blood volume for small

Table 21-1	Approximate Blood Volume by Age
Age	**Total blood volume**
Premature infants	90 to 105 mL/kg
Term newborns	78 to 86 mL/kg
>1 mo to 1 yr	78 mL/kg
>1 yr to adult	74 to 82 mL/kg
Adult	68 to 78 mL/kg

children, and these must be used to avoid the expense and risk of using blood products routinely. The pediatric nephrologist decides how much, if any, of the system prime is returned to the patient at the end of the treatment, based on the patient's specific albumin or hemoglobin deficit.

How is replacement blood transfusion volume calculated should a pediatric hemodialysis patient suffer an acute blood loss (i.e., clotted system)?

To replace acute blood loss associated with hemodynamic instability, transfuse packed red blood cells at 10 mL/kg body weight or more, depending on the estimated amount of blood lost and the child's hemoglobin before the loss.

What are the vascular access considerations in pediatrics?

The smaller the pediatric patient, the more difficult it will be to establish adequate access for hemodialysis. In patients weighing less than 10 kg, an indwelling catheter of appropriate diameter placed in a major vessel will be the only option. It is important for the catheter not to come close to or exceed the vessel size, which will lead to obstruction of normal venous flow. Dual- and single-lumen cuffed catheters are now available for even very small children (5 to 10 kg body weight). In the hands of a skilled pediatric access surgeon, an arteriovenous loop graft in the thigh may be possible for patients more than 10 kg, and a primary arteriovenous fistula in the forearm for patients more than 15 kg. In general, permanent access is extremely difficult when the patient is smaller than 20 kg and should be placed only by a surgeon or pediatric nephrologist skilled in these procedures.

Do children require special dialyzers?

In choosing the dialyzer for a pediatric hemodialysis patient, the dialyzer surface area (available from the product manufacturer) often approximates the child's body surface area. Dialyzers as small as 0.22 m^2 are available. The type chosen should be based on the blood volume of the dialyzer as well as the prescription for dialysis adequacy and the ultrafiltration coefficient. Hollow-fiber dialyzers are preferred because of their low compliance.

Are there special pediatric bloodlines?

Many manufacturers offer neonatal or pediatric-size bloodlines, which offer a substantial decrease in volume over adult lines. As these specialized bloodlines tend to be shorter, caution should be taken to secure the lines so that there is no tension on the patient's access site.

Are there hemodialysis machines specifically for children?

Volumetric hemodialysis equipment that is used for adults can be safely used for children. Volumetric equipment decreases the margin of error for fluid removal. Note that all hemodialysis system manufacturers warn of the potential variance from target of

10% for fluid removal, which is especially important in the small patient, where 10% can be a substantial amount compared with the patient's total body water.

Can reprocessed dialyzers be safely used for children undergoing hemodialysis?

Only a few pediatric care facilities practice reuse. Reuse is more widely practiced in larger integrated pediatric and adult care facilities.

How is pain associated with hemodialysis managed in children?

For the discomfort of fistula needle insertion, pain management options include topical anesthetics (e.g., EMLA cream) or subcutaneous 1% lidocaine at the needle insertion sites. Some children, often preschoolers, find topical anesthetics ineffective and subcutaneous 1% lidocaine "just another stick." For these patients a fistula needle insertion without anesthetic may be the best-tolerated option. Additional pain management techniques include deep breathing, distraction (e.g., blowing bubbles or inverting a glitter wand), or visual imagery, such as focusing on a soft-colored light. Remember that crying is a normal response to pain or to fear a needle before there is pain. The key to pain management success includes a consistent approach and good communication with the patient/family. The team should take every opportunity to soothe anxieties, to offer an array of pain management options, and to positively reinforce desired behavior, such as holding still.

If a child must be immobilized for needle insertion, minimize the personnel involved and focus on immobilizing the child's joints to prevent movement that will interfere with successful needle placement. Children less than 10 kg are best swaddled. Only rarely should a child require restraints, and then only for a short time period. When restraint is deemed necessary, a medical order should be written and refreshed with each hemodialysis treatment for which restraint is used.

Is sequential ultrafiltration (UF) used in children?

UF is only appropriate in older children and adolescents. Small infants requiring 5% albuminized saline or reconstituted whole blood prime should not have sequential UF. Prolonged UF in a small child can lead to hypothermia because the blood compartment will not be warmed by dialysis fluid.

How does one determine the target weight for a child on hemodialysis?

If the patient is growing, his or her weight should be gradually increasing. Target weight is the weight at which a patient with an adequate Kt/V is normotensive and euvolemic. Noninvasive inline monitoring devices, such as the Crit-Line, can help refine target weight determinations during a dialysis treatment. In growing children target weight should be reassessed at least monthly or more often when indicated by hypertension. Fluctuations in weight can occur frequently in children due to changes in dietary intake, compliance with fluid restrictions, or vomiting and diarrhea. Chronic fluid overload in children may masquerade as false weight gain and fool even the experienced dialysis nurse.

What is the optimal blood flow rate for a pediatric hemodialysis patient?

The optimal blood flow rate (Q_b) is a function of what the access will allow as well as the desired Kt/V. A Q_b of 200 to 350 mL/min/1.73 m^2 has been optimal to achieve these goals in our pediatric unit.

How does intradialytic monitoring differ in children?

The advent of volumetric hemodialysis equipment has made the procedure much safer in children. Blood pressure monitoring intervals should match the individual patient's care requirements. Blood pressure should always be done immediately after initiating the hemodialysis and at least hourly thereafter. When a patient is perceived to be unstable, monitoring intervals should decrease. Resist the urge to take blood pressure measurements every 15 minutes or half hour just because the patient is a child. The child may just become agitated and uncooperative, creating technical difficulty obtaining reliable readings. Monitors designed to noninvasively and automatically measure systolic and diastolic pressure, mean arterial pressure, and pulse rate for neonatal or pediatric patients are effective and versatile. They continue to monitor during most clinical crises when other indirect measurement methods may fail. Acute hemodialysis treatments in unstable patients nearly always require continuous arterial pressure monitoring for safety.

In addition to blood pressure measurement in patients weighing less than 20 kg, continuous monitoring of heart rate (electrocardiogram [ECG]) and oxygenation (pulse oximeter) is required to detect deterioration in patient condition, which is most often related to acute fluid removal. Continuous nursing assessment is also needed to pick up subtle changes of impending hypotension, like irritability or yawning or fidgety movements. Since these subtle signs vary from patient to patient, their inclusion in the individual patient's plan of care will facilitate communication of a particular patient's care to the entire team.

What is high blood pressure (HBP) in children?

Blood pressure differs by gender and increases with age and size, so parameters for hypertension will be different from adults as shown in Table 21-2 for boys. Girls and shorter children at a given age have slightly lower blood pressure than boys and taller children for age. Blood pressure must be taken with an appropriately sized cuff, the air-filled bladder of which should have a width equal to approximately 40% of the circumference of the arm, measured at a point midway between the olecranon and acromion, and a length sufficient to extend around the arm at least 80% of the circumference. Cuff size is not standardized by industry, so the name "infant," "child," or "small adult" on the cuff should be disregarded, and the above parameters should be followed for proper sizing. If a cuff is

Table 21-2	High Blood Pressure (BP) (>95 Percentile for Age)	
	SIGNIFICANT BP* BASED ON HEIGHT (HT) PERCENTILE	
Age group (Boys)	**Ht 5%**	**Ht 95%**
BP percentile	95%	95%
1 Year	98/54	106/58
2 Years	101/59	110/63
4 Years	106/66	115/71
6 Years	109/72	117/76
8 Years	111/75	120/80
10 Years	115/77	123/82
12 Years	119/78	127/83
14 Years	124/80	132/84
16 Years	129/82	137/87

Prehypertension in children is defined as average systolic blood pressure (SBP) or diastolic blood pressure (DBP) levels that are ≥90th percentile by <95th percentile.
Adapted from The Fourth Report on the Diagnosis, Evaluation, and Treatment of High Blood Pressure in Children and Adolescents, Pediatrics 114(2):555-576, 2004.

too small, the blood pressure measurement will be falsely high. An oversized adult cuff or large thigh cuff will be needed for obese adolescents.

What is the significance of latex in the pediatric hemodialysis setting?

Certain groups of children are at high risk for developing latex allergy. Children with spina bifida have a 10% to 60% risk of developing an allergy to latex. Other children who require clean intermittent urinary catheterization are also at high risk. Repeated exposure to latex products is purported to be a significant risk factor to trigger a reaction, which can begin as contact urticaria or can be as dramatic as an anaphylactic reaction. There are two basic exposure routes: direct mucosal contact and airborne latex particles. Treatment of latex allergy is best directed to preventing exposures from the numerous items, like gloves and catheters that contain latex. In addition to identifying pediatric patients at risk, each facility should develop protocols for latex precautions.

Are there any differences in heparin requirements during a pediatric hemodialysis?

The adult guidelines for heparinization and activated clotting time (ACT) monitoring can be used for children. To achieve a target ACT of 1.5 times normal, begin with a loading dose of 25 to 50 units/kg and a continuous infusion of 10 units/kg/hr. Increase the loading dose by 10 to 25 units/kg and the continuous infusion by 5 units/kg/hr as needed to achieve the desired ACT. Once the usual heparin requirement is established for a given patient, one should resist the temptation to sample blood unnecessarily for ACTs. Heparin requirements may be different if a chronic patient receives new vascular access or has surgery or gastrointestinal bleeding. Neonates, especially premature infants, who require hemodialysis or continuous renal replacement therapy need tight heparinization because they are at high risk for cerebral hemorrhage.

How does anemia management differ in children?

Two multicenter trials have shown that pediatric patients younger than 5 years old frequently require initial recombinant human erythropoietin in higher doses, approximately 300 units/kg/wk, than older pediatric patients and adults. Achieving target iron levels to support erythropoiesis requires the administration of supplemental iron, either orally or intravenously. When administering intravenous iron dextran, heed the differences in pediatric test doses, such as 10 mg for patients weighing less than 10 kg and 15 mg for those weighing 10 to 20 kg, and pediatric dosing by body weight. The Kidney Disease Outcomes Quality Initiative (K-DOQI) clinical practice guidelines note the differences in anemia management in children and are a good guideline to follow for pediatric care. (See page 338 for additional information on the National Kidney Foundation NKF-K/DOQI.)

Why are children with CKD short in stature?

Growth retardation is a significant consequence of CKD in children. The age of onset is an important variable affecting growth—the younger the patient at the onset of CKD, the greater the potential for growth retardation. Many factors contribute to poor growth, including chronic metabolic acidosis, sodium wasting and chronic dehydration, chronic fluid overload, poorly controlled renal osteodystrophy, anorexia and malnutrition from poor caloric intake, steroid therapy for underlying renal disease control, and disturbances of normal growth hormone regulation. To best achieve normal or catch-up growth, efforts should be made to correct as many of these abnormalities as possible before the patient needs chronic dialysis.

How can growth be maximized in a pediatric hemodialysis patient?

To maximize growth potential during chronic hemodialysis, efforts should continue to include correcting acidosis, minimizing fluid overload, controlling renal osteodystrophy, and promoting optimum nutrition, and should also include optimizing dialysis adequacy. Each patient's height and target weight should be monitored closely (at least every 3 months) until the bone growth plates close. Head circumference as well as length and target weight should be measured in children younger than 3 years of age. Gender-specific growth charts should be maintained and plotted quarterly, or more frequently if the patient is falling off his/her percentile on the growth chart. When height falls below the fifth percentile for age in a child more than 1 to 2 years old, initiation of recombinant human growth hormone therapy should be considered. Children with CKD and ESRD are relatively resistant to normal levels of growth hormone, so supplementation can help normalize their growth and improve muscle mass.

What are the toileting concerns in the child with ESRD?

Facilitate toilet training when the child is developmentally ready. The child with ESRD may have no urine output or a small amount of urine daily. Some children, usually those with congenital renal disease, like dysplasia or obstructive uropathy, may have a large volume of urine output daily and little concentrating ability. Young children with large urine volumes often continue to have nighttime bed wetting because they are too sleepy to feel the need to get up and urinate in the toilet.

Can children who are receiving hemodialysis treatments go to regular school?

Most school-aged children on hemodialysis are able to attend school regularly with their peers. Missing school is often related to hospitalizations or the hemodialysis treatment schedule. When scheduling hemodialysis, every attempt should be made to facilitate school attendance. School constitutes a framework for daily behavior that imposes discipline and regularities, skills that are essential to achieving adult independence and ultimately entering the job market.

What are options for measuring functional status in children?

Denver II Developmental Screening Tests are easy to perform and recommended for the assessment of children less than 6 years of age. Developmental delays are not uncommon in this chronically ill population. Another functional status tool for older children is the Children's Health Questionnaire, which is the pediatric version of the Short Form 36.

How does emergency preparedness need to be adapted when caring for children?

Medical emergency. The facility must be equipped with the appropriate pediatric-sized airways, airmask bag units (AMBUs), and endotracheal tubes. Because most pediatric drug doses are based upon weight, it is wise to have an emergency drug list with precalculated doses for each individual pediatric patient. A pediatric advanced life support (PALS)–certified nurse and nephrologist should always be readily available.

Fire. Fire drills must be adapted to each child's developmental understanding. Many child-friendly resources, such as coloring books and fact sheets, are available through the National Fire Protection Association (NFPA) or the fire divisions of the local department of public safety.

Disasters. When local disasters such as floods, tornados, hurricanes, or earthquakes strike, pediatric hemodialysis treatment becomes a priority. If a disaster can be anticipated, some pediatric patients may benefit from preemptive hospitalization.

Does pediatric hemodialysis cost more than adult hemodialysis?

Pediatric hemodialysis costs are higher because of the increased cost of supply items and services. Pricing is not as competitive for disposables in this low volume specialized market. Staffing for the increased patient dependency in pediatrics demands increased caregiver skills or more nurses. Exception requests based on atypical service intensity are available through the Centers for Medicare and Medicaid Services (CMS) to enable pediatric centers to increase their center-specific Medicare reimbursement rate to compensate for more costly operating conditions.

When do children transition to adult care?

Optimally, early preparation should begin during the stage of late adolescence (ages 17 to 21 years), which is characterized by a teenager's having developed the ability to define future goals, make close and intimate friendships, and begin rapprochement with parents and other authoritative adults. During the stage of midadolescence (ages 14 to 17 years), a teenager is at the height of risk-taking behavior, peer conformity, poor future orientation, and parental conflict, which is a very difficult time to implement the transition to adult responsibilities. Some patients who are developmentally delayed may not be ready at age 17 years. Transition preparation includes teaching self-care skills, such as taking responsibility for adhering to a medication schedule, arranging clinic visits, and arriving for treatments on time. Ideally, late preparation should also incorporate a visit accompanied by a trusted nurse and/or social worker to the adult dialysis center. Actual transfer to adult care should occur between 18 and 21 years of age, depending on patient readiness, disease management, and availability of service. Being in an integrated pediatric and adult care facility should not preclude having the adolescent participate in a defined transition preparation program to be sure the patient is ready for the demands of adult-oriented care.

22 End-Stage Renal Disease (ESRD) in the Elderly

Since the early 1990s, at least 45% of new patients entering the ESRD program in the United States each year have been more than 65 years old. This percentage is increasing; the figure for 2003 was 49%. The same trend appears in dialysis programs all over the world. Regardless of the treatment modality selected, some changes are required to adapt the therapy to the special needs of geriatric patients. As will become clear during the course of this chapter, besides presenting some limitations, older adult patients bring certain assets to their treatment regimen. All ESRD treatment modalities are available to the older adult patient, subject to the usual considerations, such as adequate vascular access or an intact peritoneal membrane.

Are the causes of ESRD different in elderly patients?

Not really. The most common cause is nephrosclerosis secondary to either diabetes or hypertension. Causes such as chronic glomerulonephritis and pyelonephritis are as common in older patients as in younger, although there may be slightly more older adult patients with an "unknown" renal diagnosis (biopsies are rarely done in elderly patients with renal failure of undetermined cause).

How do older patients differ from younger ESRD patients?

Comorbid conditions are much more common in older patients and can complicate the treatment of ESRD. Examples of significant comorbidities include an impaired cardiovascular system, osteoporosis, type 2 diabetes, delayed protein synthesis/reduced protein intake, impaired pulmonary function, impaired cognitive function, poor vision, poor mobility, and/or poor coordination.

Although not physical factors, adverse psychosocial and socioeconomic factors also complicate treatment regimens for a larger proportion of older than younger patients.

Can elderly patients benefit from renal replacement therapy?

Many, perhaps most, elderly people can benefit from renal replacement therapy, often returning to a level of physical functioning and quality of life that is either equivalent to that of people their age without ESRD or at least acceptable to the patient.

Some patients, usually but not necessarily elderly, may not benefit from treatment. Examples include those with irreversible dementia or extremely debilitating or imminently terminal comorbid conditions, such as cancer or advanced congestive heart failure. However, there are few firm medical or community standards with respect to withholding treatment and decisions regarding initiating therapy vary with individual physicians and/or family members.

What is trial dialysis?

The concept of trial dialysis is gaining favor in some areas. A patient in whom the value of therapy is questionable may be given treatment (usually hemodialysis) for a clearly defined period to see whether explicitly described clinical goals can be achieved. Examples of such patients might include those with unexplained dementia, potentially reversible acute renal failure, unexplained worsening of congestive heart failure, personality change, and adult failure-to-thrive syndrome. The duration of treatment, specific goals, and subsequent actions (continue/discontinue) are agreed to in advance by the medical team and family and, in some cases, the patient. This allows the patient every opportunity to benefit from treatment, if that is possible, and if not, provides the family and patient time to adjust and the knowledge that every effort was made.

Can elderly patients be successfully transplanted?

Certainly. Although the proportion of older adult ESRD patients who qualify for transplantation is not as high as that of younger patients, graft survival in those who do receive transplants is about the same. Kidneys are becoming more available to elderly recipients because some transplant surgeons believe that organs donated by an older person should go to an older person. Elderly patients often require less intensive immunosuppressive therapy, due to the fact that their immune systems may already be compromise by age.

Although patient survival is not as good at that of younger patients, because of an increased number and severity of complications, data show satisfactory results for transplantation in elderly patients. By the same token, dialysis is also safer than ever for the elderly, so making a decision between modes of therapy is not simple.

What are the advantages for elderly patients in being on peritoneal dialysis (PD)?

PD, unlike hemodialysis at the present time, is a home dialysis therapy. Patients benefit from being at home in a number of ways. They are spared the considerable time, effort, and expense of being transported to and from a dialysis center, for one. The transportation effort is, in itself, very debilitating for some older patients. Home dialysis patients are in full charge of administering their own therapy, for another. This not only fosters independence but also preserves their usual lifestyle, allowing patients to perform exchanges at their convenience, within reason, rather than conform to a rigid in-center schedule.

Patients on PD do not need a vascular access, with its attendant problems (although they must have a peritoneal access catheter, with its attendant problems), and many elderly patients have inadequate peripheral vessels. Because PD is a continuous—or at least daily—therapy, blood chemistries and fluid status approach a steady state; thus PD patients do not suffer the effects of the rapid biochemical and fluid changes common in hemodialysis. This can be a significant advantage because elderly patients are more prone to adverse reactions to these changes. For example, PD patients with diminished cardiac reserve experience less orthostatic hypotension or other cardiac symptoms in response to fluid removal. Slow, continuous therapy allows better correction of brain electrophysiologic and cognitive function abnormalities, which incurs less risk of destabilizing the fragile mental equilibrium of some elderly patients.

Another advantage of daily therapy is that dietary and fluid restrictions are less rigid, which can be important for those with diminished appetites or impatience with restrictions.

Can elderly patients learn to do PD?

Yes, many can do very well by themselves, and others can do PD with assistance from family members. In addition, several assistive devices are available that allow patients who are blind or have limited dexterity to perform their own fluid exchanges. Automated, overnight dialysis systems eliminate all but a single connection and disconnection procedure.

What are the disadvantages of PD for older patients?

The incidence of certain complications (dementia, hernias, *Staphylococcus epidermidis* peritonitis, abdominal and catheter leaks) is higher in elderly PD patients compared with younger PD patients and compared with elderly hemodialysis patients.

If the patient frequently requires significant ultrafiltration, the resulting increased dialysate glucose concentration can significantly suppress the appetite, resulting in substantial malnutrition. This can be difficult to diagnose, at least initially, because dry weight may be stable or even increase (dextrose provides many calories but little nutrition). This can be a special problem with elderly patients, who are already at higher risk for malnutrition.

Loss of the opportunity to socialize during in-center therapy may also be a drawback, because many elderly people are socially isolated.

What are the advantages of hemodialysis (HD) in treating elderly ESRD patients?

Most hemodialysis in the United States is provided as an in-center therapy. There may be psychosocial advantages for elderly patients in the human interactions of dialysis center treatment, as mentioned earlier.

Another advantage is frequent observation by trained personnel. Elderly patients are more prone to complications of both ESRD and dialysis. When they develop such complications, these patients often exhibit less obvious symptoms. Earlier recognition and intervention (with resulting reductions in patient discomfort and healthcare costs) is more likely in a dialysis center setting.

Modern HD equipment, with its sophisticated monitoring and ultrafiltration (UF) control systems, is better able to provide controlled rates of biochemical and fluid removal and thus provide safe and comfortable treatments for a larger range of elderly patients than was possible in the past. Some patients prefer short, thrice-weekly treatments rather than continuously being on dialysis, as with PD. Treatment "burnout" is less common in the HD population. Also, many older adult patients grew up in an era when physicians and nurses—not patients—were expected to provide healthcare. Self-treatment, whether in a dialysis center or at home, is not acceptable to every older person.

Is HD more complicated in elderly patients?

Some practitioners claim that elderly patients are easier to dialyze. They tend to have lower fluid gains, lower creatinine, and lower urea generation rates; thus they do not necessarily require extremely aggressive treatment, with its higher risk of intradialytic complications. Also, older people are generally more compliant with all facets of the treatment regimen and express higher life satisfaction than younger patients.

With one exception, the nature and frequency of intradialytic complications are similar to that of younger HD patients. The exception is hemodynamic instability, which is more common in elderly people; thus intradialytic cardiac arrhythmias and hypotensive episodes are likely in this group. In most cases, episodes of hemodynamic instability can be minimized, and often prevented, if staff members are properly trained in the methods to achieve this.

Measures to prevent hypotensive episodes include using an extracorporeal circuit with the smallest possible priming volume, equipment with a volumetric ultrafiltration control system, and a bicarbonate dialysate with sufficiently high sodium, calcium, and dextrose levels to help maintain blood pressure during UF. UF and/or sodium modeling can help, as can using cool dialysate (35.5° to 36.0° C). No patients, especially the elderly, should be allowed to eat during dialysis because blood is diverted from the peripheral circulation (where it maintains blood pressure) to the digestive organs immediately after a meal. As a result, hypotension is usually inevitable. There is now ample evidence that a brief episode of simple exercises, especially if performed during the last hour of dialysis, is an effective way to support blood pressure and minimize muscle cramping. Dietary sodium, protein and fluid intake, and an antihypertensive medication regimen should be reevaluated on a regular basis.

Arrhythmias are common in elderly hemodialysis patients and may not be associated with any detectable symptoms. They arise in conjunction with anemia, hypokalemia, hyperkalemia, acidosis, hypoxia, hypotension, hypertension, digoxin, or cardiac abnormalities due, for example, to metastatic calcifications, amyloid deposition, or cardiac hypertrophy. Arrhythmias that are associated with symptoms such as weakness or hypoxia should be reported to the physician, who may elect to adjust the patient's diet, dialysate composition, or medication prescriptions. Nasal oxygen may provide symptomatic relief for hypoxia. Transfer to PD may be necessary, if feasible, for patients who do not respond to the aforementioned measures.

What are the disadvantages of HD in the elderly?

As mentioned, patients with significant cardiovascular disease do not tolerate the rapid biochemical and hemodynamic changes that accompany HD procedures and are at higher risk of intradialytic complications. As also mentioned, debilitated elderly people undergo considerable physical and emotional stress in relation to the thrice-weekly transportation to and from the dialysis center. Patients in either group would probably do better with a daily home dialysis regimen, such as PD or daily home HD, if that is feasible. Elderly patients may also experience more vascular access problems.

It is important to realize that older adult patients whose comorbidities are no more severe than those seen in younger patients do as well.

What special precautions should be taken with respect to monitoring the nutrition of elderly patients?

All patients lose nutrients during dialysis, whether HD or PD. Compared with the general dialysis population, elderly patients are at higher risk of malnutrition, in addition to being less likely to replace the nutrients lost during treatment. For this reason, staff must be able to recognize, indeed regularly probe for, factors that signal poor nutrition.

In addition to the usual impediments to good nutrition, elderly people experience a number of losses that interfere with their ability to achieve good nutrition. There are physical losses, such as loss of teeth, loss of senses of taste and smell, which make eating difficult or uninteresting; or loss of mobility, making it difficult to get to the grocery store or prepare meals.

Mealtime, often an occasion of social interaction, can remind older adults of their social losses, such as loss of spouse, companions, or access to community support. Some patients have psychologic conditions, such as dementia, depression, or just mental inertia, which can impede their will to eat. Financial constraints can enter the picture because many elderly live on fixed incomes and may have to make choices between paying for heat or food, for example. Medical factors such as anorexia, constipation, and medication effects can interfere with eating. Even with adequate meals there can still be nutritional losses due to vomiting, diarrhea, or loss of protein through persistent exudates from wounds or sores. Some of the factors that impede good nutrition can be corrected if they are recognized.

Suspect malnutrition if the patient has an increase in episodes of intradialytic hypotension or symptomatic congestive heart failure, develops depression or dementia, reports episodes suggestive of hypoglycemia (when not on hypoglycemic agents), a steady decline in dry weight, or symptoms of adult failure-to-thrive syndrome.

A low predialysis blood urea nitrogen (BUN) is always due to poor nutrition, not great dialysis. Resist the temptation to decrease dialysis; such patients usually need more dialysis, not less. By the same token, patients who are unstable during dialysis should not be taken off early. This leads to underdialysis, which decreases appetite, leading to lower plasma protein levels and, shortly, to even greater intradialytic instability.

The physician or dietitian should be contacted if any of the situations discussed in this section are identified.

What are the problems with medications in elderly ESRD patients?

Dialysis patients, especially elderly ones, are likely to take a great many drugs. Geriatric patients are much more susceptible to drug reactions and interactions. Thus the dose of each drug must be carefully calibrated by the physician, taking into consideration many factors such as the poor intestinal absorption, impaired hepatic clearance, and alteration in distribution space common in the elderly. Various elements can alter the patient's response to the prescribed dosage or combination of drugs; therefore, any unexplained change in physical or mental condition should be reported to the physician.

However, the main issue for staff is to check with the patient on a regular basis (1) to determine whether the patient is having problems taking all of the prescribed medications and (2) to be alert to the possibility of polypharmacy, which is the tendency of some elderly people to see several physicians and, unknown to the physicians, acquire multiple prescriptions from each.

Does exercise play a role in the treatment of elderly ESRD patients?

It certainly does. Properly prescribed exercise can play a significant role in the rehabilitation and subsequent preservation of the ability to perform the normal activities of daily life. This not only provides a better quality of life for the patient but also reduces the need for expensive hospitalizations and/or home health aides.

Of special importance to hemodialysis dialysis staff is the ample evidence that a brief period (i.e., 10 minutes) of exercise, such as pedaling a stationary bicycle, especially during the last hour of hemodialysis, can reduce the incidence and severity of muscle cramps and hypotension. A special device can be constructed from a bicycle wheel and pedals that allows the patient to remain seated in his dialysis chair while exercising.

What are the outcomes of the various ESRD treatment modalities in elderly patients?

In terms of treatment selection, the most recent information available (US Renal Data System [RDS] 2003) offers these statistics at the end of 2001: 93.8% of US patients ages 65 or older were receiving in-center HD, less than 1% were on home HD, 5.2% were on PD, and less than 1% had a functioning transplant.

One-year mortality was 31.3% for patients ages 65 to 74 years, and 45.5% for those older than 75. This is an improvement over earlier years (in 1984, for example, the mortality figures were 38% and 53%, respectively) and may reflect not only an improvement in ESRD therapy over that period but also increasing experience with treating elderly ESRD patients. The mortality rate of elderly ESRD patients is noticeably greater than that seen in younger ESRD patient age groups (18.4% for 45- to 64-year-olds; 10.7% in 20- to 44-year-olds; and 5.3% in 0- to 19-year-olds), a trend noted in the non-ESRD population as well.

23 Management of Quality in Dialysis Care

Like all healthcare, dialysis programs are undergoing a revolution in accountability. The government, accrediting and regulatory agencies, payers, and patients are holding healthcare organizations accountable for the delivery of high-quality, low-cost healthcare. Healthcare providers are being asked to explain the rationale behind their decisions and plans of care. Increased competition in the managed care environment also demands that providers be responsive to quality and cost issues. Continuous quality improvement (CQI) is a method to address those concerns. CQI must be supported by a leadership style of total quality management (TQM), in which all members of the organization are motivated to go beyond meeting minimum standards by complying with regulatory requirements as they continually evaluate their performance with the goal of improving care and outcomes.

What is CQI?

CQI is the ongoing process of identifying opportunities to improve quality. It involves collecting data about the current situation, identifying ways to improve the performance, introducing new and better approaches and methods to achieve desired outcomes, and then evaluating the interventions. When CQI is operating as intended, important aspects of care in need of improvement are identified before problems occur. All personnel contribute to CQI by being vigilant in recognizing care practices in need of improvement. A patient-centered perspective and questioning (e.g., "What about my work interferes with my ability to do what needs to be done to have the best possible outcome for patients?") are effective ways to identify practices in need of improvement. The goal of CQI is to use data to make objective decisions without placing blame or finding fault.

What is the origin of CQI?

Quality management efforts began in manufacturing, where the focus was on product inspection. Quality management experts, such as W. Edward Deming, recognized that it was not enough to just evaluate the end product. He introduced the principles of CQI to improve and manage the production processes to achieve a quality product.

What are the basic tenets of quality management?

Efforts to manage quality in healthcare continue to be influenced in particular by three sets of guides: Deming's 14 points; Donabedian's structure, process and outcomes framework; and the Joint Commission on the Accreditation of Healthcare Organizations (JCAHO)'s 10 steps. Basic tenets of CQI/TQM are a focus on customers, broadly defined to include personnel and patients, and a commitment to gather and use data to identify opportunities to improve quality outcomes by modifying processes that result in higher quality care at less cost. Efforts to achieve quality are dynamic and continual and everyone in the organization is involved and responsible. Failures in quality are more often due to flaws in processes than the failure of people doing the work.

Why is CQI relevant for healthcare and for dialysis programs?

The healthcare industry is one of the largest and most costly industries in America. CQI was introduced to the health care industry in part as an effort to slow the ever-increasing percent of the gross domestic product devoted to healthcare. Care provided to people with end-stage renal disease (ESRD), specifically dialysis, is costly. Dialysis is provided to about 390,000 Americans at an annual cost of $22.8 billion (United States Renal Data System, 2003). The cost of dialysis care mandates efforts to decrease cost without sacrificing quality of care.

What is the connection between quality and cost?

Healthcare personnel are committed to providing high-quality care to patients. Consideration of the costs of that care has not always been attended to, and providers may not realize that poor care is costly. For example, if a satisfactory dialysis is not achieved for any number of process or system reasons, the patient may have outcomes that require hospitalization for emergency treatment and additional dialysis. The end result is increased cost and poor financial performance.

How is CQI different from Quality Assurance (QA)?

QA was an early effort to address quality care issues in health care. QA, initiated in response to requirements of accreditation organizations, tended to use retrospective data collection, in which audits of medical records identified problems. These audits evaluated documented, existing problems, but improved quality of care did not necessarily result. CQI is a more proactive method, focused on seeking every opportunity to improve processes and systems to achieve quality outcomes. Concurrent collection of data for analysis is a vital aspect of CQI. Rather than documentation of problems, the focus of CQI is evaluation of interventions to improve quality.

Does CQI meet a need in dialysis facilities?

As a high-volume, high-risk, problem-prone, high-cost healthcare program, dialysis is a model for CQI. Dialysis facilities can use CQI techniques to identify processes in need of improvement, implement interventions or corrective actions, and evaluate cost and quality outcomes.

What are some CQI concepts and terms important to know?

A *process* is a series of interrelated activities to achieve a desired outcome or goal. Processes are those things dialysis personnel do to achieve well-dialyzed patients. Preparing the dialyzer, assessing the patient, and conducting the treatment with vigilant surveillance of both the patient and the machine are examples of processes that influence how well the patient is dialyzed.

Standards define quality by specifying rules that apply to key processes and the results expected. They are written values communicated to all members of the organization. Professional organizations that establish standards for dialysis nurses include the American Nephrology Nurses' Association (ANNA) Standards of Clinical Practice for Nephrology Nursing. Such standards specify a desired patient outcome (the patient will be free of vascular access complications), identify the nursing management aspects of care including assessment parameters (assess vascular access for patency and evidence of complications) and interventions (use aseptic technique in handling vascular access), and implement patient teaching.

Clinical indicators are valid and reliable measures used to evaluate important patient care services. They are events that are compared to some specified universe of events to encourage a focus on desired outcomes. Individual providers and dialysis facilities are encouraged to identify indicators relevant for specific settings. Organizations involved in specifying indicators are the Joint Commission on Accreditation of Healthcare Organizations (JCAHO), National Committee for Quality Assurance (NCQA), and the ESRD networks. An indicator for a dialysis facility might be the number of times it is necessary for personnel to use more than one needle per venipuncture to initiate dialysis as compared with the total number of venipunctures done.

A *benchmark* is a frame of reference for clinical practice. It is an objective way to compare a facility's processes and outcomes with its own past performance or with external standards. A benchmark can be the gold standard or the industry's best practice. Benchmarking is a goal-setting process that recognizes that providers and the internal organization may not have the best answers for the problem being addressed. It is a process of comparing the care provided and its outcomes with what is considered the best. An example of a benchmark for a dialysis facility might be to compare the average delivered dose of dialysis (Kt/V) with what the industry has set as the standard.

An *outcome* is the result obtained from some action or intervention. The outcome must specify who will do what and by how much within a specific period. For instance, a dialysis facility might identify an outcome, as personnel will reduce the number of second sticks required to initiate dialysis to 5% within 3 months following a skill refinement workshop.

What are some tools used in CQI?

Quality improvement efforts use the scientific method to search for the root cause of a problem, find it, and fix it. FOCUS is a CQI tool to help examine and analyze a specific process.

The first step is to *find a process to improve* by analyzing data. Statistical control is used to distinguish between common and special causes of variation in processes. Data are displayed in control charts to track performance. Variations outside of the control limits are special cause variances and require investigation. For more detailed instruction on the use of statistical control and other tools like flowcharts, Pareto charts, cause-and-effect (fishbone) diagrams, and run charts, refer to a CQI reference text.

Then next step is to *organize a team* to work together to improve the situation.

Clarify the problem by collecting and analyzing data specific to the process being targeted for improvement. A cause-and-effect diagram might be useful in the clarifying phase.

To truly *understand*, health providers examine data for the causes of variation and the changes over time.

The final FOCUS steps are to *select a method of improving outcomes* and *initiate the PDCA cycle of CQI*.

What is the PDCA Cycle?

PDCA stands for *plan-do-check-act*, a framework for implementing the methods to improve outcomes selected during the FOCUS process.

Plan, the first step in instituting a change for improvement, requires an investment of time because a hastily determined solution may not produce the desired result. Using brainstorming techniques encourages all members of the team to contribute ideas to the plan. Reviewing relevant literature is a critical element of planning. One outcome of planning by the multidisciplinary team may be a decision to develop a clinical care pathway or to adopt a clinical practice guideline as a way to improve the quality and cost outcomes of an important aspect of care.

Once a plan is agreed upon, the second phase of PDCA, *do*, is applied. Typically, *do* means implementing an intervention and conducting a pilot study to see if the change is effective.

During the *check* phase, results of the trial are checked against the objectives of the plan and modified as needed.

The final phase of the PDCA cycle is *act*, in which the findings of the pilot study guide implementation of solutions in a more comprehensive, facility-wide initiative. Ongoing monitoring to make certain that improvement persists over time is necessary.

What role do the ESRD networks play in quality management?

A collaborative effort involving ESRD networks, the Centers for Medicare and Medicaid Services (CMS), and other organizations is designed to improve ESRD care by collecting and analyzing data about clinical characteristics of adult dialysis patients. Two of the initiatives are the ESRD Core Indicators project and the National ESRD Anemia Cooperative Project.

What are the foci of the ESRD networks' key indicators?

The care indicators are adequacy of dialysis, desirable hematocrit value, optimal nutritional status, and control of blood pressure. Reports generated can be used by dialysis facilities to compare their unit's results with national findings, or benchmarks. These data can then lead to quality improvement projects designed to improve patient care within a facility.

The ESRD networks are involved with several other CQI projects. One is the Fistula First Project, which began in 2002 with the CMS and the Institute for Healthcare Improvement (IHI) developing an ESRD network–based improvement project for vascular access. The National Vascular Access Improvement Initiative (NVAII) project is a 3-year project and involves increasing arteriovenous fistula rates in the United States.

The ESRD Clinical Performance Measures Project (CPM) is another collaborative CQI effort between CMS, the ESRD networks, and ESRD dialysis facilities. This project provides an assessment of the care provided for approximately 9000 adult in-center hemodialysis patients, and all pediatric patients on dialysis in the United States.

Does the National Kidney Foundation (NKF) have a quality improvement initiative?

In March of 1995, the NKF established a Kidney Disease Outcome Quality Initiative (NKF-K/DOQI) to develop evidence-based clinical practice guidelines to improve the care of ESRD patients. The guidelines were completed in 1997 and have been translated into practice through professional education programs. Adoption of the guidelines will be evaluated for their effect on patient outcomes.

Does everyone agree with the quality management movement in healthcare?

Some health care providers resist quality improvement efforts because they believe the quality of their practice is ensured by their professionalism. Some people resent what they perceive to be external interference and controls. Still others believe that the time required for quality improvement is counterproductive. These negative impressions and resistance will, with time, diminish when they are countered successfully with a patient-centered perspective and acceptance of the goal of CQI to use data to improve quality and cost outcomes of care, as well as positive experiences with an effective TQI program.

How can I learn more about CQI/TQM in healthcare?

Books, journals, the Internet, and professional organizations, such as ANNA, are great resources for additional information about quality healthcare and the specific techniques of CQI/TQM.

Nephrology Organizations and Resources

For healthcare providers who are practicing within a dialysis unit or nephrology program, it becomes important to know where to turn for specific information for patients or for staff. Several organizations can be good resources for the practitioner.

Knowing how to use these resources can be key to a successful practice. Most of us do not take full advantage of the educational and informational resources available to us from organizations and the manufacturers of the products we use every day. These organizations are listed by category, followed by an alphabetical listing that gives a description of each.

Product manufacturers have the best available information about their product. It is in the best interests of the manufacturer to provide as much information as possible about its product(s), how to use the product(s), and other important information. Use these manufacturers as an important resource.

This appendix provides information about voluntary and professional organizations of interest to health professionals caring for patients with end-stage renal disease (ESRD).

Credentialing Organizations

Board of Nephrology Examiners, Inc., Nursing and Technology (BONENT)
P.O. Box 15945-282
Lenexa, KS 66285
Tel: (913) 541-9077
Fax: (913) 599-5340
www.goAMP.com/bonent

National Nephrology Certification Organization (NNCO)
Inquiries to: Professional Testing Corporation (PTC)
1350 Broadway, 17th Floor
New York, NY 10018
Tel: (212) 356-0660
Fax: (212) 356-0678
email: PTCNY@PTCNY.COM
www.PTCNY.com

Nephrology Nursing Certification Commission (NNCC)
East Holly Avenue
Box 56
Pitman, NJ 08071
Tel: (888) 884-NNCC
Fax: (856) 589-7463
e-mail: NNCC@ajj.com
www.nncc-exam.org

Patient Organizations

American Association of Kidney Patients (AAKP)
3505 East Frontage Road, Suite 315
Tampa, FL 33607
Tel: (800) 749-2257
Fax: (813) 636-8122
e-mail: info@aakp.org
www.aakp.org

National Kidney Foundation (NKF)
30 East 33rd Street, 11th Floor
New York, NY 10016
Tel: (800) 622-9010
Fax: (212) 689-9261
www.kidney.org

American Kidney Fund (AKF)
6110 Executive Blvd, Suite 1010
Rockville, MD 20852
Tel: (800) 638-8299
Fax: (301) 881-0898
e-mail: helpline@akfinc.org
www.akfinc.org

Professional Associations

American Nephrology Nurses' Association (ANNA)
East Holly Avenue
Box 56
Pitman, NJ 08071-0056
Tel: (888) 600-2662
Fax: (856) 589-7463
e-mail:anna@.ajj.com
www.annanurse.org

National Association of Nephrology Technicians/Technologists (NANT)
P.O. Box 2307
Dayton, OH 45401
Tel: (877) 607-6288
Fax: (937) 586-3699
e-mail: nant@nant.meinet.com
www.dialysistech.org

National Renal Administrators Association (NRAA)
1904 Naomi Place
Prescott, AZ 86303
Tel: (928) 717-2772
Fax: (928) 441-3857
e-mail: nraa@nraa.org
www.nraa.org

Other Organizations

Association for the Advancement of Medical Instrumentation (AAMI)
1110 North Glebe Road, Suite 220
Arlington, VA 22201
Tel: (703) 525-4890
Fax: (703) 276-0793
www.aami.org

United Network for Organ Sharing (UNOS)
P.O. Box 2484
Richmond, VA 23218
Tel: (804) 782-4800
Fax: (804) 782-4817
e-mail: webmaster@unos.org
www.unos.org

What follows is an alphabetical listing of each organization, with a brief explanation about its function. Every effort has been made to provide the organizations' mission statements or purpose.

American Association of Kidney Patients (AAKP) considers itself "the voice of all kidney patients" and was founded in 1969 by kidney patients for kidney patients. The purpose of this organization is to help patients and their families cope with the emotional, physical, and social impact of kidney disease. AAKP's purpose is to promote the welfare of kidney patients through education and advocacy. Self-help and patient education are key elements of local chapter activities. AAKP publishes *Renalife* quarterly and provides access to information on issues affecting the care and treatment of kidney patients through its informational clearinghouse.

American Kidney Fund (AKF) provides direct financial assistance to needy kidney patients. This organization publishes public and patient education brochures that are provided upon request, as well as a newsletter titled "Professional Advocate: The AKF Newsletter for Nephrology Professionals," which covers the spectrum of the fund's programs and activities, as well as current nephrology issues.

American Nephrology Nurses' Association (ANNA) has as its stated purpose the obligation to set forth and update high standards of patient care, educate its practitioners, stimulate research, disseminate new ideas through the nephrology nursing field, promote interdisciplinary communication and cooperation, and address issues encompassing the practice of nephrology nursing. Association objectives center on the functional areas of education, clinical practice, representation, and research. Any registered nurse licensed in the United States, Canada, or Mexico who is interested in the care of patients with renal disease is eligible for full membership. All others interested in the care of patients with renal disease are eligible for associate membership. Publications include *Nephrology Nursing Journal* and the newsletter titled "ANNA Update." In addition to periodicals, ANNA publishes position papers and monographs devoted to nursing practice in nephrology, transplantation, and related therapies. For nurses interested in sitting for the Nephrology Nursing Certification Commission (NNCC) examination, ANNA has developed a Nephrology Nursing Certification Review Guide and a model Certification Review Course to assist nurses in their preparation.

Association for the Advancement of Medical Instrumentation (AAMI) provides continuing information needed by healthcare professionals to keep up with changes in healthcare technology. They publish *Biomedical Instrumentation & Technology,* a bimonthly peer-reviewed journal with solutions, news, and advice on aspects of medical technology; "AAMI News" is a newsletter that presents information on government policies and regulations as well as national and international technology standards development.

Board of Nephrology Examiners, Nursing and Technology (BONENT) administers separate examinations in the individual nephrology specialties of hemodialysis technology, hemodialysis nursing, and peritoneal dialysis nursing. Registered nurses, licensed practical nurses, and dialysis technicians who are actively working in ESRD and have a minimum of 1 year of experience are eligible to take the examination, for which BONENT provides a study outline that includes a comprehensive bibliography. Successful completion of the examination entitles the applicant to use Certified hemodialysis technician (CHT), Certified hemodialysis nurse (CHN), or Certified peritoneal dialysis nurse (CPDN) as a credential after his or her name.

National Association of Nephrology Technicians/Technologists (NANT) states that its mission is to promote the highest quality of care for ESRD patients through education and professionalism. Its goals are to provide educational opportunities for the technical practitioner and other members of the integrated team; represent the technical professional in the regulatory and legislative arena; continue the development of technical professionals in leadership roles; achieve recognition for the role and significant contribution of the technical practitioner to the total care of the ESRD patient; and serve as a resource for the ESRD community to accomplish each of these goals. NANT provides manuals and study guides on dialyzer reprocessing, water treatment, and dialysis technology, as well as selected reprints on technical aspects of dialysis. NANT also has audiotapes available from annual symposia, as well as multimedia packages of information on certification issues, reuse, access, standards/regulations, water, and clinical issues, among others.

National Kidney Foundation (NKF) has a mission to prevent kidney and urinary tract diseases, improve the health and well-being of individuals affected by these diseases, and increase the availability of all organs for transplantation. NKF goals include supporting research and research training, continuing education of healthcare professionals, expanding patient services and community resources, educating the public, shaping health policy, and fundraising. Publications include *American Journal of Kidney Diseases,* the official journal of the NKF, which includes peer-reviewed research papers as well as periodic position papers and proceedings from scientific symposia; *Advances in Chronic Kidney Disease,* a journal that provides in-depth, scholarly review articles about the care and management of people with early kidney disease and kidney failure, as well as those at risk for kidney disease journal; *Journal of Renal Nutrition,* the official journal of the Council on Renal Nutrition; and the *Journal of Nephrology Social Work,* the official journal of the Council of Nephrology Social Workers. Other publications include newsletters for the various councils, pamphlets for the layperson to educate the public about various kidney diseases, and other general renal topics.

NKF-K/DOQI: The complete text of the NKF-K/DOQI Clinical Practice Guidelines is available in a variety of formats. A specially designed caddy houses a boxed set of five volumes (Hemodialysis Adequacy, Peritoneal Dialysis Adequacy, Vascular Access, Treatment of Anemia of Chronic Renal Failure, and Executive Summaries); each of these volumes is also available as a separate piece. In addition to the printed volumes, the full text of the NKF-DOQI guidelines is available on CD-ROM (PC and MAC compatible). For additional information and/or to order the NKF-DOQI Clinical Practice Guidelines, contact the National Kidney Foundation.

National Nephrology Certification Organization describes itself as a fledgling certification organization with a unique mission to create and administer subject-specific certification examinations for the dialysis technician/technologist. Currently there are two specialty examinations: (1) patient care technician and (2) biomedical (nephrology) technician. Upon successful completion of the examinations, the applicant can become a certified clinical nephrology technician (CCNT) or a certified biomedical nephrology technician (CBNT). As time and resources permit, other examinations will be developed.

National Renal Administrators Association (NRAA) is a voluntary organization representing professional managers of dialysis facilities and centers throughout the United States. Through education, networking, information, and governmental representation,

NRAA aims to maintain competence and enhance professionalism throughout the renal community. Publications include the "NRAA Renal Watch" (a weekly email newsletter) and special NRAA reports to keep members informed of key legislative decisions and regulations affecting renal professionals, along with regional news from across the country.

Nephrology Nursing Certification Commission (NNCC) believes that certification serves as an added credential beyond nursing education and licensure, and therefore designs the examination to test the specific knowledge of the nephrology nurse. NNCC's purpose is to improve and maintain the quality of professional nephrology nursing care through the development, administration, and supervision of a certification program in the field of nephrology nursing. Those who successfully complete the certification process by meeting the eligibility criteria and passing a multiple-choice written examination are entitled to display the designated certification of certified nephrology nurse (CNN) or certified dialysis nurse (CDN).

United Network for Organ Sharing (UNOS) has a mission to advance organ availability and transplantation by uniting and supporting its communities for the benefit of patients through education, technology, and policy development.

By being aware of the resources that are available to the practitioner in the dialysis unit setting, the healthcare professional will be better prepared to assist patients and family to cope with living a life with ESRD. Research has shown that the patient with a considerable support system lives longer than the patient with little or no support. You play a key role in your patients' support system. Play this role wisely.

SI Unit Conversion Factors for Clinical Chemistry Values Used in Hemodialysis

Component	Present reference range	Conversion factor	SI reference range
Albumin (S)	4-6 g/dL	10	40-60 g/L
Alkaline (S) phosphatase	30-120 units/L	0.01667	0.5-2.0 μkat/L
ALT (S)	0-35 units/L	0.01667	0-0.58 μkat/L
Aluminum (S)	0-15 mcg/dL	37.06	0-560 nmol/L
Ammonia (P)	10-80 mcg/dL	0.5872	5-50 μmol/L
Amylase (S)	0-130 units/L	0.01667	0-2.17 μkat/L
Ascorbic acid (P)	0.6-2.0 mg/dL	56.78	30-110 μmol/L
AST (S)	0-35 units/L	0.01667	0-0.58 μkat/L
B_{12} (S)	200-1000 pg/mL	0.7378	150-750 pmol/L
Bilirubin (S)	0.1-1.0 mg/dL	17.1	2-18 μmol/L
Calcium (S)	8.8-10.3 mg/dL	0.2495	2.20-2.58 mmol/L
Chloride (S)	95-105 mEq/L	1	95-105 mmol/L

Adapted from Young DS: Implementation of SI units for clinical laboratory data, *Ann Intern Med* 106(1):114-129, 1987.

B, Blood; *P*, plasma; *S*, serum.

ALT, Alanine aminotransferase; *AST*, aspartate aminotransferase (SGOT); *CPK*, creatinine phosphokinase; *GGT*, gamma-glutamyl transferase; *LDH*, lactate dehydrogenase.

Component	Present reference range	Conversion factor	SI reference range
Copper (S)	70-140 ug/dL	0.1574	11.0-22.0 µmol/L
CPK (S)	0-130 units/L	0.01667	0-2.16 µkal/L
Creatinine (S)	0.6-1.2 mg/dL	88.40	50-110 µmol/L
Digoxin (S) (toxic)	>2.5 ng/mL	1.281	>3.2 nmol/L
Ethanol (P)	100 mg/dL	0.2171	22 mmol/L
Ferritin (S)	18-300 ng/mL	1	18-300 mcg/L
Fibrinogen (P)	200-400 mg/dL	0.01	2-4 g/L
Folate (S)	2-10 ng/mL	2.266	4-22 nmol/L
GGT (S)	0-30 units/L	0.01667	0-0.50 µkat/L
Glucose (P) (fasting)	70-110 mg/dL	0.05551	3.9-6.1 mmol/L
Hemoglobin (B)			
Men	14-18 g/dL	10	140-180 g/L
Women	11.5-15.5 g/dL	10	115-155 g/L
Iron (S)			
Men	80-180 mcg/dL	0.1791	14-32 µmol/L
Women	60-90 mcg/dL	0.1791	11-29 µmol/L
Binding capacity	250-460 mcg/dL	0.1791	45-82 µmol/L
LDH (S)	50-150 units/L	0.01667	0.82-2.66 µkat/L
Magnesium (S)	1.8-3.0 mg/dL	0.4114	0.8-1.2 mmol/L
β_2-microglobulin (S)	0.8-2.4 mg/L	84.75	68-204 nmol/L
Osmolality (P)	280-300 mOsm/kg	1	280-300 mmol/L

Continued

Component	Present reference range	Conversion factor	SI reference range
Phosphorus (S)	2.5-5.0 mg/dL	0.3229	0.8-1.6 mmol/L
Potassium (S)	3.5-5.0 mEq/L	1	3.5-5.0 mmol/L
Protein (S)	6-8 g/dL	10.0	60-80 g/L
Sodium (S)	135-147 mEq/L	1	135-147 mmol/L
T_3 (S)	75-220 ng/dL	0.01536	1.2-3.4 nmol/L
Thyroxine (S)	4-11 mcg/dL	12.87	51-142 nmol/L
Urea nitrogen (S)	8-18 mg/dL	0.3570	3.0-6.5 mmol/L
Uric acid (S)	2-7 mg/dL	59.48	120-420 μmol/L
Zinc (S)	75-120 mcg/dL	0.1530	11.5-18.5 μmol/L

Sodium and Potassium Content of Selected Foods

Food	Amount	Grams	Sodium (mEq)	Potassium (mEq)
Breads				
Biscuit	1 biscuit	35	9.5	1.0
Cornbread	1 piece	45	12.3	1.8
Cracked wheat	1 slice	23	5.3	0.8
Pumpernickel	1 slice	32	7.9	3.7
Rye	1 slice	23	5.6	0.8
Tortilla	6-in diameter	30	1.4	0.1
White	1 slice	23	5.1	0.6
Whole wheat	1 slice	23	5.3	1.6
Cereals/grain products				
All-bran	1 cup	56	24.7	13.3
Cornflakes	1 cup	22	9.4	0.7
Farina (instant)	1 cup	245	20.0	0.8
Farina (regular)	1 cup	245	—	0.8
Grits	1 cup	242	—	0.7
Macaroni (cooked)	1 cup	140	—	2.2
Noodles (cooked)	1 cup	160	0.1	1.8
Oatmeal	1 cup	236	—	3.3
Puffed rice	1 cup	14	—	0.4
Puffed wheat	1 cup	14	—	1.2
Raisin bran	1 cup	50	12.7	6.2
Rice (cooked)	1 cup	150	24.4	1.1
Shredded wheat (spoon size)	1 cup	45	0.2	4.5

Food	Amount	Grams	Sodium (mEq)	Potassium (mEq)
Cheese				
Cheddar, processed	1 oz	28	13.8	0.6
Cheddar, unprocessed	1 oz	28	8.6	0.6
Cottage, creamed	3½ oz	100	10.0	2.2
Cream	2 Tbsp	28	3.7	0.9
Swiss	1 oz	28	8.7	0.7
Eggs				
Egg, whole	1 (medium)	48	2.6	1.6
Egg substitute	¼ cup	604	4.7	3.3
Fats				
Butter	1 Tbsp	15	5.4	0.1
Margarine	1 Tbsp	15	6.4	—
Oil	1 Tbsp	14	—	—
Fish and seafood				
Clams, soft, meat	4 large/9 small	100	1.6	6.0
Cod, broiled	4 oz before cooked	95	4.6	9.9
Crab (canned or cooked)	½ cup	85	37.0	2.4
Oysters, raw	5-8 (medium)	100	3.2	3.1
Salmon, pink (canned)	⅖ cup	100	16.8	9.3
Sardines (canned in oil)	8 (medium)	100	22.2	14.4
Shrimp, raw	3½ oz	100	6.1	5.6
Tuna (canned)	¾ cup	100	34.8	7.7
Fruit juices				
Apple juice, canned	1 cup	240	0.1	6.2
Apricot nectar	1 cup	240	—	9.3
Cranberry juice cocktail	1 cup	240	0.1	0.6
Grape juice, bottled	1 cup	240	0.2	7.1
Grapefruit juice, canned	1 cup	240	0.4	8.9
Orange juice, canned or fresh	1 cup	240	0.1	12.3
Orange juice, frozen (diluted)	1 cup	240	0.1	11.4
Pineapple juice, canned	1 cup	240	0.1	9.2

Food	Amount	Grams	Sodium (mEq)	Potassium (mEq)
Prune juice, canned	1 cup	240	0.2	14.5
Tomato juice, canned	1 cup	240	20.9	14.0
Fruits				
Apple, raw	1 medium (2½ in)	150	—	4.2
Applesauce, canned (sweet)	½ cup	150	0.1	2.5
Apricots, canned (sweet)	3 halves (medium)	100	—	6.0
Apricots, raw	2-3 (medium)	100	—	7.2
Avocado, raw	half (3¼ × 4 in)	100	0.2	15.5
Banana, raw	1 (medium)	150	0.1	14.1
Blueberries, raw	½ cup	70	—	1.5
Cantaloupe, raw	¼ (5-in diameter)	100	0.5	6.4
Cherries, raw (sweet)	15 large/25 small	100	0.1	4.9
Cranberry sauce, canned	5 Tbsp	100	—	0.8
Dates, dried	10 (medium)	100	—	16.6
Figs, dried	5 (medium)	100	1.5	16.4
Fruit cocktail, canned (sweet)	½ cup	100	0.2	4.1
Grapefruit, raw	half (medium)	100	—	3.5
Grapes, domestic, raw	22 (medium)	100	0.1	4.1
Orange, raw	1 (medium)	206	—	7.0
Peaches, canned (sweet)	2 halves (medium)	100	0.1	3.3
Peach, raw	1 (medium)	100	—	5.2
Pears, canned (sweet)	2 halves (small)	100	—	2.2
Pear, raw	half (3 × 2½ in)	100	0.1	3.3
Pineapple, canned	1 slice (large)	100	—	3.8
Pineapple, raw, diced	¾ cup	100	—	3.7
Plums, prune type, raw	3 (medium)	100	—	4.4
Plums, purple, canned (sweet)	3 (medium)	100	—	3.6
Prunes, dried	10 (large)	100	0.4	17.8
Raisins, seedless, dried	⅝ cup	100	1.2	19.6
Strawberries, raw	10 (large)	100	—	4.2
Watermelon, balls or cubes	½ cup	100	—	2.6

Continued

Food	Amount	Grams	Sodium (mEq)	Potassium (mEq)
Meats				
Bacon, fried crisp	3 strips	23	10.9	1.4
Beef, lean (cooked)	1 slice	86	1.7	11.2
Ham, cured, lean	1 slice	60	22.5	6.1
Hamburger, lean (cooked)	1 patty	86	1.8	12.3
Liver, calf, fried	3½ oz	100	5.1	11.6
Pork, lean chop (cooked)	1 chop	68	1.8	9.9
Sausage, pork (cooked)	1 link	20	8.3	1.4
Milk/dairy products				
Buttermilk (from skim)	1 cup	245	13.8	8.8
Chocolate (2% fat)	1 cup	250	6.5	10.8
Half and Half	1 cup	240	4.2	7.8
Low fat (2% fat)	1 cup	244	5.3	9.6
Skim	1 cup	246	5.6	10.5
Whipping cream, heavy	1 cup	240	4.2	4.5
Whole (3.5% fat)	1 cup	244	5.3	9.0
Yogurt, low fat	1 cup	227	6.9	13.6
Miscellaneous				
Nuts, mixed, unsalted	8-12 nuts	15	0.1	2.2
Peanut butter	2 Tbsp	30	1.6	6.3
Sunflower seed kernels	3½ oz	100	1.3	23.6
Poultry				
Chicken, roasted	3½ oz	100	3.3	9.4
Turkey, roasted	3½ oz	100	5.7	9.4
Sweets				
Honey	1 Tbsp	20	—	0.3
Jelly	1 Tbsp	20	0.1	0.4
Molasses, light	1 Tbsp	20	0.7	7.7
Sugar, brown (dark)	1 Tbsp	14	0.1	0.8
Sugar, white	1 Tbsp	14	—	—
Vegetables				
Asparagus, canned	6 spears	115	11.8	4.9
Asparagus, fresh	5-6 spears	100	0.1	7.1
Beans, green, canned	½ cup	110	11.7	2.7

Food	Amount	Grams	Sodium (mEq)	Potassium (mEq)
Beans, green, fresh (cooked)	1 cup	125	0.2	4.8
Beans, pinto	½ cup	193	47.9	17.8
Beans, white (cooked)	½ cup	100	0.3	10.7
Beets, canned	½ cup	83	8.5	3.5
Broccoli, frozen (cooked)	3½ oz	100	0.7	5.4
Broccoli, raw	1 stalk (5½ in)	100	0.7	9.8
Brussels sprouts, frozen (cooked)	3½ oz	100	0.6	7.6
Cabbage, raw, shredded	1 cup	100	0.9	6.0
Carrots, canned	⅔ cup	100	10.3	3.1
Carrots, raw	1 large/2 small	100	2.0	8.7
Celery, raw	1 large/3 small	50	2.7	4.4
Collards (cooked)	½ cup	100	1.1	6.0
Corn, canned	⅖ cup	100	10.3	2.5
Cucumber, raw	½ (medium)	50	0.1	2.0
Kale, frozen (cooked)	3½ oz	100	0.9	4.9
Lettuce	3½ oz	100	0.4	6.8
Lima beans, canned	½ cup	115	11.8	6.5
Lima beans, frozen (cooked)	⅝ cup	100	4.4	10.9
Mushrooms, canned (with liquid)	½ cup	100	17.4	5.0
Mushrooms, fresh	4 large/10 small	100	0.7	10.6
Mustard greens (cooked)	½ cup	100	0.8	5.6
Okra, cooked	8-9 pods	100	0.1	4.5
Peas, canned	¾ cup	100	10.3	2.5
Peas, frozen	3½ oz	100	5.0	3.5
Potato, baked	2½-in diameter	100	0.2	12.9
Potato, mashed	½ cup	100	14.4	6.4
Spinach, canned	½ cup	90	9.2	5.8
Spinach, fresh (cooked)	½ cup	90	2.0	7.5
Squash, summer (cooked)	½ cup	100	—	3.6
Squash, winter, baked	½ cup	100	—	11.8
Sweet potato, baked in skin	1 (small)	100	0.5	7.7
Tomato, raw	1 (medium)	150	0.2	9.4
Tomatoes, canned	½ cup	100	5.7	5.6

References and Recommended Readings

Chapter 1

Board of Nephrology Examiners Technology Nursing (BONENT): *Candidate Handbook,* Lenexa, KS, 2000, Board of Nephrology Examiners Technology Nursing.

Headley CM, Wall B: Advanced practice nurses: roles in the hemodialysis unit, *Nephrology Nursing Journal* 27(2):177-184, 2000.

National Association of Nephrology Technicians (NANT): *Three Credentialing Programs for Dialysis Technicians/Technologists* (On-Line), 2003. Available at: http://www.dialysistech.org.

National Nursing Centers Consorium (NNCC): *Hemodialysis Technicians, States with Existing Legislation* (On-Line), 2002. Available at: http://nncc-exam.org/leg/.

Parker J, Gallagher N: The Certified Dialysis Nurse examination, *Dial Transplant* 31(5):313-315, 2002.

Chapter 3

Brundage DJ: Renal disorders. In Mosby's Clinical Nursing Series: *Cancer and the Kidney,* St Louis, 1992, Mosby.

National Kidney Foundation: K/DOQI Clinical Practice Guidelines for Chronic Kidney Disease: Definitions and classification of stages of chronic kidney disease, *Am J Kidney Dis* 39(2 Supp 1):S46-S75, 2002.

National Kidney Foundation: *Nephrotic Syndrome,* New York, 2001, National Kidney Foundation.

Orthobiotech Nephrology: *Chronic Kidney Disease (CKD) Practice Management Tool: A Reference Guide for Best Care Practices* (On-Line), March, 2002. Available at: http://www.beactive.info/eddownld/ckdtool/index.jsp.

Torra R: *Polycystic Kidney Disease* (On-Line), 2003. Available at: http://www.emedicine.com/med/topic1862.htm.

Chapter 4

American Diabetes Association: Clinical Practice Recommendations 2001: Position Statement: Aspirin therapy in diabetes, *Diabetes Care Online* 25(suppl 1):S78-S79, 2002.

Bliss D: Calciphylaxis: What nurses need to know, *Nephrol Nurs J* 29(5):433-444, 2002.

Bro S: How abnormal calcium, phosphate, and parathyroid hormone relate to cardiovascular disease, *Nephrol Nurs J* 30(3):275-278, 2003.

Daugirdas JT, Blake PG, Ing TS: *Handbook of Dialysis,* ed 3, Philadelphia, 2001, Lippincott.

Smith SH: Uremic pericarditis in chronic renal failure: nursing implications, *ANNA J* 20(4):432-436.

Chapter 5

Ahmad S: *Manual of Clinical Dialysis,* London, 1999, Science Press, Ltd.

National Kidney Foundation: K/DOQI clinical practice guidelines for hemodialysis adequacy: update 2000, *Am J Kidney Disease* 37(1 Suppl 1):S7-S64, 2001.

National Kidney Foundation: K/DOQI-TM Clinical Practice Guidelines for anemia of chronic kidney disease: update 2000, *Am J Kidney Disease* 37(suppl 1):S182-S238, 2001.

Polymedco: *Polymedco Introduces Full Range CRP Test* (Press Release), Courtland Manor, NY, February 25, 2003. Available at: polymedco.com/press_releases.html.

Spectra Renal Management: *C-Reactive Protein: A Test for Assessing Infection and Inflammation,* Lexington, MA, 2000, Spectra Renal Management.

Chapter 7

Ikizler TA, Pupim LB, Brouillette JR, et al: Hemodialysis stimulates muscle and whole body protein loss and alters substrate oxidation, *Am J Physiol Endocrinol Metab* 282(1):E107-E116, 2002.

Schiffl H, Fischer R, Lang SM, et al: Clinical manifestations of AB-amyloidosis: Effects of biocompatibility and flux, *Nephrol Dial Transplant* 15(6):840-845, 2000.

Chapter 8

U.S. Environmental Protection Agency: *Potential Drinking Water Contaminant Index.* Available at: http://www.epa.gov/OGWDW/swp/vcontam3.html.

Chapter 9

Association for the Advancement of Medical Instrumentation: *AAMI Standards and Recommended Practices: Dialysis,* Arlington, VA, 2001, Association for the Advancement of Medical Instrumentation.

Occupational Safety and Health Administration: *Formaldehyde: OSHA Fact Sheet,* Washington, DC, 2002, U.S. Department of Labor.

Chapter 10

Brouwer DJ: Cannulation camp: basic needle cannulation training for dialysis staff, *Dial Transplant,* 24(11):606-612, 1995.

Daugirdas JT, Blake PG, Ing T: *Handbook of Dialysis,* ed. 3, Philadelphia, 2001, Lippincott.

Dialysis Outcomes Quality Initiative: *Clinical Practice Guidelines for Vascular Access,* New York, 2000, National Kidney Foundation.

Hayes DD: Caring for your patient with a permanent hemodialysis access, *Nurs 2000,* 30(3):41-46, 2000.

LifeSite Hemodialysis System: *Instructions for Implantation and Use for the LifeSite Hemodialysis Access System,* Tewksbury, MA, 2002-2004, Vasca Inc.

McCann RL: Basilic vein transposition increases the rate of autogenous fistula creation. In Henry ML, editor: *Vascular Access for Hemodialysis,* vol VII, Chicago, IL, 2001, W.L. Gore & Associates, Inc. and Precept Press.

Dialysis Outcomes Quality Initiative: *Clinical Practice Guidelines for Vascular Access,* New York, 2000, National Kidney Foundation.

National Kidney Foundation: K/DOQI Clinical Practice Guidelines for chronic kidney disease: evaluation, classification and stratification. *Am J Kidney Dis* 39(2 suppl 1):S1-S246, 2000.

Wilson SE: *Vascular Access: Principles and Practice,* ed 4, St Louis, 2002, Mosby.

Chapter 11

Collins-Hill MB: Dialysis disequilibrium syndrome, *Nephrol Nurs J* 28(3):348-349, 2001.

Chapter 13

Aronoff GR, Erbeck KM: Prescribing drugs for dialysis patients. In Henrich WL, editor: *Principles and Practice of Dialysis,* Baltimore, 1994, Williams and Wilkins.

Aweeka FT: Dosing of drugs in renal failure. In Young LY, Koda-Kimble MA, editors: *Applied Therapeutics: The Clinical Use of Drugs,* ed 6, Vancouver WA, 1995, Applied Therapeutics, Inc.

Bailie GR: Acute renal failure. In Young LY, Koda-Kimble MA, editors: *Applied Therapeutics: The Clinical Use of Drugs,* ed 6, Vancouver, WA, 1995, Applied Therapeutics, Inc.

Bennett WM, et al: *Drug Prescribing in Renal Failure: Dosing Guidelines for Adults,* ed 4, Philadelphia, 1999, American College of Physicians.

Brater DC: Dosing regimens in renal disease. In Jacobsen HR, Striker GE, Klahr S, editors: *The Principles and Practice of Nephrology,* ed 2, St Louis, 1995, Mosby.

Cutler RE, Forland SC, Hammond PGS: Pharmacokinetics of drugs and the effect of renal failure. In Massry SG, Glasscock RJ, editors: *Textbook of Nephrology,* vol 2, ed 3, Baltimore, 1995, Williams & Wilkins.

Davidman M, Olson P, Kohen J: Iatrogenic renal disease, *Arch Intern Med* 151(9):1809-1812, 1991.

Gibbs MA: Antihypertensive medications and renal disease, *Nephrol Nurs J* 29(4):379-382, 388, 2002.

Golper TA, Bennett WM: Use of drugs in renal failure. In Massry SG, Glasscock RJ, editors: *Textbook of Nephrology,* vol 2, ed 3, Baltimore, 1995, Williams & Wilkins.

Goral S: Levocarnitine's role in the treatment of patients with end-stage renal disease: a review, *Dial Transplant* 30(8):530-538, 2001.

Jick H: Adverse drug effects in relation to renal function, *Am J Med* 62(4):514-517, 1977.

Liponi DF, Winter ME, Tozen TN: Renal function and therapeutic concentrations of phenytoin, *Neurology* 34(3):395-397, 1984.

Matzke GR, Frye RF: Drug therapy individualization for patients with renal insufficiency. In Dipiro JT: *Pharmacotherapy: A Pathophysiological Approach,* ed 3, Stamford, CT, 1997, Appleton & Lange.

National Heart Lung and Blood Institute: *Diseases and Conditions Index. High Blood Pressure.* Available at: www.nhlbi.nih.gov/hbp.

National Kidney Foundation: *Guidelines for Anemia of Chronic Kidney Disease, V: Inadequate Epoetin Response,* New York, 2001, National Kidney Foundation.

Skidmore-Roth L: *Mosby's Drug Guide for Nurses 2004,* ed 5, St Louis, 2004, Mosby.

Sommadossi JP, et al: Clinical pharmacokinetics of gancyclovir in patients with normal and impaired renal function, *Rev Infect Dis* 10(suppl 3):S507-S514, 1988.

Swan SK, Bennett WM: Use of drugs in patients with renal failure. In Schrier RW, Gottschalk CW, editors: *Diseases of the Kidney,* vol 3, ed 6, Boston, 1997, Little, Brown, and Co.

St Peter WL, et al: Chronic renal failure and end stage renal disease. In Dipiro JT: *Pharmacotherapy: A Pathophysiological Approach,* ed 3, Stamford, CT, 1997, Appleton & Lange.

Winchester JF, Kriger FL: Hemodialysis and hemoperfusion in the management of poisoning. In Massry SG, Glasscock RJ, editors: *Textbook of Nephrology,* vol 2, ed 3, Baltimore, 1995, Williams & Wilkins.

Zarama M, Abraham PA: Drug-induced renal disease. In Dipiro JT, editor: *Pharmacotherapy: A Pathophysiologic Approach,* ed 3, Stamford, CT, 1997, Appleton & Lange.

Chapter 14

Allen D, Bell J: Herbal medicine and the transplant patient, *Nephrol Nurs J* 29(3):269-274, 2002.

Bickford A: *Herbal therapies for kidney patients* (On-Line). Available at http://www.aakp.org/AAKP/renalife.htm.

Dahl NV: Herbs and supplements in dialysis patients: Panacea or poison? *Semin Dial* 14(3):186-192, 2001.

Hauschildt E: Herbal supplements can affect drug interactions in transplant recipients, *Transplantation* 71:239-241, 2001.

Myhre MJ: Herbal remedies, nephropathies, and renal disease, *Nephrol Nurs J* 27(5):473-478, 2000.

Nephrology Pharmacy Associates: Serious toxicities from "natural" products, *Med Facts* 2(3):6, 2000.

Yap H, Chen Y, Fang J, et al: Star fruit: A neglected but serious fruit intoxicant, *Dial Transplant* 31(8):564-567, 2002.

Chapter 16
Drugs Approved by the FDA: Rapamune (sirolimus), Boston, 2000, CenterWatch, Inc.

Chapter 17
Curtis J: Daily short and nightly nocturnal home hemodialysis: state of the art, *Dial Transplant* 33(2):64-71, 2004.

Hoy CD: Remote monitoring of daily nocturnal hemodialysis, *Hemodial Intl* 5:8-12, 2001.

United States Renal Data System: *USRD 2003 Annual Data Report,* Bethesda, MD, 2003, National Institute of Diabetes and Digestive and Kidney Diseases, National Institutes of Health, U.S. Department of Health and Human Services.

Chapter 18
National Institute of Diabetes and Digestive and Kidney Diseases: *National Diabetes Statistics Fact Sheet: General Information and National Estimates on Diabetes in the United States, 2003,* Bethesda, MD, 2003, U.S. Department of Health and Human Services, National Institutes of Health.

United States Renal Data System: *USRD 2003 Annual Data Report,* Bethesda, MD, 2003, National Institute of Diabetes and Digestive and Kidney Diseases, National Institutes of Health, U.S. Department of Health and Human Services.

Chapter 19
Centers for Disease Control and Prevention: Recommendations for preventing transmission of infections among chronic hemodialysis patients, *MMWR Morb Mortal Wkly Rep* 50(RR-5):1-43, 2001.

Centers for Disease Control and Prevention: *Hand Hygiene Guidelines Fact Sheet,* Atlanta, 2002, U.S. Department of Health and Human Services, Office of Communication: Media Relations.

Centers for Disease Control and Prevention: *Reported Tuberculosis in the United States, 2002,* Atlanta, 2003, U.S. Department of Health and Human Services.

Centers for Disease Control and Prevention: Overview: *Workbook for Designing, Implementing, and Evaluating a Sharps Injury Prevention Program,* Atlanta, 2004, U.S. Department of Health and Human Services, Division of Healthcare Quality Promotion.

Occupational exposures to HBV, HCV, and HIV and recommendations for postexposure prophylaxis, *MMWR Morb Mortal Wkly Rep* 50(RR-11):1-42, 2001.

The Needlestick Act: Getting the point. *Nephrol News Iss* 24:3, 2001.

Chapter 20

Benko L: HIPAA: How dialysis providers will be affected, *Nephrol Nurs J* 30(2):253-256, 2003.

Crampton K: Professional boundaries in the dialysis setting, *Dial Transplant* 30(9):592-596, 2001.

National Council of State Boards of Nursing, Inc: *Professional Boundaries*, Chicago, IL, 1996, National Council of State Boards of Nursing, Inc.

Robinson K: Does pre-ESRD education make a difference? The patients' perspective, *Dial Transplant* 30(9):564-567, 2001.

Chapters 22 and 23

United States Renal Data System: *USRD 2003 Annual Data Report*, Bethesda, MD, 2003, National Institute of Diabetes and Digestive and Kidney Diseases, National Institutes of Health, U.S. Department of Health and Human Services.

Glossary

AAMI (Association for the Advancement of Medical Instrumentation) This organization set the standards and recommended practices for dialysis machines, reuse of dialyzers, electrical safety, monitoring and culturing of machines and water systems, cleaning of machines, quality of water used for dialysis, and methodology for bacteriology and culturing samples.

Activated clotting time (ACT) ACT is a test to measure the clotting time of the blood.

acute Adjective used in two ways: to indicate that something is of short duration or sudden onset and to indicate a high degree of severity.

adsorb To cause particles or molecules in solution to stick to the surface of a solid material.

air embolus Air bubble carried by the bloodstream to a vessel small enough to be blocked by the bubble.

albumin A protein found in many body tissues. It disperses in water as a colloid and is an important fraction of blood plasma. Molecular weight is approximately 68,000 Da.

allograft A graft, such as a kidney, taken from another person (Greek *allo*, "other"). The donor may be a blood relative or unrelated.

amino acids Building blocks of protein. Amino indicates that one or more hydrogen ions of an acid have been replaced by the radical (NH_2). Amino acids also contain carbon, oxygen, and frequently sulfur.

amyloid Abnormal protein material occurring in certain disorders as deposits in various body tissues. In end-stage renal disease (ESRD) patients, it results from longtime accumulation of β_2-microglobulin.

analog A structure whose function is similar to that of another organ or structure of a different kind and origin.

anaphylaxis A particularly severe type of systemic reaction to a foreign protein or other substance. It results from previous sensitization to the particular substance and can be fatal.

aneroid Pressure gauge (positive or negative) that contains no fluid.

aneurysm A blood-filled sac formed by stretching and dilation of the wall of an artery.

angiogram X-ray film of a blood vessel obtained by injecting a liquid contrast material into the vessel.

anion Ion carrying a negative (–) electric charge. Unlike electric charges attract one another, hence the negatively charged particle is attracted to the positive pole (the anode).

anterior In front or toward the front position.

antibody A protein substance made by the body's immune system in response to a foreign substance.

anticoagulant Medication or chemical to prevent clotting.

antigen A molecule capable of combining specifically with antibody, resulting in either an immune response or a specific tolerant state.

antiseptic Chemical that stops the growth and reproduction of bacteria or germs; it does not necessarily destroy them.

anuria Complete cessation of urine flow.

APTT/PTT Activated partial thromboplastin time.

ARF Acute renal failure.

arrhythmia Any variation from the normal rhythmic heartbeat.

arterial Anything that has to do with an artery or arteries.

arteriovenous Involving both artery and vein.

artery Blood vessel carrying blood under pressure from the heart to the various parts of the body.

ascitic fluid (ascites) An accumulation of fluid in the abdominal cavity. Usually contains protein to a varying degree.

aseptic Free of bacterial or infectious organisms; sterile.

aspirate Remove something by suction or negative pressure.

atherosclerosis A type of arteriosclerosis (hardening of the arteries) caused by degeneration and fatty changes in the walls of the arteries.

ATN Acute tubular necrosis.

atony Lack of normal tone or strength.

autoclave Device for sterilization of materials, using saturated steam under pressure.

autogenous Produced within the organism itself.

azotemia Retention of nitrogenous wastes (urea, creatinine) in blood and body fluid.

bacteremia Presence of bacteria in the bloodstream.

bacteria Small one-celled plantlike organisms; widely prevalent everywhere. Many kinds are harmless or beneficial; certain ones cause infections and may be dangerous.

biocompatible Not causing change or reaction in living tissue. A biocompatible membrane would not damage blood cells, cause clotting, or release pyrogenic matter.

blood cells Cellular elements of blood. Red blood cells are vital for transport of oxygen from lungs to tissues; white blood cells act to combat infection and destroy bacteria.

β_2M β_2-microglobulins.

bradycardia Slow pulse rate or heart rate.

bruit An abnormal sound or murmur heard by listening over a blood vessel with a stethoscope; expected sound heard over a vascular access of a dialysis patient produced by the blood flowing through it.

BUN (blood urea nitrogen) A chemical determination of the amount of nitrogen, derived from urea, present in the blood. Actual urea is 2.2 times the BUN value. Normal BUN is 9 to 15 mg/dL (3-6.5 mmol/L).

BUN-creatinine ratio Normal ratio is 10:1.

cachexia General ill health and malnutrition. Wasting.

calcium-phosphorus product Calcium (in mg/dL) multiplied by phosphorus; product should be less than 70.

calibrate Adjust or accurately set a measuring device by comparison with a known standard.

cannula Tube that is inserted into a body opening.

CAPD Continuous ambulatory peritoneal dialysis.

carbohydrate One of the three main categories of basic foodstuffs; composed of carbon, hydrogen, and oxygen and readily used by the body for energy. Starches and sugars are carbohydrates.

cardiomyopathy Any weakness or dysfunction of the heart muscle. Usually there is dilation and enlargement of the heart.

catabolism Breakdown of body tissue at a rate faster than its restoration.

catheter A hollow tube for withdrawing or introducing fluid into a cavity or passage of the body.

cation Ion carrying a positive (+) charge that is attracted to the oppositely charged electric pole, the cathode.

caudad Toward the tail or the tailbone.

CAVH Continuous arteriovenous hemofiltration.

CAVHD Continuous arteriovenous hemodialysis.

CAVU Continuous arteriovenous ultrafiltration.

CCPD Continuous cycling peritoneal dialysis.

CVVH Continuous venovenous hemofiltration.

CVVHD Continuous venovenous hemodiafiltration.

CDC Centers for Disease Control and Prevention.

cellulose A complex carbohydrate polymer of form $(C_6H_{10}O_5)N$. It is the fibrous support structure of plants. Treatment with heat and chemicals produces a semipermeable membrane.

cephalad Toward the head.

CHF Congestive heart failure; also HF for heart failure.

chloramine Chemical compound containing chlorine attached to nitrogen, forming NC1 groups.

CHT Certified hemodialysis technician.

clearance Mathematic expression of the rate at which a given substance is removed from a solution, for example, the clearance of urea from blood by the natural or an artificial kidney. It is defined as the number of milliliters of solution that would be completely cleared of a given solute in 1 minute.

CLIA Clinical Laboratory Improvement Act.

CNN Certified nephrology nurse.

coagulation Formation of a blood clot.

colloid A very finely divided substance, larger than a molecule, that spreads throughout a liquid as tiny particles. A colloid does not actually dissolve in the liquid or cross a semipermeable membrane. It does exert an osmotic effect proportionate to its concentration. Serum albumin is a colloid.

comorbid A coexisting illness or disease process not directly related to the primary disorder. It may make the overall course more complicated or adversely affect the outcome.

compliance Capacity to yield or stretch. Also the adherence to a plan of care such as dietary and fluid restrictions.

compound A distinctive substance formed by the chemical union of two or more elements in definite proportion by weight.

concurrent As applied to a dialyzer, dialysis fluid and blood flow are in the same direction.

conductivity Ease with which an electric current is carried or conducted through something. The conductivity of dialysate solution is proportional to its electrolyte content.

congestive heart failure (CHF) A condition in which the heart pumps less effectively due to excess body fluid.

contaminate Make dirty, impure, or unsterile.

convection Movement of solute across a membrane caused by bulk flow of solution.

countercurrent In a dialyzer the direction of flow of dialysis fluid and of blood are 180 degrees opposite one another.

CQI Continuous quality improvement.

creatinine One of the nitrogenous waste products of normal muscle metabolism. It is produced at a fairly constant rate in the body.

creatinine clearance A test that measures how efficiently the kidneys remove creatinine from the blood.

Crit-Line monitor An arterial inline medical instrument that provides continuous measurement of absolute hematocrit, percent blood volume change, and oxygen saturation in real time. It measures blood volume change based on the hematocrit because these two values have an inverse relationship. As fluid is removed from the intravascular space, the blood density increases. This is displayed in percent of blood volume change on a gridlike graph on the instrument's screen. With this device, it is possible to maximize ultrafiltration safely and prevent hypotension, cramping, and other intradialytic complications associated with volume depletion. A disposable blood chamber is attached to the arterial side of the dialyzer and a photometric technology is utilized. This device also measures access recirculation.

CRF Chronic renal failure.

crossmatching The testing of blood and tissues to check for the compatibility of a donor organ with a recipient. A positive crossmatch indicates the donor and recipient are incompatible.

CTS Carpal tunnel syndrome.

cyclosporine A An immunosuppressive medication, technically an undecapeptide. It is highly effective in controlling transplant rejection. However, it adversely affects kidney function.

cytomegalovirus (CMV) A group of species-specific herpetoviruses that infect humans and other animals. Often asymptomatic, but tends to exacerbate in immunosuppressed individuals, causing illness with cellular enlargement, cytoplasmic inclusions, and damage to various organs.

dalton (Da) One atomic mass unit. Named for John Dalton, a developer of the atomic concept.

debris An accumulation of fragments of miscellaneous material; rubbish or junk material.

degassing Process of importance in proportioning-delivery systems; removing the gases (largely air) normally dissolved in tap water.

deionize Remove the various solute ions from a solution. Usually it refers to a water treatment process that removes all the electrolytes from the water.

delta The Greek letter D (Δ) used in mathematics to indicate a differential or change between two points.

dementia Progressive decline in cognitive function due to damage or disease in the brain beyond what might be expected from normal aging.

dextran A glucose polymer

dextrose A simple sugar, readily used by body cells for metabolism.

dialysance Expression for the capability of a dialyzer to clear a given solute. It represents the net rate of exchange of a substance between blood and bath per minute per unit of blood-bath concentration gradient.

dialysate Dialyzing fluid that has been used; it contains solutes not originally present. Often applied loosely to any dialyzing fluid.

dialysis-quality water Water that by LAL testing is less than 1 ng/mL (negative) for mycobacteria and meets AAMI chemical analysis standards for water used for dialysis.

diastole Period of relaxation of the heart; its filling phase.

diffusion Spreading out or scattering of different kinds of particles among each other.

dilate Expand or make wider.

dilute Thin out or weaken. A solution is diluted (made less concentrated) by the addition of more solvent. Chemical that destroys bacterial organisms.

distal In a direction away from the center of the body or from the point of attachment.

diuresis Increased output of urine.

diverticulum A pocket or pouch off the side of a tube or hollow vessel.

DOQI National Kidney Foundation's Disease Outcomes Quality Initiative.

dry weight The weight of a dialysis patient when the blood pressure is normal and all excess fluid has been removed.

dwell time Length of time the dialysis solution stays in the peritoneal cavity during peritoneal dialysis.

dyspnea Shortness of breath.

dyspraxia Partial loss of ability to perform coordinated movements.

ecchymosis An extravasation or oozing of blood into the skin, as with a bruise.

edema Collection of fluid in body tissue; swelling, often soft and compressible.

effluent The outflow from something (usually liquid).

electrolyte Substance that separates into ions after going into solution.

embolus Clot, or portion of a clot, carried by the blood flow from a distant vessel and forced into a small vessel and blocking it.

encephalopathy Any gross dysfunction of the brain, temporary or permanent, that may result from anatomic damage, metabolic imbalance, or toxic agents.

endocarditis Inflammation of the endocardium, or interior lining of the heart. A serious condition that can be fatal.

endogenous Originating within the body. Metabolism of the nitrogenous constituents of cells and tissues.

endotoxin A toxic substance produced and held with the cells of bacteria until they die or are destroyed, whereupon it may be released.

EPO Recombinant erythropoietin.

equilibrium State of balance between opposing forces.

erythrocyte Red blood cell.

erythropoiesis Process of making red blood cells by the bone marrow.

erythropoietin A hormone, normally produced by the kidneys that causes the bone marrow to produce red blood cells (erythrocytes). A synthetic form of the hormone, recombinant human erythropoietin, is used to treat anemia.

ESRD End-stage renal disease.

ethylene oxide A gas that may be used for sterilization of objects that might be damaged by heat. Articles must be dry and must be "aired" after sterilization.

euglycemia Normal blood glucose value.

euvolemia Normal intravascular volume.

exogenous Originating outside the organism. Due to external causes.

extracorporeal Outside the body.

febrile Feeling feverish; having an elevated temperature.

fecal Relating to a bowel movement or excretion from the bowel.

fibrin Protein product formed during the clotting of blood, usually threadlike strands.

fibrinolysin A substance that lyses, or breaks up, fibrin.

fistula Unnatural opening or passage. As related to dialysis, a surgical opening between an artery and vein to fill the vein with arterialized blood for blood access.

flowmeter Device for indicating rate of flow of a liquid past a given point.

flux The rate of flow or change across or through a surface.

formalin Disinfectant consisting of 40% formaldehyde gas in water.

gamma irradiation Gamma rays are a form of high-frequency, high-energy radiation emitted from radioactive atomic nuclei. They are very penetrating for a short distance and kill all bacteria, spores, and viruses that they strike.

gastroparesis A disorder in which the stomach takes too long to empty its contents. It often occurs in people with type 1 or type 2 diabetes; also called delayed gastric emptying.

globulin A class of proteins found in serum and tissue and of much larger molecular size than albumin. Certain serum globulins are involved in the immune response of the body and are called immunoglobulins (IgA, IgG, IgM, and so on).

Glomerular filtration rate (GFR) Rate at which a given compound passes through the glomerulus in a given time.

glucose Same as dextrose.

gradient Rate of increase or decrease between two variables.

half-life The time it takes for the amount of drug in the body to decrease by one half.

hematocrit The cellular proportion of blood expressed as a percentage when blood is separated into its liquid and cellular elements by spinning in a centrifuge.

hematoma Accumulation of blood that has escaped from a blood vessel into surrounding tissue.

hematuria The presence of red blood cells or blood in the urine.

hemofiltration Removal of water from the blood by ultrafiltration without dialysis. A volume of water with its solute load is removed by convective transfer. No osmolar gradient between body fluid compartments, which might cause symptoms, is generated.

hemoglobin Red protein portion of the red blood cells that has the capacity to bind oxygen temporarily while it is carried throughout the body.

hemolysis Breakup of red blood cells so that the hemoglobin is released into the surrounding fluid. Hemolysis may result from mechanical, chemical, or osmotic injury.

hemolytic-uremic syndrome An acute illness, most common in children and usually brought on by toxic bacterial diarrhea. Involves breakup of red cells (hemolysis) with release of hemoglobin, thrombocyte destruction, vascular endothelial injury, and acute kidney damage with azotemia and uremic symptoms and findings.

hemoperfusion Removal of noxious substances by passing blood over a column of charcoal or special resin that has high binding capacity. No dialysis or ultrafiltration is involved.

hemothorax A collection of blood in the space between the chest wall and the lung (the pleural cavity).

heparin Chemical that slows the natural clotting of blood.

hepatitis Inflammation of the liver, often caused by a viral infection but can result from toxic agents or medication.

HFAK Hollow-fiber artificial kidneys.

Hg Mercury (Latin, *hydrargyrum*).

high-efficiency dialysis Nonconventional dialysis performed with a special dialyzer that uses a membrane of very large surface area, which allows middle-molecular-weight solutes (up to 5000 Da) to be diffused across the membrane in significant amounts.

high-flux dialysis Nonconventional dialysis performed with a special dialyzer that uses a highly permeable synthetic membrane that allows low- and high-molecular-weight solutes (up to 12,000 Da) to be convected across the membrane.

human leukocyte antigen (HLA) Molecule found on cells in the body that characterizes each person as unique. Determines whether a recipient will accept a donor organ.

hydrolysate A substance produced from the breakdown of another substance by the addition of the elements of water.

hydrophilic Water loving; a substance that blends or combines well with water.

hyper- Prefix to indicate higher than or greater than some standard.

hyperglycemia A blood sugar level higher than normal.

hypertension Blood pressure that is higher than normal.

hypertrophy Abnormal enlargement of a body part or organ.

hypo- Prefix to indicate lower or less than the normal.

hypobaric Less than normal atmospheric pressure.

hypocalcemia Serum calcium value less than normal (normal: 9-11 mg/dL).

hypokalemia Serum potassium (Latin, *kalium*) less than normal (3-5 mEq/L).

hyponatremia Serum sodium (Latin, *natrium*) less than normal (135-145 mEq/L).

hypotension Blood pressure that is abnormally low.

hypovolemia Low volume within the vascular system.

iatrogenic A condition resulting from therapy or medical treatment.

icterus Jaundice.

idiogenic Something separate or independent, originating with an organ or cells.

IDPN Intradialytic parenteral nutrition.

immunosuppressant A drug used to suppress the natural responses of the body's immune system; in transplant patients prevents organ rejection.

in vitro A test done not in a living organism but in a synthetic environment for the particular test.

in vivo A test done in a patient or in a living experimental animal.

infarction An area of tissue destruction resulting from obstruction of the local circulation usually from embolism or thrombosis.

infuse Introduce a fluid into something.

intima (tunica intima) The inner lining of blood vessels.

intravenous Within a vein (abbreviated IV).

ion Atom, or group of atoms, that has an electric charge.

IPD Intermittent peritoneal dialysis.

ischemia A temporary deficiency of blood supply.

isotonic Having the same concentration or the same osmotic pressure (Greek *iso,* "same" or "equal").

jaundice Deposition of bile pigments in the skin, producing a yellowish tinge, caused by liver disorder or disease.

K Potassium (Latin, *kalium*).

kinetic Having to do with motion or movement.

kinetic modeling Sometimes called urea kinetic modeling (UKM). A mathematic tool used to prescribe and monitor dialysis therapy and to assess protein intake.

Kt/V A calculation result derived from UKM. The Kt/V goal for adequacy of hemodialysis is not less than 1.2 for three times weekly and 1.9 for twice weekly. The goal for peritoneal dialysis is greater than 1.5.

k_{UF} The ultrafiltration coefficient, which ranges from 0.5 to 80 mL/hr/mm Hg, depending on the membrane.

labile Unstable or easily changeable.

LAL Limulus amebocyte lysate. An assay for endotoxin that uses a protein extract from the horseshoe crab *(Limulus)*. Values are given in nanograms or in endotoxin units (EU) (1 ng/mL = 5 EU/mL).

lateral To one side or the other.

lesion Any injury or wound or local area of degeneration.

leukocyte A white blood cell.

lipid A group of substances including fats and esters, a fatty or organic oily substance.

lot In manufacturing terminology a group of units manufactured at the same time, from the exact same material, or to the same specifications.

lumen The open space within a tube or container.

lyse To destroy or break up cells.

macerate To soften or break up by immersion in water.

malrotate To rotate or turn incorrectly or inappropriately.

manometer Instrument or gauge to indicate pressure.

medial Toward the middle or midline.

metabolic acidosis Decreased pH and bicarbonate concentration in the body caused by the accumulation of acids.

metabolism Chemical and physical processes by which living organisms produce and maintain their own substance and develop energy for their use.

metastatic Disease or disorder that is transferred from one organ or tissue to another area not directly related to the primary site.

methemoglobin Hemoglobin in which the iron is in the ferric form rather than the ferrous form of normal hemoglobin. In this ferric form it cannot combine with oxygen to transport it in the normal way.

microalbuminuria Screening tests for the presence of albumin, or other protein in the urine, such as the widely used "dipstick," generally do not detect protein in amounts less than 200 mg/dL. Sensitive analytic testing methodology measures much smaller or "micro" amounts.

microglobulin β_2-microglobulin is a protein (MW-11,800 Da) produced by normal turnover of nucleated cells in the body. It is catabolized by normal kidney tubules. In ESRD, β_2-microglobulin accumulates, leading to deposits of an abnormal protein—amyloid—in bone, joints, tendons, and elsewhere.

modeling Mathematic simulation using probability analysis to predict outcome from changes in the known variables of a particular process. Usually done by computer.

module Self-contained unit that may be combined with others of the same type to form a larger unit.

mole One molecular weight of any given substance expressed in grams.

molal Solution containing 1 mole of solute in 1 kg of solvent.

monitor To supervise or check on something; a mechanical or electronic device that checks or supervises some operation.

mono- Prefix indicating one.

mycotic A disease or disorder caused by a fungus rather than by bacteria.

NCDS National Cooperative Dialysis Study. It was a multicenter study to correlate patient outcome with amount of dialysis delivered.

necrosis Death of tissue.

nephrectomy Surgical removal of a kidney.

nephrologist Physician who specializes in kidney diseases and their treatment.

nephron Basic functioning unit of the normal kidney.

nephropathy Abnormal functioning of kidney. It may result from trauma, inflammation, toxic agents, or metabolic disorder.

neuropathy Damage to or disease of nerves.

NPD Nocturnal peritoneal dialysis.

obtund Dull, stupid; poorly responsive.

obturator Metal rod or stylus that fits inside the tube of a trocar. It carries a sharp point and can be withdrawn from the trocar after insertion.

occlude Close off or shut off.

oliguria Daily urine output less than 400 mL, which is the minimum amount of normal urine that can carry away the daily load of metabolic waste products.

omentum Fold of peritoneum that hangs like an apron between the stomach and the anterior abdominal wall.

oncotic Osmotic pressure resulting from the presence of nonionic solutes and suspended materials such as plasma proteins.

OSHA Occupational Safety and Health Administration; a federal agency that edicts safety and health issues.

osmolality Osmotic effect of a solute based on the molal concentration of the solution.

osmometer Instrument for determining the osmolality of a solution. It operates by determining the precise depression of the freezing point of a solution, which is directly related to the concentration of particles of solute per unit amount of solvent.

osmosis Passage of solvent through a semipermeable membrane that separates solutions of differing concentrations.

osteitis fibrosa cystica Bone rarefaction with fibrous degeneration and cyst formation; a result of parathyroid overactivity.

osteoblast A cell that lays down new bone structure.

osteoclast A cell that resolves and removes bone structure.

osteodystrophy General term for defective bone formation; it includes osteomalacia, osteoporosis, and so forth.

osteomalacia Softening of bone caused by lack of calcium deposition.

osteoporosis Bone rarefaction or thinning caused by inadequate new bone formation.

palpitation Irregular jumping or pounding of the heart.

PAN A dialyzer made of polyacrilonitrile (synthetic) membrane.

parameter Quantity to which arbitrary values may be assigned, as distinguished from a mathematic variable, which can assume only values determined by the form of the mathematic function. Parameters measured in dialysis work are blood pressure, flow rates, conductivity, temperature, and so on.

panel reactive antibody (PRA) The percentage of cells from a panel of donors with which a potential recipient's blood serum reacts.

parathyroid glands Four small glands located on the posterior surface of the thyroid gland (*para*, "beside," "adjacent to"). The parathyroid hormone is concerned with regulation of calcium in body fluid.

patent Open.

pathogenic Causing a disease or abnormal process.

peptide A compound of two or more amino acids in which the carboxyl group of one is linked to the amino group of the other. A polypeptide is a chain of such peptides connected in special sequence.

percutaneous Through the skin.

pericarditis Inflammation of the pericardium, the sac surrounding the heart.

peritoneal equilibration testing (PET) Measures the characteristic of the peritoneum in terms of solute transport and ultrafiltration.

peritoneum The smooth, serous (and permeable) membrane that lines the abdominal cavity and covers the loops of intestine, the liver, and other organs.

petechia A small spot or freckle formed by blood leaking into skin; usually occurs in crops (petechiae).

phlebitis Inflammation involving the walls of a vein.

phlebotomy Release of blood from a vein.

photocell Electronic device sensitive to light. An electronic circuit may be closed or opened by its response to light.

physiology Life processes and functioning of living organisms.

plasma Fluid portion of blood (without cellular elements) before clotting occurs.

plasmapheresis *Pheresis* denotes "taking something away," derived from Greek. Special filter units, usually hollow fibers, permit removal from serum of elements such as antibodies and immunoglobulins.

platelet A small circulating white blood cell, about 25% as large as a red blood cell, primarily concerned with instituting clot formation on contact with any abnormal surface of the circulatory system or a defect in the integrity of the system.

PMMA A dialyzer made of polymethylmethacrylate (synthetic) membrane.

pneumothorax The presence of air in the chest cavity between the wall of the cavity and the lung. Large volumes can constrict the movement of the lungs and lead to respiratory failure.

polymer A compound of the same elements in the same proportion as another but of differing molecular weight: (CNOH), $C_2N_2O_2H_2$, $C_3N_3O_3H_3$, and so on. Many plastics are polymers of simple compounds.

pore A very small opening or hole.

posterior Behind or toward the back of something.

premorbid Before an illness.

protamine Substance that neutralizes the anticoagulant action of heparin by combining with it.

protein An essential constituent of all living cells that is formed from complex combinations of amino acids.

proteinuria A condition in which the urine contains large amounts of protein.

protein catabolic rate (PCR) Refers to a given patient's protein metabolism expressed in grams of protein per kilogram.

proteinaceous Proteinlike, or material derived from protein.

proximal Near to a point or near to the central area.

pruritus Intense itching.

pseudoaneurysm (false aneurysm) Sac or outpocketing on the wall of a vein.

Pseudomonas Genus of bacteria found in soil, water, sewage, and air. They are often highly pathogenic and resistant to many antibiotics.

pulsatile Rhythmic throbbing; a rhythmic forward thrust.

pyrogen Any substance or agent that causes a fever.

QB Indication of blood flow rate.

QD Indication of dialyzing fluid flow rate.

qualitative Identifying a substance as to kind.

quantitative Identifying a substance by amount present.

radial Located on the side of the forearm near the radius, the forearm bone that ends at the wrist near the base of the thumb.

recombinant Something manufactured by inserting the deoxyribonucleic acid (DNA) of a chosen or desired gene into the DNA of a bacterium, which reproduces itself generating more of the desired gene.

red blood cells See *blood cells.*

renal Pertaining to the kidneys (Latin *ren,* "kidney").

renin A hormone produced in the kidney with important effects on sodium and potassium balance and on blood pressure.

resin Substance capable of binding, chemically or physically, some other substance and rendering it inactive.

reticulocyte Immature red blood cell.

retrograde In a backward manner, or opposite to the usual direction.

reverse filtration During high-flux dialysis a gradient from dialysate to blood may occur, a reversal of the usual blood-to-dialysate gradient. This reversal of flow may carry bacterial or pyogenic material into blood.

reverse osmosis (RO) The process of removing almost all solute from a solution by applying high pressure on it against a membrane permeable only to the solvent; used to purify water.

rhabdomyolysis Breakdown of muscle tissue with release of myoglobin into the circulation that may result from trauma or toxic substances. Myoglobin is toxic to the kidney and a cause of acute renal failure.

sclerosis An unusual hardening.

semipermeable membrane (SPM) A selective membrane allowing some substances to pass through while not allowing others.

septicemia Bacteremia with growth and multiplication of organisms in the blood. It is usually severe and may be life threatening.

serum Fluid portion of blood remaining after a clot has formed.

shunt Short circuit or bypass; in dialysis usage, the system of tubing that connects the flow of blood from the arterial cannula to the venous cannula when they are not needed for actual dialysis.

SI units An extension of the metric system used by clinical laboratories. The amount of substance is reported as moles/L rather than g/L or mg/dL.

sodium modeling/variation Technique of raising the sodium concentration in the dialysis bath for part of the treatment to minimize hypotension during fluid removal.

solute A dissolved substance.

solvent A liquid capable of dissolving a substance.

sorbent An agent that acts by its adsorption effect.

sphygmomanometer Device for measuring the blood pressure by means of an inflatable cuff placed around an extremity.

spores Certain bacteria, in an inactive or resting stage, that are highly resistant to antiseptic effect.

Staphylococcus Genus of bacteria, some of which normally inhabit skin or other body surfaces. Some are pathogenic and may cause serious infection.

sterile Completely free of any living microorganisms.

subcutaneous Underneath the skin.

sump Depression, or low point, for collecting fluid.

syndrome A complex or set of symptoms occurring together.

synthetic Manmade; not occurring naturally.

systemic Affecting the entire body as a whole.

systole Contraction of the heart; its emptying phase.

tachycardia Excessively rapid heartbeat.

tamponade Compression or pressure on. Pericardial tamponade compresses the heart by pressure of fluid in the pericardial sac.

thermistor Small sensitive metal device that changes its electrical characteristics with temperature change. These changes are sensed by electronic circuitry and displayed on an indicator or recorder.

thermocouple Measuring device using a pair of coupled dissimilar metal conductors that bend when a temperature difference exists.

thrombosis Clot formation.

thrombus Clot formed in a blood vessel or a blood passage.

tight heparinization Monitoring ACT to maintain a clotting of 90 to 120 seconds. This is used in managing the patient at risk for bleeding during the hemodialysis treatment.

tissue typing The matching of blood cells of transplant candidates with donors.

tortuous Full of twists or turns; winding.

TPD Tidal peritoneal dialysis.

transducer Device that transmits power from one system to another. For example, a pressure transducer converts the pressure (power) at its sensing surface to an electronic force that can be shown on an indicator or recorder.

trauma Injury or wound.

Trendelenburg position A body position in which the head is placed at a 45-degree incline down on a table with the legs elevated.

trocar Tube with a sharp point for making puncture wounds.

turbulent Characterized by agitated or irregular mixing action.

ulnar Toward the ulna, the forearm bone on the inner side when the arm is held in the classic anatomic position.

ultrafiltration Filtration by a pressure gradient between two sides of a porous (filtering) material.

urea One of the chief nitrogenous waste products formed by metabolism or breakdown of protein in the body.

urea reduction ratio (URR) Another method to calculate adequacy of dialysis. The formula is percentage of urea reduction = $100 \times (1 - Ct/Co)$.

uremia The symptoms manifested when there is a buildup of excess water and waste products in the body as a result of renal failure.

uric acid Breakdown product of certain proteins, known as nucleotides. Excessive amounts in blood may cause acute inflammation of joints known as gout.

urticaria An allergic skin reaction; hives.

vascular Having to do with the blood vessels.

veins Blood vessels that return blood from various parts of the body to the heart. Usually they are under lower pressure and have thinner walls than arteries.

venospasm Involuntary contraction or narrowing of a vein.

venous Anything related to the veins.

vestibular Having to do with the vestibule of the inner ear, which is concerned with maintaining balance.

virus Submicroscopic, infectious living agents that are causative factors of many illnesses. They are completely dependent on the cells of the host that they infect. They are not sensitive to antibacterial medications.

white blood cells See *blood cells.*

xenograft A graft of tissue or an organ taken from a different animal species.

Index

A

Absorption of medications, 172–173

ACE inhibitors, 189

Acid, 19

Acid–base balance, 70, 231

Acidosis
 acute dialysis for, 213
 metabolic, 48–49

Activated clotting times, 166, 167b, 215

Acute dialysis, 212–217

Acute rejection, 246–247

Acute renal failure (ARF)
 causes of, 36–37
 CAVH for, 220–221
 CAVHD for, 221–222
 in children, 313
 vs. chronic renal failure, 31
 complications of, 214
 CRRT for, 218, 226
 CVVH/CVVHD for, 225–226
 dialysis in relation to transplant, 231
 dialytic precautions, 215–216
 diet for, 205
 disequilibrium syndrome, 216–217
 etiologies of, 210–211b
 first-use syndrome, 215
 hemofiltration for, 227–228
 hemoperfusion for, 228–229
 hypotension in, 216
 isolated ultrafiltration for, 217–218
 plasmapheresis, 229
 poisonings in, 230
 SCUF for, 219–220
 SLED for, 226–227
 transient, 170
 treatment of, 212–213
 types of, 209, 211
 urine output in, 211–212
 vascular access for dialysis in, 214

Acute tubular necrosis, 37, 209, 239–240

Adequacy
 of dialysis, 58–60
 of home peritoneal dialysis, 268–269
 of peritoneal dialysis, 256–257, 259t

Adjustment stages for ESRD patients, 302–303

Adsorptive capacity of cartridges, 228–229

Advance Directive, 309

Advanced practice nurse, 3

Air bubble detectors, 86

Air embolism, 152–153

Air removal from dialyzer, 110

Alanine aminotransferase, 291, 296

Albumin, 53–54

Aluminum
 phosphate binder based on, 192
 phosphate-binding gels containing, 43
 toxicity, 54

American Association of Kidney Patients, 336–337

American Kidney Fund, 337

American Nephrology Nurses Association, 4, 337

Ammonium ions, 82

Amyloidosis, 35
 dialysis, 46

Anastomoses, 119f

Anemia
 in ESRD, 41–42
 management in children, 320
 medication in relation to, 185–188

Anesthetics, prior to needle placement, 129

Aneurysm, due to AV fistula, 125

Angiotensin-receptor blockers, 189–190